Religion and AIDS in Africa

Religion and AIDS
in Africa

JENNY TRINITAPOLI
and
ALEXANDER WEINREB

OXFORD
UNIVERSITY PRESS

OXFORD

UNIVERSITY PRESS

Oxford University Press is a department of the University of Oxford.
It furthers the University's objective of excellence in research,
scholarship, and education by publishing worldwide.

Oxford   New York
Auckland   Cape Town   Dar es Salaam   Hong Kong   Karachi
Kuala Lumpur   Madrid   Melbourne   Mexico City   Nairobi
New Delhi   Shanghai   Taipei   Toronto

With offices in
Argentina   Austria   Brazil   Chile   Czech Republic   France   Greece
Guatemala   Hungary   Italy   Japan   Poland   Portugal   Singapore
South Korea   Switzerland   Thailand   Turkey   Ukraine   Vietnam

Oxford is a registered trade mark of Oxford University Press in the UK and certain other countries.

Published in the United States of America by Oxford University Press
198 Madison Avenue, New York, NY 10016

Library of Congress Cataloging-in-Publication Data
Trinitapoli, Jenny Ann.
Religion and AIDS in Africa / Jenny Trinitapoli and Alexander Weinreb.
p.   cm.
Includes bibliographical references and index.
ISBN 978-0-19-533594-1 (hardcover : alk. paper)
1. AIDS (Disease)—Religious aspects.
2. AIDS (Disease)—Africa, Sub-Saharan.
3. Africa, Sub-Saharan—Religion—21st century.
I. Weinreb, Alexander. II. Title.
RA643.86.A25T75   2012
362.196'97920097—dc23   2011051888

1 3 5 7 9 8 6 4 2

Printed in the United States of America
on acid-free paper

CONTENTS

PART FOUR   RESPONDING

ACKNOWLEDGMENTS

The work described in this book was made possible by an enormous number of people and institutions.

Throughout its long gestation we benefited from our relationship to several exceptionally supportive (public) research universities: the University of Texas at Austin, Penn State University, Arizona State University, and Hebrew University. Core funding for data collection was provided by the National Institute of Child Health and Human Development to the Malawi Diffusion and Ideational Change Project for many years (5R01-HD041713) and the Malawi Religion Project (1R01-HD050142). The Population Research Center at the University of Texas at Austin and the Society for the Scientific Study of Religion funded early trips to Malawi, including the collection of sermons data. We also made extensive use of publicly available data sources: Demographic and Health Survey data; Afrobarometer data; World Values Survey data. If there is a single theme running through all of these, it is associated with the word "public." We work at research universities and use data whose collection is funded by the public. We hope that funding streams will continue to make this type of work possible. Learning about the world is not a luxury. It is vital and necessary.

The list of people to whom we are indebted is long. Susan Watkins has been our most trusted mentor and critic. Her thoughtful but candid feedback on early drafts of this manuscript pushed us to develop much needed clarity in our thinking and writing. She is also unmatched as a fieldwork companion, constantly plying us and the gaggle of young researchers around her with things that make their work better: thoughtful and skeptical questions, caffeine, and cigarettes. We know she will not agree with all our claims, but we hope she recognizes her influence on the better parts of our work.

There were other important players. Susan Newcomer at the National Institutes of Health (NIH) recognized the pressing need for high-quality empirical work on the role of religion in the AIDS epidemic, if only to cut through the counterproductive polemics growing out of U.S. culture wars. Mark Regnerus had the initial idea to turn what would have been a series of little-read articles in academic journals about the relationship between AIDS and religion into a book that we hope will reach a wider audience. He made the initial contacts with our editor at Oxford University Press, Cynthia Read—who has remained enthusiastic and patient during the book's very long gestation—and then stepped out, moving back to better and brighter stuff on sex and marriage in the United States.

Many others have contributed, knowingly and unknowingly, to our thinking on AIDS and religion and our analyses. Sara Yeatman, jimi adams, and Anat Rosenthal have been excellent conversation partners about the social dimensions of AIDS for several years. David Ansari generously shared the data he collected with Imams in Senegal, and the Guttmacher Institute provided us with access to the survey and focus group data they collected from adolescents in four African countries. The GIA Core at Penn State's Population Research Institute prepared the maps that appear in Chapter 1. Sam Mchombo engaged in a very helpful correspondence on the meaning of *kudziletsa* in Chapter 5. Kyle Longest provided practical advice on executing the qualitative comparative analyses that appear in Chapter 7. Nicolette Manglos and Emily Smith provided research assistance. We also received constructive criticism and intellectual support from Adam Ashforth, Jennifer Johnson Hanks, Joe Potter, Francis Dodoo, Roger Finke, Victor Agadjanian, James Pfeiffer, and Sarah Hayford.

Over the course of a decade we have worked with dozens of interviewers, supervisors, field scouts, data entry clerks, translators, typists, drivers, nurses, cooks, and countless others in Malawi and Kenya. It would be impossible to recognize each of them by name here, but a few key figures stand out: Abdul Chilungo, Stawa Shaibu, and Sydney Lungu in Malawi and Francis Ayuka and George Auko in Kenya. Much of the foundation of what we know about AIDS and religion was laid through their efforts.

We are also indebted to our respondents. Like other field researchers, we rely on the goodwill of people who do not know us, who give of their time to answer our questions, often very invasive ones. For most of our respondents in Malawi, time spent answering questions for "the purpose of research" (whatever that means) chips away at tasks that are critical to household functioning: working the field, shelling maize, fetching water, caring for children, selling goods at the market—and all this in a setting where no one has much extra time to give. We (and they) are under no illusions that this type of research helps them in the short-term. But we hope that in the long-term it may push things in a better direction. Either way, our respondents didn't have to consent to be interviewed. We gave them very little for their efforts.

Finally, the work reported in this book took us to exotic places for extended periods, easy when single and childless, much harder when not. For this we are deeply indebted to our spouses, Gregory and Amy, each of whom has made our careers possible while also pursuing their own. We're also deeply indebted to our children—in order of age: Maya, Max, Cassia, Boaz, Luce, and Sophia—for handling our absences and their own associated international trips with such aplomb. We note—with some embarrassment—that four of them were born during the work reported here. We hope this is less evidence of our laziness than a testament to the life-affirming nature of our experiences in Africa, even, or perhaps especially, an Africa with AIDS. We also hope that in their lifetime, if not in ours, the problems associated with AIDS and its effects can be significantly reduced, if not resolved entirely. In Africa we believe they will be, in part through the religious mechanisms that we describe here, even if those have the sting evoked in Ecclesiastes 1:18: "In much wisdom is much grief; and he who increases knowledge increases sorrow."

ACRONYMS AT A GLANCE

ABC   Abstain, Be faithful, use Condoms. It represents the central approach to HIV prevention in SSA.

AGI   Guttmacher Institute, a research-friendly nonprofit working to improve reproductive health in the United States and developing countries.

AIC   African Independent Churches, African Instituted Churches, or African Indigenous Churches. The term is used to represent a heterogeneous grouping of African-led churches that emerged during the mass exodus of white missionaries from Africa.

ART   Antiretroviral therapy (therapies), a variety of drug regimens used to manage HIV and prevent or delay the development of AIDS.

DHS   Demographic and Health Surveys, an ongoing data collection project that has collected waves of nationally representative data on health and population in more than 90 (mostly developing) countries since the late 1980s. It is largely funded by USAID. More on the DHS can be found in Appendix A.

HBM   Health Belief Model, a conceptual model that treats knowledge and perceptions as key factors in promoting positive health behaviors and the uptake of health services. The HBM is a dominant paradigm within the field of public health.

IAA   Islamic Approach to HIV/AIDS formalized by the IMAU in 2001 and turned into a global model via a series of meetings held by the International Muslim Leaders Consultation on HIV/AIDS (2001 in Kampala, 2003 in Kuala Lumpur, 2007 in Addis Ababa).

IMAU   Islamic Medical Association of Uganda, the first to articulate an Islam-friendly approach to AIDS, subsequently formalized in 2001 as the IAA.

MDICP Malawi Diffusion and Ideation Change Project, now called the Malawi Longitudinal Study of Families and Households (MLSFH). Details about this and other data sources can be found in Appendix A.

MRP Malawi Religion Project. More on the MRP can be found in Appendix A.

NGO Nongovernmental organization, an amorphous category of legally constituted groups that pursue social goals but not as political parties.

PEPFAR The U.S. President's Emergency Plan for AIDS Relief, established in 2004 and committed to spending US$15 billion over its first five years. Its reauthorization in 2008—to run from 2009 to 2013—increased its budget to a maximum of US$48 billion and broadened its scope to include the coverage of malaria and tuberculosis in addition to HIV/AIDS.

SSA Sub-Saharan Africa, that is, all African countries barring the Arab North. Also includes island states like Madagascar and Cape Verde.

STI Sexually transmitted infections.

USAID United States Agency for International Development, a government agency that administers civilian foreign aid under the authority of the secretary of state.

VAC Village AIDS Committee, the lowest rung among the slew of organizations spawned by AIDS.

Religion and AIDS in Africa

Introduction

Our initial exposure to the AIDS epidemic in Africa came during the late 1990s, first in Kenya and then in Malawi. Of course, we'd read about AIDS in popular literature and somewhat more systematically in graduate courses prior to ever setting foot in Africa. But it was only after first setting foot on "that Dark Continent" (as one of our mothers tactlessly put it) that we became aware of the magnitude of the presence of AIDS. Conversations about AIDS, or casual references to it, began to take place wherever we were, as if shadowing us: on the street, in offices and small businesses, while waiting in line at the bank or post office, on crowded *matatus* (minibuses). These conversations included an increasingly diverse cast of characters: local researchers, village headmen, teachers, hazy-eyed drunks drinking homebrew (sometimes these three were one and the same), a gamut of African women—from reserved and traditional to vocal and flamboyantly modern—and religious leaders. And all were set to a backdrop of rapidly expanding AIDS-related campaigns and growing public awareness. This is not to say that people talked only about AIDS—far from it. It was simply that they talked about it a lot.

A few themes emerged very clearly from our conversations. One, which didn't surprise us, included heartfelt laments about the deaths of friends or family members, in particular people in their 20s and 30s, the age groups most affected by AIDS in terms of mortality. "Today's world has turned against younger people," said one elderly informant in Kenya in 1997. "We are left dying of hunger in front of our houses while younger energetic people die," said another. Other themes, which surprised us more but in retrospect shouldn't have, moved far beyond these lamentations. We heard people speak about friends' and family members' deaths not having been in vain because they had been "saved." We heard that people who had been "born again" were less sexually active outside marriage, implying that a personal religious state could lower the likelihood of infection. We began to hear new care-centered discourses, often framed in profoundly religious vocabulary and emanating from churches and mosques. We also heard that extended families and community-based networks were reconstituting themselves to more effectively care for surviving orphans and others affected by an AIDS-related sickness or death, sustained by these new, religious, care-centered discourses. Increasingly, we became convinced that our informants experienced AIDS and responded to it, whether individually or communally, less as a medical issue than as a religious one.

At first, we resisted this impression. Both of us had been intellectually socialized into demography and sociology, two disciplines whose ideas about religion and its trajectory are strongly steeped in secularization theory. A popular version of this theory uses the metaphor of a *sacred canopy* (Berger 1967) to refer to a shared set of assumptions about the spiritual world. At first blush, the metaphor fit our early impressions of religious life in Africa to a T. Africa is characterized by extraordinarily high levels of religious belief and participation, an unbelievably dense and diverse religious marketplace, and fervent prayer. Combined with heavy reliance on traditional healers and persistent fears of witchcraft, it seemed to us that daily life in Kenya and Malawi was deeply affected by the spiritual realm but that in time the march of "development" would reduce those effects. It would weaken and eventually tear apart the sacred canopy. In other words, the superstitions and religious enchantment described by dozens of anthropologists working across Africa would not—could not—hold up to an expanding educational system, new technologies, economic prosperity, or an increasingly functional state apparatus. Africans would become less dependent on the precarious weather. They would adopt Western biomedical models of health. In line with this view, we imagined that the religious responses to AIDS in the context of sub-Saharan Africa (SSA) were a vestige of antiquated ideas about health, illness, germs, viruses, witches, and spirits. Or else they were a product of the largely impoverished state of the local medical system or absence of formal, public safety nets. Such circumstances force people to step in and help each other in lieu of the outside institutions on which we, in richer countries, can fall back.

An emerging culture war in the world of AIDS policy bolstered this view. At its center, of course, lies the heated debate about the relative value of abstinence/faithfulness versus condoms as the best strategy for preventing the continued spread of HIV. In the public health literature, the authoritative voice of science on these topics, religion is systematically cast as the Bad Guy in this culture war. It is the superstitious enemy of progress, enlightenment, and, therefore, condoms. That view was supported by some early interactions. In one informal interview conducted in Kenya, for example, a middle-aged Catholic missionary with decades of experience in Africa expressed satisfaction in the prospective "return to natural values"—he meant monogamy and faithfulness—that AIDS, in his view, would inevitably bring about.

With time, however, our skepticism was slowly swept aside by two things. The first factor was the sheer weight of our own observations. We became convinced that local responses to AIDS in this part of the world are animated by the deeply embedded nature of religious life. In this regard, the Pew Foundation's 2010 "Global Religious Futures" project, which has identified the area between the southern border of the Sahara and the tip of South Africa as "the most religious place on Earth," completely fits our own assessment of religious life in Africa. Given this, it would not be surprising if these religious ideas and narratives provided both the sick and the healthy with interpretive frames that allowed them to imbue the experience of AIDS with meaning and, often, comfort. Or that these same narratives strengthened local models of care and provided people with models of prevention. Or, equally intriguing, that AIDS itself might be quietly altering religion and religious life in Africa. We saw signs of each of these.

Reading about epidemics historically emboldened us to study and write about AIDS as a "religious thing." For although religion and AIDS in Africa is a late 20th- and early 21st-century issue, bounded by the technologies, politics, and sensibilities of our time—we cover these in Chapter 1—debates about how to interpret plagues are age-old. Work by sociologist Rodney Stark (1996) on the 3rd-century Plague of Cyprian and its effects on the popular adoption of Christianity in Rome is well-known. The 6th-century Plague of Justinian did much the same for the adoption of Christianity in Gaul (Reff 2005). Somewhat lesser known, however, is the fact that, in each of these instances, plagues gave rise to heated debates between Christian theologians of different stripes. Some favored interpreting the plague using a "punitive theology" in which God was depicted as "capable of virtually annihilating mankind for the purpose of morally reforming it" (Kaldellis 2004: 10). Others were reluctant to impose this type of "moral interpretation of the plague" (Kaldellis: 10).

These two perspectives have a familiar ring to people tracking religious leaders' pronouncements on AIDS, even if 1500 years separates the Plague of Justinian from AIDS. They suggest that religious responses to human suffering are much less unitary than the existing professional and (non-African) journalistic literature suggests. Indeed, these two interpretive sides can be seen in the type of language—"registers" in social science terms—that clinicians and clerics in Malawi use to talk about the epidemic. They often frame AIDS in both material and spiritual terms, even if our assumption is that a clinician's primary register should be material and a cleric's spiritual. One of our Malawian research assistants, for example, is a nurse responsible for training adolescents to serve as peer educators about AIDS in their communities. She told us, "As a nurse, I know that HIV is contracted; it is sexually transmitted. But there is also a spiritual side to it." She went on to describe the importance of spiritual healing and comfort for her patients, the rapid growth of a controversial healing ministry in her home district, and her ideas about how spiritual forces can alter susceptibility to illnesses that have clear, biomedical causes. Days later, another informant in the same area, a Pentecostal minister from whom we fully expected to hear an allegory about AIDS and Old Testament plagues, told us this: "AIDS is not a punishment; AIDS is a syndrome caused by a virus." It was difficult to explain, he continued, but it certainly wasn't as simple as being punishment.

Dozens of historical examples helped us place the relationship between religion and AIDS in Africa in perspective. Among our favorites is the literature on the perceived spiritual benefits of illness (and suffering in general), rooted in the ancient wisdom literature (e.g., the Book of Job). Along these lines, we were especially taken with the writings of early 17th-century French Jesuit Etienne Binet, whose books dealt with care and consolation of plague victims or other sick people. Binet treated plagues as a "happy necessity" since "illness is the mistress of virtues and the purgatory of our sins." Plagues inspire devotion and saintliness, he claimed, by drawing sick individuals closer to God, by providing the healthy with an opportunity to practice charity and love, and by providing many more opportunities for positive communal rituals such as processions, the intercessions of plague saints, or the dedication of a new hospitals or some other infrastructure to one of those saints (Rittgers 2007; Worcester 2007). This literature on the positive aspects of plagues resonated with our impressions of the effects of AIDS in SSA. People were not simply lamenting the deaths of their friends and family members. They were looking for—and often finding—meaning and comfort in these painful events.[1]

This tension between what we'd initially come to Africa "knowing" about AIDS and religion, on one hand, and our observations and casual reading of the historical record, on the other, persisted. Increasingly, we became aware of empirical puzzles in the AIDS literature—detailed in the following chapters—that we suspected could be resolved by investigating the relationship between religion and AIDS more thoroughly. This became our goal. With funding from the National Institute of Child Health and Human Development (NICHD), we were able to piggyback on an existing research project established in Malawi in 1998.[2] We called ours the Malawi Religion Project (MRP).

The MRP is a unique study. Initiated in 2005 its research sites comprised tens of villages in each of Malawi's three regions, and it employed a mix of data collection strategies across time—in social science speak it was a longitudinal, mixed-methods research project. More specifically, the MRP was explicitly designed to help us understand the relationship between religion and AIDS in a sub-Saharan setting with high HIV prevalence in three ways:

1. *Systematically*: We wanted to compare the experiences of AIDS, and responses to AIDS, across a large range of congregations, representing multiple denominations and factions within both Christian and Muslim religious traditions. Some of these congregations were as small as 10 individuals. Others contained thousands of members.

2. *In-depth*: Beginning with our observation that actual behavior on the ground often differs markedly from official doctrine and party lines— condom-distributing Catholic priests are everyone's favorite example, but

there are many others—we wanted to look at variation in these experiences and responses both *within* individual churches and mosques and *between* them. We began at the lowest possible level of organization: local religious congregations. Within each congregation we spoke both with lay members and the leaders. We also moved up the organizational ladder and approached denominational leaders in cases where congregations belonged to larger organizations. Sometimes these relationships were strongly hierarchical (e.g., bishop of a diocese with direct oversight of local clerics) and sometimes loosely organized (e.g., a fellowship of Charismatics). Layering different types of informants allowed us to incorporate individual, community, and organizational perspectives on religious responses to AIDS.

3. *Over time*: Rather than measuring these experiences and responses at a single point in time, we wanted to establish how, if at all, these relationships were changing. The MRP therefore included waves of data collection, allowing us to identify trends over several years—these include the very years of increasing AIDS mortality and stabilization—which lets us speak to the dynamics of religion in this epidemic.

As a mixed-methods research project, our data were collected in face-to-face interviews using structured questionnaires—the kind of data demographers are well-known for. In addition, we used a range of qualitative "semi-ethnographic" methods, including the following: having some of our local informants attend churches and mosques as participant observers on our behalf, then tape and transcribe services and sermons; arranging for the same local informants to complete hundreds of in-depth semistructured interviews with laypersons and clerics; and analyzing local journals in which AIDS-related gossip was recorded by a select group of local diarists (as heard in markets, bars, bus stops, boreholes, and other settings)[3].

In spite of this wealth of data from Malawi, our analysis of the relationship between religion and AIDS is not restricted to Malawi, nor are our claims. As the MRP began to provide answers to some of our questions in one national setting, we began to think about the relationship between religion and AIDS in SSA in general. We visited a number of other African countries during the writing of this book (Ghana, Mozambique, Tanzania, South Africa). We talked to colleagues working in those countries and others. We expanded the scope of our analyses by using secondary data from many other countries in SSA, including nationally representative Demographic and Health Survey data from across SSA, and materials generously shared by colleagues with an interest in religion who work in other African contexts—in particular urban Senegal and rural Mozambique.

Overall, then, this book is about religion and AIDS in SSA as a whole. Data from across SSA allow us to confidently make assertions about broad-brush religious differences in things like HIV prevalence, AIDS-related worry, and condom use as well as to provide some information about the correlates of these trends. But only our Malawi data are rich enough to allow us to describe the relationship between religion and AIDS as thickly as we think the relationship deserves. For example, only in the MRP data can we match accounts of hundreds of Malawian laywomen with the sermons we observed in their churches and mosques and the interview data from the leaders of their congregations. These data uniquely provide us with multiple angles from which to assess the moralization of AIDS across major and minor denominations, the capacity of religion to circumscribe sexual behavior and family life, and the impact of AIDS on religion. Throughout, we pay particular attention to differences between official doctrine, the views of local religious leaders and actual lay perspectives and behavior.[4]

Our general approach to the relationship between religion and AIDS is also largely empirical. We have already described how our interest in this relationship was triggered by the apparent inconsistencies between, on one hand, our own observations on the ground and our reading about historical epidemics, and on the other, the dominant views of religion and its effects in our natal academic disciplines. A related motivation for focusing on religion and AIDS empirically stems directly from fieldwork.[5] After many years of fieldwork, we think of the politics of sex and foreign aid—which have dominated public discourse on AIDS in Africa—as largely non-African debates. They are far removed from—even irrelevant to—the daily lives of the people in Africa living with HIV and AIDS as well those worrying about HIV and AIDS, those caring for sick family members, and those burying their family members and friends. By choosing to privilege local perspectives on the experience of AIDS, including how people are interpreting it and what they're doing about it behaviorally, we hope to bypass as much of these foreign debates as possible. This is not to say that we ignore these things completely. We are not radical behaviorists. Like Mary Douglas, we believe that "in all places and in all times the universe is moralized and politicized" (Douglas 1992: 5). But we also believe that the most relevant conversations for understanding religion and AIDS in Africa are those happening on the ground, not at a nongovernmental organization (NGO) roundtable in Washington, D.C. or at an international AIDS conference. Conversations about AIDS in Africa and religion in Africa are difficult to have in those places. Conversations about AIDS are steeped in actual sex and ideas about sex. Conversations about religion get sidelined by culture wars. Conversations about both are impacted by problems of representation, neocolonial compulsions, and postcolonial perspectives. Given this, we wanted our contribution to be first and foremost an empirical one. After all, we set out to assess how religion structures societal responses to what is arguably the most serious global health crisis of our time.[6] As the project progressed, we began asking about the consequences of an epidemic for the way people believe and behave religiously, including how they institutionalize those behaviors and beliefs in religious organizations. These are largely empirical questions.

Our approach is not wholly atheoretical, however. Our discussion of strictness and social control in churches and sects draws on Max Weber. Emile Durkheim figures prominently in our description of the extrareligious functions of religious communities and the "moral communities" hypothesis. More recent theorizing about diffusion informs our questions about how religious congregations facilitate the spread of AIDS-related information and gossip, sometimes with important implications for the behavior of members. Indeed, we see the relationship between public health messages about AIDS and religious messages about AIDS primarily as a diffusion story, with each centering on the transmission of information across a population and the subsequent adaptation of innovations in prevention measures.

So what is the relationship between religion and AIDS in sub-Saharan Africa, that subcontinent of 48 countries that fascinates some, repels others, but in general remains poorly understood by people in the West? We found quite a bit of truth in many of our initial perceptions. In broad terms, religion in Africa has affected and continues to affect the spread of HIV and the care of those affected by HIV. On both of these dimensions, religion often has desirable effects—fewer infections, fewer deaths, and reduced suffering in general. Likewise, there are also some signs that AIDS is actually changing religion in Africa itself.

Our initial impressions were not always on target, however—we're not that good. As social scientists are wont to say, things are more complicated than they first appeared. Depending on the particular dimension of belief or behavior, we sometimes found surprising differences in the relationship between religion and AIDS across countries and across denominations. Likewise, we found equally surprising parallels and consistencies.

Of course, sex occupies a central role in the story of the relationship between AIDS and religion. But religion is relevant to AIDS in ways that extend far beyond the sexual realm. In *Religion and AIDS in Africa*, we take a more comprehensive approach to understanding how and why religion matters for AIDS (and vice versa) than studies that focus exclusively on religion as it relates to sexual behavior. We begin in Chapter 1 by laying out the key religious and AIDS-related patterns of the past 30 years in relation to a few other major shifts and events. Our aim here is to firmly situate AIDS in an appropriate historical context. In Chapter 2, we navigate the epidemiological terrain, with an emphasis on religious patterns in HIV prevalence—both in broad strokes (e.g., across the subcontinent) and in considerable depth by examining particular communities. Part 2, the beginning of the book's main analytic section, focuses on understanding AIDS. By *understanding* we refer both to the meaning of AIDS in high-prevalence contexts (in Chapter 3 we explore the existential and semantic side of AIDS) and to a more concrete manifestation that is of particular interest to public-health types, that is, the levels and sources of knowledge about HIV and AIDS (Chapter 4). Part 3 addresses questions of how religion influences the behavior of individuals, with an emphasis on prevention strategies. This is the sex part. Here we explore traditional prevention measures, as guided by the ABC campaign (Chapter 5), before providing an account of local prevention strategies that are not on the radar of most public health experts (Chapter 6) and demonstrating that religious organizations combine strategies in innovative, and sometimes very effective, ways (Chapter 7). The question of religion and AIDS mitigation has been the subject of considerable speculation, including by anecdote-loving journalists. In Part 4, we empirically examine the consequences of AIDS with particular attention to stigma, caregiving for the sick, and the issue of AIDS orphans. Our final chapter (Chapter 10) then flips the causal direction between religion and AIDS. Here we look for signs that AIDS has changed religious behavior and the religious landscape in SSA. Our concluding chapter serves as both a synthesis and extension of the most important thing we learned while writing this book: AIDS in Africa cannot be understood without reference to religion.

PART ONE

THE BASICS

1

AIDS in Context

[They] fell sick daily by thousands . . . Some breathed their last in
the streets, and others shut up in their own houses . . . And,
indeed, every place was filled with the dead.
—Bocaccio, *The Decameron, p.xxiii.*

The relationship between religion and AIDS in Africa is played out on a large
stage. But it is not an empty stage. AIDS is only one of a number of things that
has happened in Africa—or, some would say, *to* Africa—over the last three
decades. Likewise, and we say this only half in jest, although some people and
institutions discovered Africa only because of AIDS, Africa, and its religions,
clearly predate AIDS. Understanding the relationship between religion and AIDS
in Africa requires some familiarity with these contextual factors, some historical, others changing alongside the AIDS epidemic.[1] Only by taking these contextual factors into account is it possible to make sense of the stage on which the
relationship between religion and AIDS in Africa plays out. The central point
here is that the set changes over time, affecting both religion and AIDS in themselves and also altering the dynamic between them. We begin with a brief introduction to the main protagonist, AIDS itself.

Chief Protagonist: AIDS

The following facts are widely circulating. Sub-Saharan Africa (SSA) is the center
of the AIDS pandemic. Conventional scientific opinion is that the virus first
emerged somewhere in Central Africa in the 1950s and then spread through heterosexual contacts—still the principal pathway for infection in SSA. Due to a
number of factors—chief among them the high prevalence of sexually transmitted infections and variable rates of male circumcision—HIV prevalence is
highest in SSA. In fact, 65% of all global infections are in SSA, including 90% of
all infections among infants and young children, who in the absence of intervention have a roughly 40% chance of "vertical" infection from their HIV-positive

mothers during delivery and subsequent breastfeeding. Likewise, in 2008, 72% of *all* AIDS-related deaths occurred in SSA (UNAIDS 2009). This can be seen clearly in Figure 1.1, which maps adult HIV prevalence—the proportion of adults aged 15–49 who are HIV positive—globally. It demonstrates not only that HIV is heavily concentrated in this part of the world but also that the magnitude of its spread between 1990 and 2000 has been particularly dramatic here.

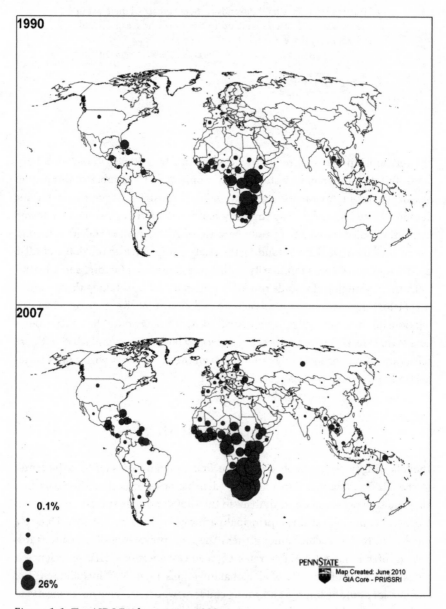

Figure 1.1 The AIDS Epidemic since 1990

Less well-known outside academic and public health circles is the fact that there is extremely high variation in HIV prevalence across the continent. This, too, can be seen in Figure 1.1. But it is clearer yet in Table 1.1, which ranks 44 countries in SSA by adult HIV prevalence. Most of the prevalence estimates in Table 1.1, including all from high-prevalence countries, are drawn from nationally representative samples—sometimes called "population-based sero-prevalence" surveys—the new gold standard for such estimates. Where no such data exist or have been made publically available, estimates are derived from antenatal clinic data and other non-population-based samples. The latter are generally considered less reliable (see, for example, Boerma et al. 2003; Ghys, Kufa, and George 2006; Reniers and Eaton 2009).

Immediately apparent is the fact that HIV is concentrated in southern African countries. This is Africa's "AIDS Belt." The highest HIV prevalence is found in smaller ethnically homogenous countries like Swaziland, Botswana, and Lesotho. Here, adult HIV prevalence is in the range of 20–30%. In neighboring South Africa and Zimbabwe, adult prevalence is a little lower, between 14 and 19%. Prior to the recent scaling up of antiretroviral therapy (ART) in these countries, AIDS had led to an unprecedented three- to fourfold increase in age-specific mortality rates among adults in the 25–39 age range. Likewise, prior to the wide distribution of single-dose nevirapine to pregnant women, the standard protocol for preventing vertical infection (i.e., mother-to-child transmission), AIDS had also led to dramatic increases in infant mortality in these high-prevalence settings, even while progress was being made in reducing infant and child mortality from other causes (Handa, Koch, and Ng 2009; UNICEF 2009). Not surprisingly, the wider effects of AIDS are thought to be most pronounced in these settings. Other presumed effects, some verifiable and verified and others more speculative, include increased levels of orphanhood, impoverishment of families and communities, loss of skilled labor, and the slowing of economic development.

Moving north—into Zambia, Malawi, and Mozambique—adult prevalence drops a little, into the 10–15% range. A little more north yet, from Kenya in the east to Côte d'Ivoire in the west—and ironically including the regions of Central Africa in which HIV first emerged—we find still lower HIV prevalence, usually in the 3–8% range. And to the north and west of this, from Ethiopia in the east to Benin in the west, adult prevalence falls to the 1–2% range, even dipping below 1% in Senegal and Niger.

HIV prevalence in SSA also varies dramatically within countries. For example, although national prevalence in South Africa is 16.9%, it exceeds 35% in Kwazulu-Natal Province (UNAIDS 2008). Likewise, a population-based sero-prevalence survey in a single area of Kenya's Nyanza Province in 2001 showed an HIV prevalence in excess of 20% (Auvert et al. 2001) while Kenya's own National AIDS Control Council estimated 2006 adult prevalence in Eastern Province at 2.8% and 1.1%

Table 1.1 **Estimated Adult HIV Prevalence in SSA (%)**

Country	Estimate	Lowest	Highest
Swaziland	25.9	24.9	27.0
Botswana	24.8	23.8	25.8
Lesotho	23.6	22.3	25.2
South Africa	17.8	17.2	18.3
Zimbabwe	14.3	13.4	15.4
Zambia	13.5	12.8	14.1
Namibia	13.1	11.1	15.5
Mozambique	11.5	10.6	12.2
Malawi	11.0	10.0	12.1
Uganda	6.5	5.9	6.9
Kenya	6.3	5.8	6.5
United Republic of Tanzania	5.6	5.3	6.1
Cameroon	5.3	4.9	5.8
Gabon	5.2	4.2	6.2
Equatorial Guinea	5.0	3.5	6.6
Central African Republic	4.7	4.2	5.2
Nigeria	3.6	3.3	4.0
Cote d'Ivoire	3.4	3.1	3.9
Chad	3.4	2.8	5.1
Congo	3.4	3.1	3.8
Burundi	3.3	2.9	3.5
Togo	3.2	2.5	3.8
Rwanda	2.9	2.5	3.3
Djibouti	2.5	1.9	3.2
Guinea Bissau	2.5	2.0	3.0
Ethiopia[a]	2.1	1.8	2.2
Angola	2.0	1.6	2.4

Table 1.1 **(continued)**

Country	Estimate	Lowest	Highest
Gambia	2.0	1.3	2.9
Ghana	1.8	1.6	2.0
Sierra Leone	1.6	1.4	2.1
Liberia	1.5	1.3	1.8
Guinea	1.3	1.1	1.6
Burkina Faso	1.2	1.0	1.5
Benin	1.2	1.0	1.3
Mauritius	1.0	0.7	1.3
Mali	1.0	0.8	1.3
Democratic Republic of the Congo	—	1.2	1.6
Senegal	0.9	0.7	1.0
Eritrea	0.8	0.6	1.0
Niger	0.8	0.7	1.0
Mauritania	0.7	0.6	0.9
Somalia	0.7	0.5	1.0
Madagascar	0.2	0.2	0.3
Comoros	0.1	< 0.1	0.1

[a] Ethiopia data from 2007.
Source: UNAIDS, 2010.

in sparsely settled North Eastern Province (NACC 2007). The same high levels of within-country variation can be found in many sub-Saharan countries, even "low prevalence" ones. Among certain regions and subpopulations in Ghana (national prevalence < 2% in 2007), for example, prevalence exceeds 8% (USAID 2010).

Understanding these patterns of variation—across and within states—is important for a number of reasons. First, it makes analysis possible. The questions "why is y higher here than there?" and "does that variation in y have something to do with x?" are the ones that animate all science. This book is primarily devoted to describing how, if at all, religion affects variation on these phenomena.

Second, and more generally, these patterns of variation in HIV prevalence evoke long-standing debates in social science about how to characterize SSA or "Black Africa" in general and how to characterize the nature of states in SSA. For example, how cohesive or undifferentiated are African states? To what extent does the level of internal cohesion affect the ability of African states—as well as nonstate actors such as nongovernmental organizations (NGOs)–to influence the trajectory of AIDS? These types of questions are not our central focus, but they are inescapably related to our enquiry. The magnitude of the differences in HIV prevalence across SSA, or within African countries, highlights substantial social and structural fissures, a point we address at greater length in Chapter 3. For example, HIV prevalence is six times higher in Zimbabwe than in the Democratic Republic of Congo, even though the latter is thought to be the area in which HIV first emerged. Prevalence is also lower in much of West Africa than it is in Haiti or areas of Thailand and India. Together, these two examples show that the conditions and pace at which HIV spreads vary within SSA. There is something about societies in the south and east of Africa that has made it much easier for HIV to spread than in the west and north; these societies are different in fundamental ways. Moreover, the same line of thinking can be applied to within-country differentials. Like other aspects of within-country inequality, disparities in HIV-related phenomena tell us something about the internal constitution of African states, in particular about connections between different subpopulations (Lieberman 2009). We argue here that religion and its institutions are crucial components in establishing and sustaining these connections. Religion provides one of the central building blocks for social identity and civil society in most sub-Saharan African states, often overlapping with ethnic identity. Consequently, religion affects belief and behavior in structured ways.

Because AIDS is most intense in areas of southern and eastern Africa, our empirical focus privileges those areas. But we cannot and do not ignore other areas of SSA. Religious developments in one region often echo those in another. The same is true of development paradigms, political processes, and intellectual trends. These are among the contextual factors implicated in the relationship between religion and AIDS.

The Stage: The Historical Period

Three major transformations have taken place in Africa during the AIDS era: democratic transitions; general ideological changes that have affected African and global relations; and changes in international aid. All three have affected both religion and AIDS. To situate the changing relationship between religion and AIDS, we briefly describe them.

Stage Right: Democratic Transitions

Democratization is relevant to AIDS for a couple of reasons. The first and most obvious is a matter of timing. Africa's democratic transition occurred at exactly the same time that HIV prevalence was rising sharply, that the effects of AIDS were becoming apparent, and that local and international responses to AIDS were being initiated and rapidly scaled up. As of the late 1980s, for example, all but five of SSA's 48 states were dictatorships, either civilian or military. By 2000, the majority of these countries had introduced political reforms that turned them into "multiparty" democracies or were in the process of doing so. This includes countries in the heart of the AIDS belt, such as South Africa, as well as countries in the second and third tier of HIV prevalence, such as Mozambique, Namibia, Malawi, Kenya, Angola, and Zambia. Today, even though this process of democratization has stagnated (Bates 2008; EIU 2009) and in certain cases has reversed (Zimbabwe is the prominent example among high HIV prevalence countries), African states in general are more democratic and open than they have been since the beginning of the Independence era.

The second reason that African democratization is relevant to understanding AIDS and religion relates to the underlying motivations of this political transition. Africa's democratic transition resulted, in part, from major global geopolitical shifts—in particular, the collapse of the Soviet Union and the end of the Cold War (Bates 2008; Huntington 1993). These events ended the (direct) coddling of unsavory regimes in Africa, in particular by Western leaders' Cold War *realpolitik*—Eastern Bloc leaders had fewer qualms. It also led to changes in development paradigms and altered the conditions accompanying international aid (Van de Walle 2001), in particular by placing much more emphasis on good governance and accountability. In turn, these changes have affected the international community's response to AIDS. Like development interventions in general, those directed at AIDS are now supposed to be *participatory*, involving all *stakeholders* including representatives of affected communities (Swidler and Watkins 2009). Although this new model is difficult to enact in practice, there is no mistaking its underlying democratic flavor. We review changes in international aid practice in more detail at the end of the chapter.

Africa's democratic transition was also brought about by increasing internal pressure from within African states. This is relevant to religion and AIDS since religion played a key role in the transition. In multiple countries, the leaders of Mission Protestant churches, in particular, played major roles in pressuring long-time autocrats to open up their political systems and allow for multiparty democracy (Philpott 2004; Sabar-Friedman 1997; Van Hoyweghen 1996). The hallowed walls of their churches—almost always churches, rarely mosques—provided some of the only legitimate spaces in which people could meet and engage in quiet forms of protest (Gifford 2005). Likewise, the transnational funding streams of these Mission Protestant churches protected them from state sanctions—a danger to which African Independent Churches (AICs), large and small, were not immune.

Religiously based funding streams are particularly significant for understanding how the relationship between religion and AIDS has played out over time. As AIDS became increasingly visible from the late 1990s, AIDS-related funding streams also ballooned, and a wide array of religious leaders—Christian and Muslim—joined the struggle against AIDS. Some religious leaders became involved at the behest of local and international public health activists. Others engaged in response to local needs without having to be "mobilized" by the international community. In either case, their increasing participation in the struggle against AIDS occurred at a time when the new, more competitive multiparty system had opened up space for civil society, that amorphous set of institutions that act collectively outside formal state parameters. This had implications for the range of AIDS-related activities that could be legitimately undertaken. In particular, it allowed religious groups to fight AIDS using a completely different strategy from the one they'd used to fight autocracy. Most importantly, it placed many African religious leaders squarely in opposition to Western messages, for, in relation to AIDS, those Western prevention messages were based in biomedical and public health discourses. African religious leaders, as we shall see, often see AIDS differently.

Stage Left: Ideological Transitions

Another fluke of historical timing has also affected the way the world intervenes in Africa. Simply put, AIDS is the first major epidemic of the postcolonial era. Responses to AIDS are, therefore, the first to take into account key elements of postcolonial thought. First and foremost this has changed what comes to Africa from outside. Contemporary non-African experts attempt to persuade Africans to adopt different—better—types of behavior just as their predecessors did 50 or 100 years ago, and they are no less likely to use the authority of science to justify their efforts. However, in general, contemporary efforts to impose policy are more manipulative than they were during either the colonial period or early independence—back then efforts were much more openly coercive. African voices and perspectives—once "subaltern," as postcolonial theory describes them—are to be listened to and taken into account. African actors' agency is to be acknowledged and legitimized. Along with the increasing space available to stakeholders and civil society, this means that a wider array of groups, positions, and voices can be heard. Had AIDS emerged 40 years earlier, the response would have been different.

The change in what comes from outside also interacts with an ideological trend from within Africa. African leaders and elites of the 1950s and 1960s, limited in number, occupied an existential no-man's-land between African and European cultures and identities. This is one of the principal themes in African literature in both its Francophone (e.g., Cheikh Hamidou Kane) and Anglophone (e.g., Ngugi wa Thiongo) forms as well as in reflective writing by early African political leaders. "I find myself more at home with French friends than with my own elder brother who has never been to school," claimed Ahmed Sékou Touré, Guinea's long-time president. "We were trained to be inferior copies of Englishmen . . . neither fish nor fowl," wrote Kwame Nkrumah about African elites' "pretensions to British bourgeois gentility [and] . . . grammatical faultiness" (cited in Hapgood 1965: 21–22).

In the half-century since African independence, African political and religious leaders have become much more comfortable and self-confident. In other words, the "colonial alienation" (Thiong'o 1986: 17) described in the previous passages is largely a thing of the past. This new self-confidence expresses itself across many domains. Critical to the story of religion and AIDS, this includes a readiness to express views that are contrary to Western norms, legitimating those views in what are called "authenticity claims"—claims that these are related to genuine African principles or beliefs. There are notable contrasts, for example, between contemporary views of sexual orientation and polygyny that prevail in Africa—among African leaders at least—and those we see among their Western counterparts. With the possible exception of South Africa, African leaders' views, as well as political discourse in general, are much more antihomosexual and pro-polygyny than views and discourses in the political mainstream in the west. And while this contrast would have been quietly asserted 40 years ago, now it is done more assertively, as if it, too, is part of the ". . . ceaseless struggles of African people to liberate their economy, politics and culture from that Euro-American-based-stranglehold . . ." (Thiong'o 1986: 4).

A parallel set of ideological changes has also affected African Muslims through a slightly different mechanism, the growth of Islamist reform movements. Like their counterparts outside Africa (Ajami 1992; Burgat and Dowell 1997), African Islamist movements define themselves in opposition to what they see as Western modernity, secularism, and its products. They are suspicious of non-Muslim interventions and their motives. Geopolitical tensions between the West and Islam—alongside the end of the Cold War, the other major geopolitical change that co-occurred with the AIDS pandemic—entrench these suspicions further. In turn, Islamist leaders more readily assert what they see as an authentic Muslim pathway. In Nigeria, for example, nine Muslim-majority states have instituted *Sharia*—broadly defined as jurisprudence based in Islamic texts—as their main body of civil and criminal law since 2000.

These new forms of cultural and political self-confidence are directly relevant to the relationship between religion and AIDS. For starters, many of the debates between purported Western and non-Western (African or Muslim) models reference some aspect of sexuality, which is often the target of Western AIDS-related interventions. Is it more authentically African, for example, to use a condom or to abstain from nonmarital sex? Is it more authentically African to interpret AIDS as a moral–ethical problem or as a biomedical condition? These debates are taking place across Africa—in formal venues like the op-ed pages of national newspapers, public health workshops, and National AIDS committee meetings. They're also taking place in informal venues: men arguing over beers in the trading centers, women at the village well, and parents and children in the family compound. We address several of these debates in the following chapters.

This new cultural self-confidence is relevant to the religion–AIDS nexus for a second reason: African cultural expression tends to be more religious than its Western—or at least European—counterpart. Indeed, many of the changes in African religious life stem, at least in part, from a related ideological transition: "Africanizing" Christianity and, ironically, de-Africanizing Islam (Gifford 1995; Robinson 2004). Among African Christians, this process of Africanization has roots in a nascent cultural assertiveness vis-à-vis the West. In particular, while African Christian leaders will readily admit that Christianity was introduced to SSA by Europeans—Ethiopia is the exception—they are equally quick to assert that Jesus was not European, that some positions of established Western churches are alien to authentic Christian values, and that African churches are closer to those values than most Western ones. Among African Muslims, the embrace of a new non-Western cultural identity involves the adoption of more standard, "reformist" forms of Islam. This is the latest in a repeated cycle of reform movements to have affected African Islam over the last 1000 years (Robinson 2004).

Upstage: Changes in International Aid Practice

The final wide-ranging change of relevance to religion and AIDS is in the scale and structure of international aid over the last 30 years. Developed countries and multilateral donors now pour more than $5 billion per year into AIDS-related programs in developing countries.[2] As with the democratic and ideological transitions described already, the rapid growth in this funding has altered the relationship between religion and AIDS. Of the many general changes in international aid practice over the last few decades, three relevant factors stand out.

The most important is the way that the intervention occurs. In the first decades after the African independence era (late 1950s to early 1960s), bilateral and multilateral assistance to SSA countries went almost entirely to newly independent African governments. From the early 1970s until the late 1980s, however, two changes began to occur. First, skepticism about the quality of African governance grew—it was increasingly seen as autocratic, corrupt, and "rent-seeking." Second, *development* became a profession: the first graduate programs in international development were established in the 1970s, and subfields and professional associations emerged in areas of economics and public health shortly thereafter. These two changes substantially altered the way aid flows. Problematic governments were bypassed as much as possible, and development funds were increasingly channeled through professionalized NGOs and international nongovernmental agencies (INGOs) (Maren 1997; Waal 1997).

By the time AIDS became an object of international assistance, aid flows had been thoroughly consolidated in the NGO sector. Local, national, and international organizations became the primary institutions charged with administering interventions. NGOs, referred to as the "third sector" because they lie somewhere between the private and public sectors, were a central component of the administrative structure that emerged within the newly democratized African states of the 1990s. They became the natural partners and *stakeholders* for donor organizations, and their reach often extended from the capital cities, where all larger NGOs and INGOs maintained offices from which they could interact easily with each other and with national leaders, to remote villages through their connections to local groups.

Accompanying this broad shift from government to NGO was another important change: the emergence of faith-based organizations (FBOs), a specific type of NGO rooted in religious organizations. The emergence of FBOs also affected the relationship between religion and AIDS, particularly aspects of prevention and care. Even before the George W. Bush administration's acceptance of FBO-based prevention programs, elements of religion-based interventions were already present throughout SSA. This reflected the long-term involvement of religious groups in development work—broadly defined—in Africa, going back to early missionary activity. It also reflected the essentially moral and spiritual aspects of African society. But the Bush administration's willingness, through PEPFAR, to work with and through FBOs both within Africa and internationally did, in all likelihood, accelerate this trend. In so doing, it may have increased the overtly religious tone of prevention messages, legitimizing what many observers—especially those coming from overtly secular public health—characterized as the moralization of the fight against AIDS. In fact, as we show in our discussion of the abstinence campaign (Chapter 5), things are not that simple. A given behavior can be promoted on either moral or instrumental grounds. In the case of abstinence, it is much more frequently the latter.

Relationship to Religious Leaders

The backdrop to each of these parts of the set—democratic transition, ideological transitions, and changes in international aid practice—is general discomfort with religion's role in the fight against AIDS on the part of the public health community and the mainstream high-quality Western press (e.g., the *New York Times*, the *Guardian*, National Public Radio). People who Geoffrey Nunberg (2006) playfully characterizes as "latte-drinking, sushi-eating, Volvo-driving, *New York Times* reading" see Christian and Muslim religious organizations as barriers to more effective and just responses to AIDS. This is evidenced by a fixation on religious prohibitions against condom use (which we address at length in Chapter 5) and by abundant references to the role of religion in perpetuating AIDS-related stigma. In light of these attitudes—the accuracy of which we treat empirically in Chapter 8—it is no surprise that many AIDS scholars and activists bemoaned the shift in priorities that took place when FBOs came to the center of AIDS prevention efforts. PEPFAR program funds are sizable; they are also accompanied by a set of recommendations, for example, that 20% of funds be spent on prevention, and requirements, such as that 33% of funds *must* be spent on promoting abstinence and faithfulness. Critics have characterized the PEP-FAR plan as "ill-informed" and "ideologically driven" (*Lancet* 2006). Their discontent is rooted primarily in the perception that condoms have been sidelined. This has occurred directly—through mandates that condoms be promoted only among "high-risk adults." It has also occurred indirectly. Ambiguous guidelines caused confusion about whether or not PEPFAR-funded programs would lose their support—or individuals their jobs—for distributing condoms. African leaders, however, tend to interpret PEPFAR differently. Many see it as the West's first big investment in an "African" solution. This view builds on the widely held belief—technically inaccurate, as we show in Chapter 5—that the "ABC" campaign (Abstain. Be Faithful. Use Condoms.) was designed by President Yoweri Museveni of Uganda, making it an African solution. From this perspective, a disproportionate emphasis on condoms reflects the primacy of foreign over African interests (Kamwi, Kenyon, and Newton 2006).

The decision to integrate religious organizations in the fight against AIDS by loosening religious restrictions on eligibility for receiving US federal funds mirrored the patterns of trust in authority figures in SSA.[3] These trust patterns can be seen in Afrobarometer data collected between 2002 and 2004.[4] They show that religious leaders are the most trusted authority figures in SSA. This is largely in line with what Westerners would expect based on stories of widespread corruption in the public sector. But what is notable is that there is not a single country in which even NGO officials or teachers are seen to be as trustworthy as religious leaders (see Appendix C). Similar results are evident in analyses of the role that African leaders play in advising and assisting members in their communities. For example, the third round of the Afrobarometer survey asked respondents: "During the past year, how often have you contacted any of the following persons for help to solve a problem or to give them your views?" The problems ranged from paying school fees for children to fixing uncovered wells to resolving marital disputes. As shown in Table 1.2, of the types of leaders mentioned, religious leaders topped the list in 13 of 17 countries. Across the

Table 1.2 **Percent of Population That Sought Help or Advice from Leaders in the Past Year**

Country	Local Government Councilor	Member of Parliament	Official of Government Ministry	Political Party Official	Religious Leader	Traditional Ruler	N
Benin	21	6	4	8	22	16	1195
Botswana	26	12	13	12	26	36	1200
Ghana	14	16	13	21	48	30	1187
Kenya	33	16	18	13	61	23	1277
Lesotho	28	15	23	23	49	71	1123
Madagascar	17	5	1	7	26	14	1346
Malawi	8	12	9	14	36	35	1200
Mali	30	9	4	17	28	23	1244
Mozambique	9	8	15	22	44	33	1140
Namibia	17	9	16	15	26	18	1193
Nigeria	19	8	11	16	46	27	2359
Senegal	25	11	11	19	37	23	1190
South Africa	22	5	6	14	30	14	2375
Tanzania	29	17	17	18	47	13	1299
Uganda	61	14	15	11	56	14	2399
Zambia	20	12	10	15	57	24	1190
TOTAL	25	10	11	15	49	23	

Source: Afrobarometer, Round 3 (2005–2006).

region, 49% of individuals reported seeking help from religious leaders. The next most trusted authority figures—traditional rulers (typically local chiefs) and government councilors—were called upon by only half as many people. Political party officials or parliamentary representatives scored much lower.

Religious Transitions

What makes these facts about African religious leaders so remarkable—that they are perceived as the least corrupt leaders across the subcontinent and, overall, are considered the best target for requesting assistance or advice—is the fact that religious leaders are not a monolithic group. As we show in the following chapters, religious leaders lead a tremendously diverse collection of groups and denominations, and they do so with quite varied leadership styles and religious messages.

This diversity is the product of the rapid religious transitions occurring in Africa over the last 120 years or so. We do not provide any in-depth historical background on either Christianity or Islam in this book—we'd prefer not to offer a hack history where so many good accounts are readily available (Hastings 1979, 1996, 1999; Isichei 1995; Robinson 2004). But it is useful to provide a snapshot of religious change on the Continent from 1900 to 2010 for the three major religious traditions: Christianity, Islam, and traditional African religions (commonly referred to as ethnoreligions) as well as for Pentecostalism, the most rapidly growing variety of Christianity. The trends depicted in Figure 1.2 are constructed using data from the World Christian Database, the gold standard for mapping religious trends across the globe. We see that over the course of the twentieth century the percentage of Africans who are Christian increased from about 10% to almost 50%, and the percentage of Africans who are Muslim increased from about 32% to 42%. Making each of these changes possible was a dramatic reduction in the proportion of Africans associated with an ethnoreligion. Also notable is the precipitous rise of the Pentecostal share of Christianity beginning in the 1970s.

Like HIV prevalence itself, these overall trends conceal large regional variation. Signs of this can be seen in Figure 1.3, which shows the very substantial differences in religious distribution across SSA. Briefly, Islam dominates the Sahel, the area just to its south, into such places as northern Nigeria, Ghana, and Cameroon, and the Horn of Africa, including almost half of the Ethiopian population. There are also sizable Muslim populations along the coast of the Indian Ocean to the south of Somalia (Kenya, Tanzania and northern Mozambique). These distributions are largely the product of Islam's spread along trading routes, beginning in the eighth century. In contrast, Christianity is concentrated throughout southern, eastern, and central Africa, including a broad strip along the Atlantic shore in West Africa up to Liberia. With the exception of Ethiopia,

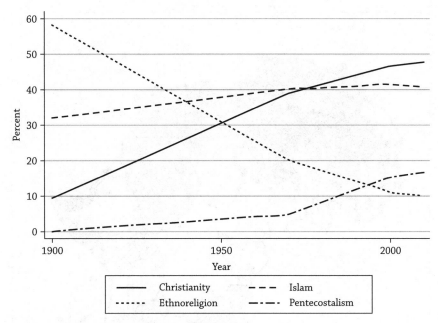

Figure 1.2 Religious Change in Africa, 1900-2010
   Source: The American Religion Data Archives

these distributions closely reflect the intensive missionary activity that began in the 1850s in these areas.

All the current survey data we have seen (and our experiences working in Africa) tell us that nearly everyone in Africa identifies with a religious group that would be recognizable to Westerners. This is not to say that traditional religious practices have died out completely. On the contrary, notwithstanding the attempts of many missionaries and, in the Islamic tradition, "reformists"—see Robinson (2004) on the influence of Uthman dan Fodio on Islamic thought in Nigeria—contemporary elements of traditional religion have been either seamlessly incorporated into the two dominant religious traditions or are practiced outside or in addition to normative religious practice. Much has been written about this mixing of traditions in both Christianity and Islam, but we do not deal with this theme extensively.

The point here is that the two dominant religious traditions in contemporary SSA are Christianity and Islam. This can also be seen in African Demographic and Health Surveys (DHSes).[5] We used data from these surveys to estimate the proportion "unaffiliated" in each country (see Appendix D). In 10 of the 27 countries, 1% or less of the population does not identify as belonging to a Christian or Muslim religious tradition; note that in seven countries, no (as in *zero*) respondents to the DHS survey indicated they had no religion. According to these data, Swaziland and Gabon might be characterized

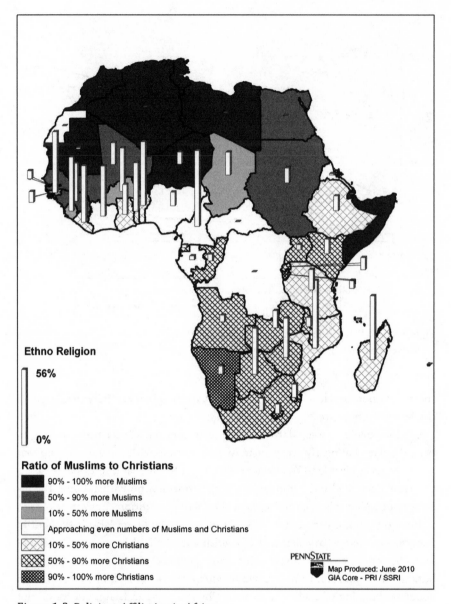

Figure 1.3 Religious Affiliation in Africa

as the most "secular" countries—about 11% of their populations do not identify with any religious tradition. However, this is lower than in the United
States—currently estimated at 14% (Baker and Smith 2009)—and far lower
than in secular European countries like France, where 31% are unaffiliated.

Not only are African countries characterized by high levels of religious
affiliation—that is, few people claiming to be unaffiliated or practicing only

ethnoreligion—but they also score high on what sociologists refer to as *religiosity*, the intensity of religious behavior or participation within those established traditions. In subsequent chapters, we will show that religiosity is often a much more salient dimension of religion than affiliation. The problem is that, in contrast to the abundant, though not always detailed, data on religious affiliation, data on religious participation are much more difficult to come by. One of the best contemporary sources of comparable, cross-national data on religion is the World Values Survey. A total of 11 of its 90 countries are located in SSA, and these data clearly demonstrate the remarkably high levels of religiosity in the region.

Figure 1.4 shows us that a majority of individuals in these 11 (highly diverse) countries attend church or mosque at least once a week—note that the first category demonstrates the proportion that attends more than once a week. The percentages reach 80% or higher in Rwanda and a few countries with large Muslim populations (Ghana, Nigeria, Uganda, Tanzania). The biggest "secular" outlier is South Africa. There, only 20% report at least weekly church or mosque

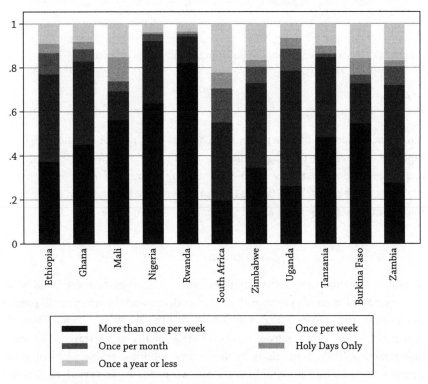

Figure 1.4 Frequency of Attendance at Religious Services (Proportion)
Source: World Values Surveys, 1999–2007

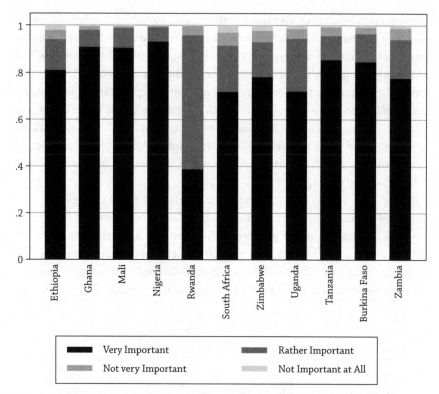

Figure 1.5 Reported Importance of Religion in Daily Life (Proportion)
   Source: World Values Surveys, 1999–2007

attendance. Figure 1.5 presents parallel analyses on religious "salience"—the reported importance of religion in a respondent's daily life—in these same countries. It demonstrates the overwhelmingly spiritual outlook of most Africans. In all countries between 1% and 10% report that religion is not very important or not important at all to them.

Conclusions

To situate our inquiry into the relationship between religion and AIDS in SSA, we have provided an overview of the AIDS epidemic and the diversity in prevalence within and across countries in SSA. During the period in which AIDS took root in Africa and then moved to center stage, many other transitions were under way: political transitions to democratic regimes, profound ideological changes, the transformation of international aid practices, and religious change. Each of these has affected the way the relationship between religion and AIDS is playing out.

In the chapters that follow we explore the profoundly religious nature of AIDS-related discourse at the local level, in particular as it concerns questions like "How do we stop this disease from spreading?" and "What is our obligation to the suffering people around us?" We use a classical sociological approach, describing official, international, and institutional responses to AIDS but giving primary weight to local discourses and local institutional responses. We begin, however, by describing the religious contours of HIV prevalence across SSA.

2

Religious Patterns

Awkwardly do health and holiness fraternize together.
—Binet, *Consolation, 1617*[1]

The existing scholarly literature on religion and HIV prevalence in Africa is tiny, at least relative to other areas of research on AIDS in Africa or research on African religion.[2] What does exist can be placed in one of two main categories. The first focuses on broad differences in HIV prevalence[3] between religious traditions and denominations—this is the more "macro" literature. The second tries to explain these differences using measures of individual behavior. The goal of each, in its own way, is to explain the enormous differences in adult prevalence across sub-Saharan Africa (SSA).[4]

The macro literature builds on a simple expectation: because HIV in SSA is primarily transmitted through heterosexual sex, religious constraints on sexual behavior or related risky behaviors should translate into differences in HIV prevalence. One focus of this macro literature has been on Muslim–Christian differences. Gray (2004), for example, suggested that HIV prevalence should be lower in countries with large Muslim populations for three reasons: the strict regulation of sex outside marriage; prohibitions against alcohol consumption that further reduce risky sexual behavior; and male circumcision, which reduces transmission probabilities per sex act.[5] An equivalent macro literature has looked at differences in HIV prevalence among Christian denominations. Here, too, scholars have suggested that HIV prevalence should be lower in theologically conservative denominations and congregations since these often have more developed social mechanisms for regulating sex, marriage, and alcohol consumption (Garner 2000; Hill, Cleland, and Mohamed 2004; Trinitapoli and Regnerus 2006).

Aggregate patterns of HIV prevalence are consistent with these expectations. Using 1999 data from 38 African countries, for example, Gray (2004) found HIV prevalence to be lower in countries with large Muslim populations. Likewise, there is strong suggestive evidence that HIV prevalence is lower among members of theologically conservative traditions in Zimbabwe (Gregson, Zhuwau, Anderson, and Chandiwana 1997) than in Mission Protestant and Catholic churches. These patterns coincide with what Garner refers to as "safe sects," religious groups whose strict norms about sex and other risky behaviors offer members some protection from infection.

The Problem with Aggregate Analyses

These strong aggregate relationships between national HIV prevalence and the proportion of the population that is Muslim, or the variation in HIV prevalence across strict and lax Christian denominations in southern Africa, are suggestive. They hint at one important type of religious variation in the AIDS epidemic. The problem is that, like aggregate data in general, they are difficult to interpret.

A useful illustration of this difficulty can be seen by extending Gray's (2004) analysis. We combined more recent data on HIV prevalence from UNAIDS with data on men's sexual behavior from 29 countries from which Demographic and Health Surveys (DHS) data are available and religious composition data from the World Christian Database. We then tested the relationship between three variables at the aggregate level—as Gray did. Figure 2.1 displays our results. Consistent with Gray's hypothesis, we found that the proportion of men reporting an extramarital partner is slightly lower in countries where Muslims

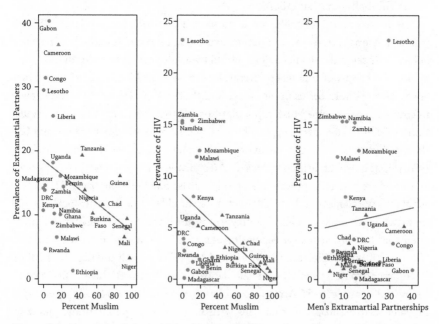

Figure 2.1 Aggregate Relationships between HIV Prevalence, Percent Muslim, and Men's Extramarital Sex

   Source: African Demographic and Health Surveys

make up a large share of the population and that HIV prevalence is slightly lower in countries with large Muslim populations. However, in extending the logic of the differential sexual behavior argument one step further, we did not find any relationship between the number of men reporting extramarital partners and HIV prevalence. In other words, the negative relationship between the prevalence of Islam and the prevalence of HIV does not appear to be explained by differences in sexual behavior. It must be the product of one of the other factors suggested by Gray or by some other unobserved factor.[6,7]

There are, in fact, two central problems with these types of aggregated macro analyses. The first is that they cannot tell us much about the actual mechanisms through which a given characteristic affects individuals. In the case of Muslim–Christian differences, for example, is it differential sexual behavior, circumcision, or some other unobserved factor that just happens to be correlated with Muslim–Christian residential patterns (e.g., predominantly Muslim countries in Africa are further from the virus's origin point)? Second, just because there is an association between group averages of two different variables does not mean that one can generalize from that association to the individual. This type of inference is a classic scientific pitfall known as an *ecological fallacy*. In this case, noting that HIV prevalence tends to be lower in countries where a large proportion of the population is Muslim does not mean that individual Muslims are at lower risk. Indeed, though unlikely, it *could* be the case that Muslims are disproportionately affected in these very settings.

Microdata: Differences in HIV across Major Religious Blocs

The best way to both avoid falling into ecological fallacies and identify actual mechanisms that generate differences among groups is to use microdata—data on individuals. In relation to the question at hand, this boils down to asking how an *individual's* likelihood of being HIV positive varies by religious group. We did this by looking at the relationship between individuals' declared religious affiliation (across the major religious traditions) and HIV biomarker data from DHS data collected in 17 African countries (Table 2.1). To the extent possible, we standardized religious groups across countries to compare prevalence patterns in each country. We also replicated analyses with and without statistical controls for confounding factors like individuals' education, sexual behavior, and ethnicity.

All our analyses produced similar findings. Specifically, Muslims have the lowest HIV prevalence in 7 of these 17 countries; they also have the highest in a few (Liberia, Rwanda, and Malawi, the last of these representing a high-prevalence population) and are roughly equal to other religions in a few others.

Table 2.1 **HIV Prevalence by Denomination (%)**

Country, Year	Catholic	Protestant	Muslim	Pentecostal	Other	None	Total
Burkina Faso, 2003	2.4	2.8	1.7	—	1.5	1.0	1.9
Cameroon, 2004	5.7	6.1	4.8	—	3.8	1.7	5.4
Cote D'Ivoire, 2005[a]	4.0	6.9	3.4	—	4.6	—	4.2
Ethiopia, 2005	0	1.6	0.7	3.0[b]	0	—	1.92
Ghana, 2003	2.2	2.4	1.5	—	2.1	1.9	2.1
Guinea, 2005	3.5	—	1.3	—	0	0.9	1.5
Kenya, 2004	7.1	7.2	2.3	—	0	5.7	6.6
Lesotho, 2004	23.4	22.7	—	—	33.3	19.4	22.9
Liberia, 2007	1.7	—	2.5	—	0	0.8	1.8
Malawi, 2004	13.3	12.0	14.3	—	7.1	3.3	12.5
Mali, 2006	1.3	—	1.3	—	0.8	1.7	1.3
Niger, 2003	0	—	1.0	—	0	2.4	1.0
Rwanda, 2005	3.3	3.1	7.3	—	5.5	1.3	3.3
Senegal, 2005	0	—	0.5	—	0	—	0.5
Swaziland, 2006	26.9	22.9	37.5	23.1	28.3	26.7	26.0
Zambia, 2005	14.1	14.9	6.5	—	11.9	—	14.7
Zimbabwe, 2005	18.3	17.0	17.2	17.2	18.2	20.9	17.9

[a] Data from women only.
[b] This is Orthodox, not Pentecostal.
Source: African Demographic and Health Surveys.

Likewise, among the major Christian blocs, HIV prevalence among Protestants tends to be higher than that of Catholics in relatively low-prevalence countries (e.g., Burkina Faso, Ghana, Cote D'Ivoire, Ghana) but lower than Catholics in high-prevalence settings (e.g., Swaziland, Malawi, Zambia). Overall, then, our analyses of microlevel data point to few general patterns and suggest that there are no consistent differences in HIV prevalence across the major religious blocs. Rather, the burden of AIDS across major religious blocs varies by country and setting.

HIV Prevalence by Denomination

DHS data also have a critical weakness for this type of analysis. They don't differentiate between the diverse streams and denominations that make up larger religious traditions. This is because the standard approach used by DHS and many other household surveys conducted in SSA asks respondents to select their religious affiliation from a limited number of choices. Sometimes there are just three: Protestant, Catholic, and Muslim. In predominantly Muslim countries, Protestantism and Catholicism sometimes remain undifferentiated within a single "Christian" category. In predominantly Christian countries like Kenya and Ghana, "Pentecostal" was added as an option to recent survey rounds. In all cases, however, this limited number of response categories reduces DHS data's utility for our purposes. Although they contain rich data on sexual behavior and a host of AIDS-related outcomes, we cannot use these data to identify differences between more and less conservative Protestant denominations, much less congregational differences *within* a given denomination. Yet to evaluate the hypothesis that members of "safe sects" have distinctive behaviors that reduce their risk of being infected with HIV (Garner 2000; Hill, Cleland, and Ali 2004; Trinitapoli and Regnerus 2006), analyses need to be conducted *precisely* at the congregational and denominational levels.

Our data from Malawi allow us to examine HIV prevalence across denominations and religious traditions in a more refined way. Through the Malawi Diffusion and Ideational Change Project (MDICP), we gathered detailed information from over 3000 rural respondents about the specific congregation to which they belong and the specific denomination with which they identify. Figure 2.2 summarizes the typology of religious traditions we created to make meaningful comparisons between religious blocs in Malawi. We distilled these six from the enormous list the survey responses generated, making distinctions along two dimensions: each denomination's theological characteristics (e.g., speaking in tongues easily differentiates most Pentecostal groups); and the historical conditions of its establishment (e.g., while the first wave of Mission Protestant congregations were established by 19th-century European missionaries, the New Mission Protestant churches were established nearly a century later and currently occupy a distinct position along the church–sect continuum).

The resulting typology for Malawi represents a marked improvement over other available sources. First, the MDICP data explicitly focused on capturing diversity within Protestant Christianity—in particular, measuring growth within the Pentecostal tradition and distinguishing between old and new Mission Protestant churches. A second improvement is our inclusion of the "independency" as its own religious category. Variably referred to as African Independent Churches, African Indigenous Churches (see, e.g., Githieya 1997; Thomas 1994), or African Instituted Churches (e.g., Ositelu 2002), the term AIC is used to represent a heterogeneous grouping of African-led churches that emerged during the mass exodus of white missionaries from Africa.[8] A third improvement is one we do not leverage extensively here; the MDICP data distinguish between two diverging branches of Islam: the Qadiriyya, which is older "Africanized" Islam, diverse, largely Sunni, and with its syncretic elements legitimized in Sufi rituals and practice; and the more recently arrived Sukuti tradition, a more austere and orthodox tradition associated with Salafi Islam.

Also contained within Figure 2.2 are simple calculations of HIV prevalence for each of these six religious groups (plus those who do not identify at all, though these are a very small number), using the biomarker data the MDICP collected in 2004.[9] HIV prevalence in this sample hovers around 7%; this is about what we find among each of Malawi's primary religious groups, with one important exception: prevalence is lower among New Mission Protestants (4%).[10] As we discuss in later chapters, this is the bloc that observes and enforces the greatest restrictions with regard to sexual behavior, dietary restrictions, family life, and general socialization (i.e., these churches provide all-consuming social networks for members.)

In addition to making these more meaningful denominational distinctions, the MDICP data are suitable for testing associations between religiosity (here, attendance at weekly religious services) and the HIV status. In contrast to the similarity in HIV prevalence we observed across denominations in Malawi, we did find significant differences by religiosity. At the bivariate level, there is a weak negative relationship between religiosity and HIV serostatus for men and a stronger negative relationship for women. This crude finding provides the starting point for a more detailed investigation into the relationship between religiosity and HIV prevalence.

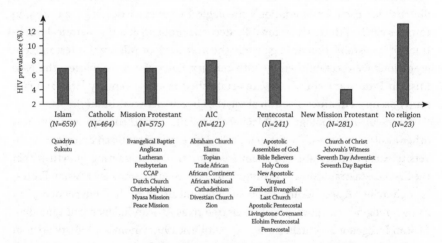

Figure 2.2 HIV Prevalence by Major Religious Bloc, MDICP 2004, with Associated Denominations

It's Not Only about Individuals

There is also another difficulty that weakens researchers' ability to explore the relationship between religion and HIV prevalence. Belonging to a strict church that more effectively limits risky sexual behavior will reduce a person's risk of being infected with HIV only if an individual's sexual behavior is a good predictor of his or her HIV status. Unfortunately, this is not always the case. To the dismay of many scholars and activists, epidemiological studies show that, *in the context of generalized epidemics*, those who acquire HIV during their lifetimes are not particularly distinct from those who do not (Lopman et al. 2008). Many of the measures of sexual behavior that "should" be associated with HIV status (e.g., lifetime number of partners, condom use, extramarital partners) are not. And where associations are found, they are weaker than expected. Understanding why this is the case provides a key entryway into understanding how religion affects the spread of HIV in SSA.

Here's the first factor. Getting HIV is not like getting tennis elbow. You can't get it by pleasuring yourself too often or too rigorously. In some sense you don't actually even get HIV from sex itself. You get HIV from a partner. In other words, at its core, the risk of HIV isn't an individual-level thing. The risk is a function of the pool of people from which individuals draw their sex partners. Sex is merely a mode of transmission.[11]

The second factor makes this even more complicated. There is an enormous stochastic element in HIV transmission. HIV, in other words, is difficult to acquire. Calculated per coitus, where one sexual partner is HIV positive and the other is not, and neither has any other sexually transmitted infection (STI), the probability of transmission is low—about 1 in 300 male to female and 1 in 1000 female to male (Gray et al. 2001; Wawer et al. 2005). This is why there are so many "serodiscordant" couples, that is, long-term couples with different HIV statuses (Bishop and Foreit 2010; Eyawo et al. 2010).[12]

Each of these facts about HIV is well-known. Researchers also recognize the importance of pooled risk on a conceptual level. The problem is that this broader epidemiological milieu is largely absent from the existing empirical research on HIV risk and prevention and from related policy initiatives. The dominant approach is the one we subsequently outline in Chapters 4 and 5, which focus on an individual's AIDS-related knowledge and the three primary outcomes emphasized by the ABC approach to HIV prevention: abstinence, faithfulness, and condom use.

This disconnect between a complex epidemiological reality and the simplicity of dominant scholarly approaches is problematic in general. But it's particularly problematic here, since the most plausible argument for an effect of religion on the risk of infection is that religion alters not only the behavior of an individual but also the pool of risk, which is a function of the behavior of other members of

the community. To understand the effects of religion we therefore need to account for both the role of individual religiosity and the broader religious context. These are two distinct dimensions.

One useful concept in this literature is the *sex market* (Laumann 2004), which
can be thought of as a spatially and culturally bounded arena in which decisions
about sexual partnering are made. The primary appeal of this concept is that it
helps us understand how community-level phenomena affect the patterns of
sexual partnering that facilitate the spread of AIDS in SSA. Certain demographic
factors like the age and sex ratios of a community place structural constraints on
the sex market (Oppenheimer 1988). Other supraindividual factors that can affect the sex market—or a person's access to it—include organizational interventions or surveillance by family members. For example, a recent study of marital
infidelity in Zambia identified a number of community-level factors that predict
extramarital sex for both men and women. Community-based interventions
were associated with reduced levels of (reported) male and female infidelity, as
were community media efforts (Benefo 2007; Gerland 2005). Increased economic
opportunities in a community were particularly important for reducing levels of
male infidelity—perhaps because it increased women's economic independence
and their bargaining power in relationships or perhaps because men's own self
worth could now be augmented in ways other than sexual conquest.

Moral Communities

Like other contextual factors that provide constraints and opportunities on the
sex market, religion also operates through these types of contextual influences.
What is known as the "moral communities hypothesis" is rooted in this line of
thought. It not only posits the existence of contextual religious influences on
individuals' behavior—regardless of their own particular commitment to the
religion—but also suggests that living with or near a considerable number of
religious people will affect how an individual's own religion influences his or her
behavior. Stark (1996: 164), for example, argues that "what counts is not only
whether a particular person is religious, but whether this religiousness is, or is
not, ratified by the social environment." Religiosity is associated with confor-
mity (i.e., obeying community norms), he argues, only in distinctly religious
contexts—among groups of people or in communities where the mean level of
religiosity is high (Stark and Bainbridge 1996).[13] In statistical terms, there are
both direct and indirect effects of living in a devoutly religious context: the
direct effects modify an individual's behavior; the indirect effects shape how
individual religiosity is associated with the behavior in question.

Our data from Malawi allow us to examine HIV prevalence across these two
distinct dimensions: the religiosity of individuals and the religious context. By

grouping respondents within their villages we can measure religiosity as both an individual and a collective attribute, and we can empirically evaluate the moral communities hypothesis by modeling the relationships between these two distinct domains and HIV prevalence or, in the following chapters, the HIV-related behavior of individuals.[14]

Like neighborhoods in the United States, all Malawian villages have their own character even if, to the outsider, they initially appear quite similar. Some are large (hundreds of households); others are tiny (around a dozen families). Some are overwhelmingly female (due to high levels of labor migration for men), while others are fairly balanced or even have an excess of males. Some villages look like a ghost town on Sunday mornings, with everyone worshipping at their respective congregations. In other villages, the markets are just as crowded as religious congregations on Friday afternoons and Sunday mornings. Table 2.2 displays a range of these features, including HIV prevalence, in 95 Malawian villages from our study.[15] Nine villages have *no* infected respondents—and can be considered relatively insulated from AIDS, even in a context of a generalized epidemic. In 11 villages, HIV prevalence exceeds 25%, representing a very different reality. In villages where average religiosity is high, over 90% of residents attend services every week, while only about half attend this frequently in the low religiosity villages.

To assess the contextual role of religion, we merged data on the characteristics of these villages with data on the HIV status and sexual behavior of the individuals living within them. In a subsample of currently married individuals, 6% of women and 18% of men reported having an extramarital partner in the past year, and our biomarker data show that 8% of women and 6% of men tested positive for HIV in 2004. We then specified a series of hierarchical linear models (HLM) that allow us to test the moral communities hypothesis in a direct way. Like standard regression, HLM estimates can tell us

Table 2.2 **Descriptive Overview of 95 Rural Malawian Villages in Three Districts**

	Mean	SD[a]	Min	Max
Respondents per Village	31	24	10	142
Average Age	33	4	23	42
Proportion Male	0.45	0.09	0.25	0.71
Proportion HIV Positive	0.07	0.08	0.00	0.33

[a] Standard deviation.
Source: MDICP-3, 2004.

whether risk behavior and HIV status vary by religiosity for individuals. But uniquely, HLM techniques also allow us to see whether these individual-level characteristics (sexual behavior or serostatus) also vary by characteristics of their village. We can also test whether key village-level factors alter the relationship between religion and individual-level outcomes like HIV status and extramarital sex.

HIV Serostatus: A Village Affair

Our Malawi data reveal important *religiosity* differences in HIV status at both the individual and village levels. Figure 2.3 shows the relationship between religious involvement and HIV positive status for women and men, respectively.[16] In each case, three lines can be seen, each representing a different level of village-level religiosity, where the darkest line represents the most religious villages (top quartile) and the lightest line estimates trends within the least religious villages (bottom quartile).

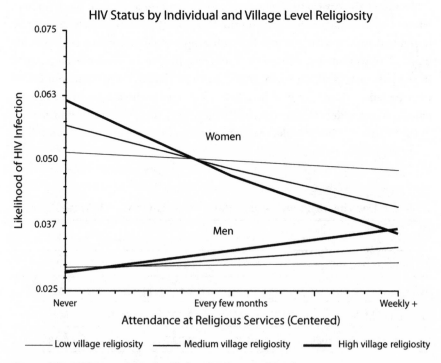

Figure 2.3 HIV Status by Individual and Village-Level Religiosity
Source: Malawi Diffusion and Ideational Change Project

As evidenced by the top three lines, for women the relationship between religious involvement and HIV-positive status is negative (evidenced by downward-sloping lines) across village contexts, but the relative impact of individual-level religiosity varies. Religious women in religious villages (located at the right-most point of the darkest line) are the least likely to test positive for HIV. In villages where religiosity is low overall, on the other hand, individual-level religiosity has only a tiny protective effect for women (this line is nearly flat). For women overall, therefore, individual-level religiosity is negatively associated with HIV infection, but the magnitude of this association depends on the religious context.

The relationship between religiosity and HIV for men tells a different story. Both village- and individual-level religiosity positively predict HIV-positive status among men. Furthermore, the two interact in a way that amplifies these associations. In highly religious villages, highly religious men are the most likely to test positive for HIV. In contrast, there is no effect of village-level religiosity on the likelihood of infection among less religious men.

There are a number of possible explanations for this counterintuitive finding among men (which is, it should be noted, net of many sociodemographic and risk factors). One is that since religious villages have stronger norms against extramarital sex, men in these villages are less likely to have extramarital sex with other women in their village—too few willing partners and too many eyes and ears. If they want extramarital sex, they are therefore more likely to seek it with women outside their own village. Where these women are drawn from a higher risk pool, including sex workers and other women who "bridge" sexual networks, rural men are more likely to become infected by going "outside" than by limiting their search for sexual partners to women in their own village.

Gender differences in selection processes may also help explain the anomaly of religion and HIV prevalence for men. Although teachings against extramarital sex are applied to both men and women, religious norms against extramarital sex may be particularly strong for women, leading women who are either engaging in risky sexual behavior or who know that they are infected with HIV to reduce their levels of religious involvement as a way of avoiding real or perceived stigma. Men, on the other hand, may be less likely to experience social sanctioning from religious leaders or fellow members; men who are infected may also be less fearful of being stigmatized. In fact, the men who are most likely to be infected may be increasing their levels of religious involvement as a strategy for avoiding HIV. This raises a secondary series of methodological questions about "selection," which has significant implications for understanding causal order in a linked series of events. We return to this question in the final chapter in the context of a more in-depth discussion of AIDS's effects on religion.

Conclusions

In examining the relationship between religion and HIV status at the ecological and individual levels, we have established some clear and important religious patterns in the shape of the AIDS epidemic. First, across countries, no single religious bloc stands out as either more protected against HIV or—on the flip side—more likely to have been infected. We will see later that this lack of difference across major religious blocs is reflected in the lack of difference across denominations. Instead, HIV clusters in particular villages, and it is also significantly affected by religiosity at both the individual and village levels.

The associations between religiosity and HIV prevalence are critically important. They show that thinking about the effects of religion on AIDS only in terms of religious identity or affiliation is an analytic dead end. It hardly matters what religion someone is. But it matters a lot how religious someone is: people who are more religious (as measured by involvement in their religious community) are less likely to be HIV positive. Moreover, this is not simply an artifact of reverse causation. Controlling for health status—whether or not a person is well enough to walk to church or mosque—mediates but does not explain this negative relationship between religiosity and HIV infection.

Beyond individual religiosity, religious context—often overlooked—independently affects a person's likelihood of being HIV positive. The most notable result here, in our view, is the fact that religious villages provide a (relatively) protective environment for women—especially for those who are religious themselves. Since women, especially young women, are at the center of most efforts to stop the spread of HIV, this is an important finding. It also underscores the analytic utility of moving back and forth between the individual and community levels to develop a clear picture of religion's role. We now explore that back and forth in a slightly different way by looking at the cognitive and moral frames that people use to interpret AIDS. These, too, are deeply affected by religion.

PART TWO

UNDERSTANDING AIDS

In this section we tackle the relationship between religion and popular understandings of AIDS across the subcontinent. In doing so, our approach deviates from the more typical one used in public health scholarship. We begin by showing how interpretive schemes across all branches of the Christian and Muslim traditions in sub-Saharan Africa (SSA) draw heavily on religious discourse, sometimes in opposition to, but sometimes in sync with, Western biomedical schema (Chapter 3). Only then do we deal with knowledge of HIV and AIDS—where knowledge is typically understood as a necessary condition for behavior change because it provides people with information that they can use to protect themselves (Chapter 4). This sets the stage for discussing HIV prevention, the principal topic of Part 3.

Interpreting the AIDS Epidemic

For there is wrath gone out against us, and the Plague is begun.
That dreadful arrow of Thine sticks fast in our flesh.[1]
—Common Prayer, *July 12, 1665*

Thinking about the ways AIDS is interpreted in Africa—which we must do before considering African responses to AIDS and its effects—leads us directly into the broad area of religion. For AIDS in Africa, like the experience of illness in religious societies in general, is often interpreted religiously. The vocabularies and scripts associated with its religions and religious institutions are the primary resources people draw on to imbue AIDS-related suffering and death with meaning (Wuthnow 1989).[2] Religious perspectives and worldviews color people's experience of AIDS—from first perceptions about it, to stereotypes about people that have it, to ways of combating it, to assumptions about the worthiness of different human lives, right down to how people endure its final agonies and manage the grief of losing loved ones. Differences in perspectives and worldviews—in particular between the understandings that prevail in SSA and the West—also help explain the origins of various prevention strategies and clarify why there remains no clear, uncontested way to avoid new infections.

In seeking to understand how AIDS is interpreted locally, we will not describe the contours of indigenous belief systems in great detail, long the turf of anthropologists (Leclerc-Madlala 1997). Rather, we focus on publicly circulating African AIDS narratives, which are embedded in people's wider social world and social experiences. First we mention some special characteristics of AIDS that shape its interpretation in SSA. We then describe perceptions of the overall risk environment, three approaches to divine judgment, and the distinction between proximate and ultimate causes of infection. We end by reviewing two more general issues that shape how AIDS is understood. The first is a brief description of views about the origins of HIV. The second deals with the relationship between attitudes to AIDS and attitudes to fertility.

"We have this disease these days called AIDS."
—Pastor, *African Independent Church, Rumphi*

HIV is distinct from most other health conditions. These differences contribute to the sense of enigma that surrounds AIDS. Understanding them helps us understand the interpretive challenges that AIDS poses in SSA and appreciate the suspicions that enshroud all interpretive discussions of AIDS (Liddell, Barrett, and Bwdawell 2005; Smith 2004b).

We think there are five core characteristics of AIDS that affect its interpretation in SSA.

- *The mysteries of infection*: HIV often seems arbitrary in whom it strikes. Compared with easily transmittable sexually transmitted infections (STIs) like gonorrhea, HIV is hard to get—all other things being equal and known, which of course they never are.[3] As noted in Chapter 2, the probability of transmission is low, which is one of the main reasons that there is no clear relationship between promiscuity or any "risky" sexual behavior and infection. Consequently, stories about a neighbor who occasionally cheats on his wife yet appears healthy could be stories of very good odds. And stories of faithful men and women who nevertheless become ill could be stories of bad odds. But where faith in randomness and luck is feeble, more culturally appropriate explanations inevitably emerge.
- *The long latent period*: Infected individuals become symptomatic nearly 10 years after contracting the virus. This long period between infection and symptoms makes it difficult to draw clear causal connections between behaviors and outcomes as these relate to AIDS. It also means that otherwise healthy-looking people transmit the infection.
- *The mysteries of science*: Despite billions of dollars and over 25 years of focused research, there is no cure for HIV or AIDS. And even though there is a pill (or set of pills—antiretroviral drugs) that can keep AIDS at bay and whose distribution is increasingly being "scaled up" in SSA, until recently, few Africans had access to them. Likewise, exactly when and how HIV morphs into AIDS remains elusive, even to scientists.
- *Relationship-based*: The most common pathway for HIV transmission in SSA is through heterosexual sex. This means that HIV is what social network scholars call "alter dependent"—an individual's own HIV status hinges on the status of a sexual partner.[4] In turn, this makes AIDS different from other serious health problems. For example, while one's own risk of cancer or heart disease can be affected by things that friends do—we're more likely to smoke if our friends do or to eat endless pots of ice cream or fatty meats if they do, too—we don't catch cancer or heart disease from our friends. We can, however, catch HIV from them.

- *International response:* AIDS has left an enormous footprint in SSA. Many of its effects are profoundly personal. In the high-prevalence areas with which we're most familiar, everyone knows that young adults live shorter lives than they used to. People bemoan the increase in funerals and, more quietly, complain about the burden of contributing to so many. Increasingly, people talk about the growing number of orphans and both the obligation and struggle to provide for them. We revisit specific examples of these effects in the following chapters—institutional effects in Chapter 7 and care of those affected by AIDS in Chapters 8 and 9. One special characteristic of AIDS compared with other health issues, however, is the strength of the international response. The megabucks spent on AIDS-related programs and interventions—a slew of new nongovernmental organizations (NGOs), omnipresent signs, radio announcements, and seminars about AIDS are among the clearest examples—have led to an institutional revolution on the ground. The NGO sector has ballooned, medical systems have been changed, school curricula reformed.

Each of these characteristics adds another layer of interpretive challenges. It's confusing to have no clear line of sight between behavior and outcome; or to officially have a condition but show no signs of being sick for years; or to be told that scientists—the all-powerful magicians of the modern era—can't figure out AIDS; or to see or hear about enormous inflows of money from donors. This confusion creates a fertile landscape for alternative narratives. Before describing those, however, we talk about one of the more surprising aspects of AIDS in Africa—at least surprising to outsiders highly sensitized to AIDS—its relatively low place on the risk-related totem pole.

Living in a Richly Risky Environment

Survey after survey confirms that nearly everyone in SSA understands how HIV is transmitted. People know how to prevent infection. They know the symptoms. And they also know how AIDS impacts those infected with the virus and their survivors. These high levels of knowledge have been observed across SSA for quite some time.[5] In Malawi, knowledge of HIV was estimated at 98% in rural areas as early as 2001, long before media coverage and formal prevention programs proliferated (Watkins 2004).

Many in the West find this hard to believe. We presume "they" *must* not know. Otherwise, why wouldn't they pull out all stops to put an end to the epidemic? The assumptions that Africans don't know and that what they need is more information drives both secular and religious donors to fund public service announcements, drama teams that go from one market town to another putting

on AIDS-related shows, the ubiquitous pamphlets and posters, and other programs designed to disseminate knowledge about HIV. At the root of the assumption lies a dogged commitment to the Health Belief Model (HBM), the conceptual
framework that has shaped health education since the 1970s (Janz and Becker
1984; Rosenstock 1966; Rosenstock, Strecher, and Becker 1988). The HBM takes
various forms (see, e.g., Redding, Rossi, Rossi, Velicer, and Prochaska 2000), but
all of these forms treat knowledge as a necessary condition for (desirable) behavior change. In other words, the HBM framework presumes that individuals will
act rationally in order to reduce the risk of infection (or ill-health) once they
know about the undesirable health consequences of a given behavior. In cases
where individuals continue to choose risky behaviors even after receiving that
knowledge—in developed societies, some people continue to smoke or to drive
without seat belts even when they know that their long-term risks of illness or
injury are higher—knowledge is still considered a *good* thing. To HBM believers,
these failures simply signal a lack of "self-efficacy"—the ability to do something
that one knows is right. In turn, this lack of self-efficacy is typically attributed to
socially embedded factors like sense of self, feeling of empowerment, or place in
the social hierarchy. Each of these implies that "doing the right thing" in terms
of health can run headlong into "doing the right thing" along some other dimension: acting in accordance with one's own moral code or community standards or
meeting familial expectations.

Applied to AIDS, the HBM implies that people will stop unsafe sexual practices once they know how HIV is transmitted and have been told or—better
yet—shown what AIDS will do to them (Rosenstock et al. 1988; Rugalema
2004). Indeed, this model underlies HIV testing and counseling (HTC) in Africa
just as it underlies public health campaigns in developed countries. The problem, of course, is that the relationships between knowledge, attitudes, and action are much more complex than the HBM allows for. This is true in Western
societies, where many people continue to "irrationally" smoke cigarettes and eat
unhealthy foods in the face of prominently placed warning labels or nutritional
information.[6] The same is true in Africa. AIDS is simply one of a long list of
things that can destabilize daily life. Eliminating AIDS would still leave poverty,
lack of access to capital, capricious authorities, corrupt bureaucracies, a complex
disease environment, and an unreliable food supply. AIDS is simply another
source of uncertainty. It needs to be situated within the broader set of factors
that people worry about and that place constraints on their readiness and ability
to act. The extent to which AIDS-related constraints are qualitatively different
from all the others remains unclear. This is something that those of us who
(have the good fortune to) live in more developed societies have a hard time fully
understanding.[7]

How pressing a problem is AIDS in SSA, relative to other problems? Data
from nationally representative Afrobarometer surveys allow us to answer this

question. Contrary to what we might expect based on the staggering statistics of AIDS-related mortality and illness, AIDS ranks pretty low on the list of concerns. Specifically, across the 20 countries that fielded this type of survey in 2008–2009, respondents were asked to list their three most pressing problems. Less than 1% (0.8%) mentioned AIDS as the most important problem in a first response, 1.3% as a second response, and 1.5% as a third response. In all cases, AIDS ranks far below the top-ranked problems, which relate to economic issues, infrastructure, drought, crime, and security. And even in high-prevalence countries, AIDS still ranks far below unemployment, crime, poverty, education, roads, food shortage, water supply, and more general health concerns.

This low ranking of AIDS is not a sign of profound irrationality. On the contrary, in the African context—or across different African contexts—it makes perfect sense. Even where HIV prevalence is high, daily life in SSA is oriented to things that are very familiar to us in the West: people want to find work, feed their families, nurture their marriages, and watch their children grow with more opportunities than they had. AIDS ranks relatively low on the list of major problems because it is only one of a number of things that can derail these hopes and ambitions and because its consequences are only rarely immediate. Ironically, this is even true for HIV-positive individuals. The Afrobarometer data don't allow us to examine this directly—they didn't test people for HIV so we can't differentiate rankings by HIV status—but they certainly imply as much given that the cumulative percentage mentioning AIDS as one of their most pressing problems is consistently lower than observed HIV prevalence rates (true across Africa and in individual states in Africa). This, too, makes intuitive sense. People's immediate concerns center on pervasive and urgent problems: food shortages for their families today, how to secure anti-malarial medication for a sick child by tomorrow, and what to do about the mediocre harvests shaping up next month (Dionne, Gerland, and Watkins 2011).

Another way to look at perceptions of AIDS in a generalized epidemic is to ask directly about its salience to daily life. We followed this strategy with our Malawi Diffusion and Ideational Change Project (MDICP) respondents in rural Malawi, asking them how concerned they are that they will become infected. Results are shown in Table 3.1. While being "worried a lot" is the modal answer at 40%, over one in three Malawians are not worried at all about acquiring the virus. In a country with 11% HIV prevalence, one in three sounds like a relatively low number. This further suggests that Malawians are less worried about AIDS than we, as outsiders, would expect them to be.[8] This pattern of AIDS-related worry is true across religious groups, even though there is also some religious variation in its intensity: high levels of worry are most prevalent among Muslims (around 47%), when compared with Mission Protestants, New Mission Protestants, and Pentecostals (all in the 38–40% range), but there are no differences in AIDS-related worry when examined by religiosity (not shown).

Table 3.1 **Level of Worry about Catching HIV/AIDS, Malawi 2004**

How Worried?	Catholic	Mission Protestant	Pentecostal	African Independent Church	Muslim	New Mission Protestant
Not Worried	36.1	34.6	37.4	35.0	31.3	39.5
Worried a Little	23.2	26.9	23.6	24.8	21.3	21.5
Worried a Lot	40.6	38.3	38.9	40.1	47.3	38.9
N	551	646	267	488	740	329

Source: MDICP-3 (*N* = 3040).

Another indicator of concern about AIDS is a person's perceived likelihood of being infected, both now and in the future.[9] Other scholars have shown this measure to be a strong indicator of actual HIV status, and it taps a more specific idea than the general questions about worry examined in Table 3.1.[10] Subjective risk perceptions have another benefit: they can be asked about varying time frames—including about the future. In our Malawi data from 2004, we find that a plurality of people who had never had an HIV test consider their chances of being HIV positive at the time of survey to be zero and that a substantial majority report either zero or low levels of concern (67% of men in general and 77% of religious leaders). In contrast, only a minority (35% of women and 39% of men) report zero chance of being infected in the future.

To test for religious differences in these perceptions, we compared the proportion of individuals who believe there is zero chance of being infected—now and in the future—by religious tradition and level of religiosity (separately for men and women). Examined by religious tradition (not shown), we find that only about 50% of Muslim men and of women belonging to African Independent Churches (AICs) report no chance of becoming infected in the future. In contrast, 72% of New Mission Protestant men express confidence in their ability to avoid infection—interesting, since this tradition is largely composed of the strictest denominations. Results for the effects of religiosity, as measured by the frequency of attendance at a church or mosque, are presented in Figure 3.1. We find a negative linear relationship between more frequent attendance and perceived likelihood of infection for both men and for women. The patterns for current and future infection run along similar tracks. Relative to their less religious peers, a larger proportion of religious men and women, men especially, see themselves as insulated from the epidemic.

So how serious a problem is AIDS for people living in high-prevalence settings? The answers are surprising. Although levels of worry about AIDS are high overall, a sizable portion doesn't worry at all or perceive themselves to be at risk,

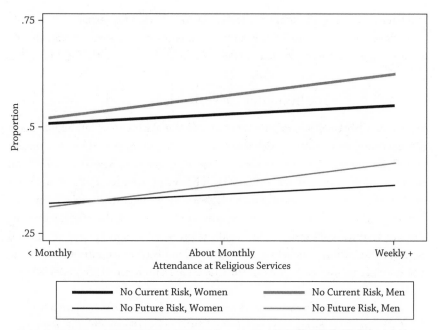

Figure 3.1 Percent Perceiving No Likelihood of Infection by Religious Attendance

even where HIV prevalence is very high. Those who do worry about AIDS are also experiencing other, more pressing problems. This includes both the vast majority of African adults who are HIV negative and those who have HIV, most of whom are still functionally healthy (which in itself allows them to worry about other things). So while few would argue against the notion that AIDS is the most pressing global health problem of our time, its salience to *daily* life in SSA is surprisingly muted.

Divine Judgment

Being cognizant of the widespread suspicion of purely scientific accounts about HIV/AIDS and its origins—more on this later in the chapter—we wondered about the extent to which Africans interpret AIDS supernaturally instead of biomedically, or supernaturally in addition to biomedically. The simplest way that this can be framed in religious terms is this: Is AIDS seen to be God's judgment upon the sexual (or other) misdeeds of people? Or is it just a virus contracted through contact with an infected individual, possibly in ways that have nothing to do with sex and certainly nothing to do with God?

We asked Malawian religious leaders these questions. Although none (i.e., not one out of more than 200) disputed the germ theory of disease, most nevertheless see God at work in the pandemic. STIs themselves, regardless of their role in a pandemic, are widely thought to reflect divine retribution for sexual sin (Caldwell, Orubuloye, and Caldwell 1999). For many, this mysterious, sexually transmitted disease, for which there is no cure, reflects the will of God at work (Ingstad 1990).

The Dominant View: The Hand of God

In general, Christianity puts little stock in traditional African beliefs about ancestors as a source of health or sickness, but Christianity does endorse the notion that God punishes sin. Numerous laws about appropriate sexual behavior and examples of punishing sexual deviance can be culled from the Hebrew Bible and the New Testament. For example, the Hebrew Bible suggests that God sent epidemics both to punish sin—a number are reported during the 40-year Exodus, another terrible one during King David's reign—and to soften hard hearts and bring people back to obedience. Several Christian leaders we interviewed made reference to the "incurable disease" threatened in Deuteronomy 28: 21–24, 27–28:

> The LORD will plague you with diseases until he has destroyed you from the land you are entering to possess. The LORD will strike you with wasting disease, with fever and inflammation, with scorching heat and drought, with blight and mildew, which will plague you until you perish. . . . The LORD will afflict you with the boils of Egypt and with tumors, festering sores and the itch, from which you cannot be cured. The LORD will afflict you with madness, blindness and confusion of mind.

While foreign to most Westerners, on a continent that has long been steeped in such stories—and in pestilence—these references are immediately relevant (Jenkins 2006). A Presbyterian elder with whom we spoke did not mince words. He directly compared their experience of AIDS to that of the days of Noah before the flood:

> The way I see it [AIDS] is the punishment from God. . . . In the way our friends died with the floods, Noah. It was a punishment. In the same way I take it as a punishment to us! . . . [Do the church members also take it as a punishment?] Yes! They take it as a punishment . . . yes! [Pause] . . . All who have a strong faith—they will be saved. In the same way our friend Noah was saved because his faith was strong enough.

A Presbyterian deacon also drew a parallel between current experiences and biblical precedent:

> . . . [In] the Bible it says there will come some diseases which will not be cured. But the Bible was written days [tr. "ages"] ago. Before AIDS.

Therefore it means the disease has come on earth, which shows the ending of the earth. Once a person gets the disease he is going to die because there is no medicine. The Bible it says it will be diseases and war. At our congregation they refer to the coming of AIDS; that is the punishment.

Mainstream Muslim views are similar. Several Muslim scholars who have written about AIDS (e.g., Bham 2008; Badri 1997/2000) draw on the following *hadith*:[11]

If *fahishah* or fornication and all kinds of sinful sexual intercourse become rampant and openly practised without inhibition in any group or nation, Allâh will punish them with new epidemics [*ta'un*] and new diseases which were not known to their forefathers and earlier generations.

Like their Christian counterparts, most of the Muslim sheikhs we interviewed expressed their belief in a divine origin to the disease, suggesting the AIDS pandemic was foreordained. One told us:

Our book of Quran says that close to the final days people will be all over, enjoying their life, and forget whatever God has told us . . . never following what our prophet Muhammad was doing and other prophets, that in the end result people will experience diseases which will not be cured. That is what I know about AIDS.

Others added a veneer of inevitability to the divine ordination. This sheikh, who doubles as a traditional healer, was particularly pessimistic:

[*What did you say about HIV to the mosque during prayers?*] I said that, gentlemen . . . God said that there will be . . . an outbreak of diseases which is incurable. This is the time. We are all getting finished. There will be nobody who will be left because now this disease has come.

We could add dozens of examples here. Together, they point to a very clear and singular message. The hand of God plays a central role in the spread of HIV. This view is consistent with deeply embedded cultural schema about experiences with the supernatural. Christian and Muslim narratives about creation, the fall of humankind, the ire of God, and promises of redemption echo anthropologist Daniel Smith's (2004b: 430) claim—based on his research in Nigeria—that "the dominant religious discourse about AIDS is that it is a scourge visited by God on a society that has turned its back on religion and morality."

These "hand of God" theories do not contradict other narratives about the origins of AIDS, such as the widespread belief that it originated in the West, as we discuss later in this chapter. On the contrary, all these views are seamlessly merged in a classical approach to Biblical exegesis: God uses people to shape history in accordance with a master plan. The merging of these two views is evident in work by other scholars. One of Smith's (2004b: 430) Nigerian informants describes AIDS as one of a number of scourges—others are crime, corruption, famine, and other illnesses—which are ". . . God's punishment, but we have brought it on ourselves." The punishment is the result of a breakdown of older ways and moralities.

This instrumental use of people is also a theme some informants use to make sense of how AIDS affects the innocent. Narratives about AIDS are rooted in the link between individual sin and collective suffering. One Muslim sheikh explained it as follows:

> As it was in the past, God afflicted the people with plague because of the sins of one or two people. But it was found that many people were afflicted by the plague.

This even puzzled the interviewer:

> [*If not mistaken, I have heard you talking about AIDS not (being) a sin and about the plague. Can you explain more and differentiate these things?*]. . . .
> Let me put it this way: a child can feed on the breast milk of an infected mother, who got the disease during adultery. The child gets the virus, but can we say that the child was involved in this act? So the child faces the problems because of the mother.

In other words, AIDS is understood fundamentally as a divinely ordained plague. But as recounted in the Biblical and Koranic stories, innocents are caught up in the suffering. A Pentecostal elder talked about plagues, comparing AIDS to drought, which certainly falls outside human control:

> Plague means a thing that cannot have any treatment . . . like drought. Drought and plague are two things that are similar, for those who have harvested and those who haven't. They all get struck by the drought.

These views are in complete contrast to those held by most people in the West. Comparatively few Americans (and even fewer Europeans) hold that God might judge and punish people for their behavior, much less bring a calamity like AIDS upon the world that punishes the guilty and innocent alike. For example, in a 1998 religion module of the General Social Survey, a major source of data on the U.S. population, less than 6% of people asked to "Think about how you try to understand and deal with major problems in your life" closely identified with the suggestion that "God is punishing me for my sins or lack of spirituality." Fully 77% of Americans strongly disagreed with the idea. Nor do Americans tend to equate HIV/AIDS in Africa with the divine judgment of God—at least not publicly, and at least not today—even if they do interpret AIDS in religious terms. (Indeed, many religious Americans may do that. We don't know and have not found any survey data that can answer that question.) The central point is that the idea of "God's divine judgment" on nations or groups has been largely suppressed in contemporary Western Christianity. Notwithstanding occasional claims by popular televangelists (e.g., Pat Robertson on 9/11, Hurricane Katrina, and the Haiti earthquake), ours has become a more individualistic religious culture. In the same way that our legal system does not countenance collective punishment, most of us don't believe in collective moral culpability.[12] In much of Africa, however, and in Islam in general, notions of collective divine punishment are woven into the social fabric. As the Pentecostal elder said, "Those who have harvested and those who haven't . . . all get struck by the drought." Even where versions of Christianity have individualistic elements—like in the increasingly popular Pentecostal tradition, in which individuals, and not communities, are "born again"—a collective relationship to the supernatural remains paramount in SSA.

We have at least one empirical indicator from Malawi to support these assertions about the importance of the collective. Even though the religious leaders we interviewed ranked many other things as more pressing problems than AIDS, and most hardly worried about their own prospects of infection (see Table 3.2), they readily spoke about AIDS as a collective problem. In particular, when we

Table 3.2 **Perceived Likelihood of Current and Future Infection in Malawi**

	Laypersons (%)		*Religious Leaders (%)*	
	Current	*Future*	*Current*	*Future*
None	60	39	70	60
Low	20	28	13	17
Medium	5	11	2	6
High	4	6	1	2
Don't Know	10	16	13	14
N	1455		187	

Sources: MDICP-3, 2004 and MRP, 2005.

asked them about how AIDS stacked up against other problems that confront their congregations, 28% of leaders listed it as *the single biggest problem*. An additional 36% list it as a "big problem" but not the largest. These responses are in a completely different ballpark than the responses about individual rankings and risks. These reports also massively exceed the national HIV prevalence in Malawi, in the 10–14% range when these data were collected.

This difference between how religious leaders and individuals rank AIDS hinges on the extent to which AIDS is interpreted as a collective problem. Groups can be punished for the actions of individuals: "all get struck by the drought." As we shall see later, this view also has implications for how religious leaders attempt to police their members' actions. Simply, where one believes that collective punishment can result from an individual's sin, helping others avoid sin is a rational and reasonable—even morally obligatory—response because it helps minimize punishment writ large.

Moralizing the Individual: AIDS as the Mark of Cain or Mark of Stupidity

A related but distinct discourse about punishment focuses on individuals. This discourse figures strongly in debates about religion's role in fostering stigma—the central focus of Chapter 8. The key idea here is that having HIV is like the mark of Cain. It's evidence of a person's immorality.

Pentecostals are widely assumed to be the group that makes the most explicit connection between sex and HIV in this type of moralistic framework (Smith 2004b). Somewhat counter to this assumption, however—ironically so—is the fact that Pentecostals are also the most market-driven Christian tradition active in Africa today. Their evangelical raison d'être shapes the Pentecostal messages about AIDS—they can't have too punitive an approach since this would preemptively exclude large numbers of people (HIV-positive individuals and their families) from their pool of potential recruits.

We tested for denominational differences in this "mark of Cain" discourse by asking our MDICP respondents to report whether their religious leaders believe that the sexually *movious*—those who "sleep around" and get infected—have gotten what they deserved. We then compared these with the reports of the religious leaders themselves.

Results can be seen in Table 3.3. The first thing to note is that there is little variation in what people think their religious leaders believe. Roughly 4 in 10 say their religious leader believes that the sexually immoral HIV-positive individuals got what they deserved. Far higher percentages of religious leaders actually say this.

More noteworthy, however, is the fact that Pentecostal leaders are not as "judgmental" as other religious leaders about sexual sin and HIV as its consequence.[13] Despite their close identification of HIV/AIDS with God's

Table 3.3 **Popular Perceptions and Religious Leaders' Self-Reports about Promiscuity and HIV Infection, by Religious Tradition in Malawi**

Religious Tradition	"The Movious Who Become Infected Deserve It" (% Agree/Strongly Agree)		
	People Report Religious Leaders in the Village Think This	Religious Leaders Actually Believe This	Difference Between the Two
Catholic	40.8	85.7	44.9
Mission Protestant	39.4	84.2	44.8
Pentecostal	37.4	53.1	15.7
African Independent	43.7	70.3	26.6
Muslim	41.5	81.8	40.3
New Mission Protestant	40.0	85.3	45.3

Sources: MDICP-3, 2004 and MRP, 2005.

judgment and people's sin, they are, in fact, the *least likely* to say that the sexually immoral deserve what they got. Those in the pews at these same Pentecostal churches grasp this position fairly accurately. Only 16 percentage points distinguish the leaders' actual reports and the laity's perceptions, well below the average 40–45% gap in perception observed for the other religious traditions.

This is not to say that Pentecostals in SSA always have warm and fuzzy views about AIDS. Far from it. A common theme in Pentecostal talk about AIDS is the destructive consequences of ignoring God's intentions for human sexual behavior. Pentecostals believe that breaking God's rules brings disorder and pain. They simply make fewer theological arguments about the particular direction or targets of God's wrath. We discuss these issues further in Chapter 8, when we describe how these perceived associations between HIV infection and God's judgment affect active discrimination and hostility against individual persons living with HIV and AIDS.

Alongside this mark of Cain talk is a second discourse. We refer to it as "playing with fire." It identifies stupidity, rather than immorality, as the underlying cause of a person's infection. A good example of this is reported by Watkins (2004), based on her record of daily conversations in Malawi over a period of several years during which AIDS was on the rise. She saw people move from confusion about a wasting disease without a known cause to consensus about the stupidity of people who did not change their behavior in light of AIDS. She explains that those who do not heed the advice to "take care"—which may suggest condom use or being choosy about sexual partners—are considered foolish and careless, throwing away their own futures as well as risking those of their spouse and children. Of course, there are no guarantees that these particular precautions will avert infection. But it's a behavioral move toward greater self-protection. Failing to do it invites infection.

Similar views fusing a person's foolish and sinful behavior as the ultimate cause of infection are widespread across the subcontinent. For example, a Senegalese imam interviewed in 2007 (more on those interviews in Chapter 8) summarizes this view in likening adultery to suicide:

> For me . . . it [adultery] resembles when someone takes a knife and cuts his own throat. Because everyone knows that the event of sleeping with someone who is not one's wife brings the *maladie*. If you do it, you wound yourself. It's suicide. God gave you a spirit, eyes, ears, etc. The person recognizes heat and cold. A person can recognize if water is cold or hot. You know if that if you do adultery, you can get HIV, so don't do it. If you do it and you get the *maladie*, it's a punishment. God said in the Koran to not do things that He doesn't want because it can bring danger. If someone comes and gets in a village and sleeps with whomever, it's he who does it. If he gets sick and dies because of it, it is he who has killed himself. It's not an act of God, it's suicide.

Likewise, during one of the most memorable religious services we observed in Malawi, a Catholic priest's homily concerned a foolish man who found a snake pit outside his house, but the message was not about a snake pit at all. One day, this foolish and boastful man curiously stuck his arm into the pit. Fortunately (this was an aggressive kind of snake), the snake did not attack the fool. But instead of being thankful for his good fortune, the man went around bragging to his neighbors, "Look! This snake cannot bite me." Every day, the man would stick his arm in the snake pit and brag about it. The neighbors counseled him that sticking his arm into the snake pit was not a good idea, but he did not heed their warnings. They became bored with his foolishness and began to ignore him, shaking their heads when he came around. On the day the snake finally did bite him, none of these neighbors were very sympathetic. The story, told to an audience that included small children, had people on the floor laughing. Yet it is not a message of fire and brimstone. It is pragmatic and good-humored. To this priest, the occasional (sexual) misstep is a completely understandable thing. But brazen risk-taking—in the era of AIDS—is just foolishness.

A Minority Position

Not all religious leaders point to sin—individual or collective—as the source of divine indignation and, therefore, AIDS. Some carefully clarify that even if it is a sin, only God can know. For example, a Church of Christ pastor described the epidemic this way:

> AIDS is not a sin. [*I see.*] AIDS on its own is a disease . . . A sin is that person who is committing adultery [pause] . . . He is just very unfortunate, because he can sin because of adultery but some of us sin through stealing. There is no difference between theft and adultery, (it's) all sin.

Consistent with this, he goes on to explain that ". . . if one sins and gets AIDS it does not mean that he has sinned most . . ."

Similar Muslim voices can also be heard. One sheikh offered no sense of divine drama, even when asked why AIDS "is on us." Instead he diverted the discussion to the primary mechanisms of infection: "AIDS is [upon] us firstly [by] adultery, secondly sharing needles and razor blade, thirdly at the hospital giving our friends blood which is not tested."[14]

For others still, the elements of unjust suffering and innocence simply mitigate the idea that a good God could be the source of the pandemic. One Presbyterian elder pointed out the common misgivings while still suggesting that God does not let sexual sin go unpunished:

> . . . maybe they were married and it's the other partner who passed it to them. So we cannot always take it as a sin, but we know for sure that God will punish everyone accordingly, so it doesn't matter if you got it after breaking the rules of the Lord or it's your husband who passed it to you.

This African Continent Mission (AIC) leader agreed:

> . . . AIDS is not related to sins because one can get it unknowingly. Not all people who are suffering from AIDS got it through sex. Maybe they got it from the injections which are commonly found in these villages, so [there's] no link between these two. If [it] is a sin, only God knows.

Although some religious leaders are hesitant to suggest that God sent the AIDS pandemic, very few would dispute that God can or does punish the sexual misdeeds warned against in the Bible and the Koran. Even leaders in religious groups that are traditionally more educated and closer to Western theological positions, like Presbyterians, do not stand out here. They are as likely as any other religious group to claim divine involvement. In fact, in analyzing over 200 interviews with religious leaders in Malawi, we identified the extent to which leaders articulate a collectivist "all get struck by drought" message as one of the most critical dimensions along which AIDS-related theodicies could be differentiated. Yet these differences did not always overlap with denomination in predictable ways. On one hand—and not surprisingly—messages of collective punishment appeared more frequently in Pentecostal and Charismatic congregations than in the Mission churches (e.g., Anglicans and Presbyterians). But on the other hand, collectivist views of divine punishment were present across traditions, and the tenor of these interpretations varied more within denominations than across them.

Proximate and Ultimate Causes of HIV

Understanding African views about the role of God and divine judgment in the spread of HIV is related to a more general discussion about the difference between proximate and ultimate causes of infection. We have already mentioned that HIV infections are hard to predict. This is true for social scientists trying to model the disease (even the best models explain only a small fraction of the variance), and it is true on the ground as well.[15] The clearest example of this is the one that we described in relation to the mysteries of infection: one person cheats on his spouse and "gets caught" by getting infected, while another does the same yet remains HIV negative and healthy.

Fear or anxiety about suffering and death—which AIDS undoubtedly constitutes in the lives of many and threatens in many more—are not only "lived through," as sociologist Peter Berger (1967: 53) suggests. Since we are inherently meaning-seeking creatures, we also seek to explain suffering "in terms of the *nomos* (or the meaningful order) established in the society in question." This interpretive process is necessary for making sense of events. It makes the emotional (and perhaps even the physical) pain of death and suffering more tolerable, less overwhelming, and thus staves off both terror and anomie.

Contrasting the HIV-positive status of a faithful wife with the HIV-negative status of a known cheat and philanderer raises difficult questions about *nomos*. Because AIDS affects a group but leaves its main mark—infection—on individuals, *nomos* vis-à-vis AIDS is distinct from the other causes of uncertainty and suffering we mentioned earlier (e.g., drought, political instability, religious tensions, everyday corruption). Only where infection is seen as a product of individual action can being HIV positive be like a mark of Cain. This type of mark is distinct from the effects of drought or political instability, broadly understood as nets cast widely from above that capture people indiscriminately.

This distinction between proximate from ultimate causes of HIV is critical for understanding how people in SSA address the interpretive challenges associated with resolving the *nomos* issue AIDS engenders. This boils down to asking why a particular person is infected. This question may seem self-explanatory to most westerners. We have internalized official Western biomedical discourses on "why?" That discourse is rooted in scientific practice and standards, is inherently materialistic, and embeds knowledge of observable phenomena in a probability-based frame. It therefore identifies an individual's HIV status as the product of proximate causes and "risk factors," each filtered through a crucial and *exogenous* stochastic element: good or bad luck.

This marks a significant difference with the interpretive frames that are dominant in Africa. Across SSA, premature death is seldom attributed exclusively to bad luck, chance, or the unknowable hand of God (Yamba 1997). This is not to deny the proximate reason of infection—usually sex with an infected person—which is well understood. But from an African perspective, these proximate causes merely explain *how* someone becomes infected. They don't explain *why*. The why is the ultimate or *real* cause of the condition.[16]

Scholarship on African health and nonwestern disease etiologies offers a useful typology for understanding how ideas about proximate and ultimate causes of disease are not necessarily inconsistent with one another (Foster 1976; Ingstad 1990; Liddell et al. 2005). Illnesses are often categorized into one of three types:

1. minor illnesses or infections that are annoying but lack any moral or social cause;
2. serious illnesses to which only Africans seem susceptible, like river blindness or Ebola;
3. modern diseases introduced in Africa by outsiders (HIV/AIDS and other STIs fit this).

Serious illnesses and modern diseases are often thought to have an ultimate cause (i.e., why the person became ill) that is distinguishable from its proximate cause (i.e., how the person became ill). Proximate causes are analogous to Western explanations. So when people know or deduce how they were infected with HIV, this does not explain why they got it. The question may strike Westerners as odd or rhetorical, but it is ever-present in African conversations about AIDS—public and private. At the risk of reifying it, we also can't imagine it diminishing substantially in the foreseeable future (e.g., with increasing modernization). It is, and will remain, a central a part of African cultural cognition.

People everywhere fish around for answers to these types of questions. In SSA, most of the fishing takes place in the religious realm—this is the domain in which explanations like "punishment from God" or "a jealous neighbor bewitched me" emerge. In fact, the so-called real causes of illness and infection fall under the following broad categories (Ingstad 1990):

- witchcraft triggered by jealousy;
- an offense against ancestors;
- having broken traditional order or wisdom—often through unacceptable sexual practices;
- divine punishment for their own or their partner's sexual missteps.

Each of these reasons represents an exercise in meaning-making over and above the biomedical facts that explain how someone got infected. Note that even though the last in the list refers to divine punishment, here the focus centers on the individual, which stands in contrast to the collective understanding of divine punishment discussed in the previous section.

In this light, the African pursuit of transcendental explanations is completely expected. The Western disinterest in the why questions is the oddity that needs explaining, for the Western approach requires people to fight against their essence as makers of meaning—to abandon the dogged pursuit of ultimate explanations—unless they choose to fall back on ideas about luck and random chance.

In the end, three types of discourses about AIDS have emerged and diffused across Africa (Yamba 1997). Each is distinct and draws differentially upon non-native influence:

1. *Biomedical discourses* take a scientific approach to the subject of HIV, offering a clear cause and effect perspective: treat STIs, change risky sexual behavior, and you too can avoid infection. The fundamental problem with these biomedical approaches is that they do not answer the types of "why" questions specified above—those that address the ultimate causes of disease. They simply give people some behavioral tools they can use to lower the risk of infection.

2. *Religious discourses* may or may not refer to the narrowly specified cause and effect perspective. Their main focus is on avoiding the sexual immorality that is associated with nonmarital sex and is at least implied by condoms. This is comparatively "new" advice—we expand on this in Chapter 6—but is nevertheless consistent with aspects of older, traditional concerns (about, e.g., sexual intercourse with a menstruating woman). These guidelines perform the additional function of making sense of survival and death. They provide a narrative that moves beyond narrowly specified cause and effect.

3. *Traditional African discourses* about social and sexual norms lack a distinctively religious component, but they are similar in lamenting the loss of the "old ways." This generates suspicions—sometimes profound—of biomedical approaches that have yet to cure such a terrible disease, despite the massive

influx of research dollars and brain power. Indeed, the difficulty of curing AIDS is evidence that ostensibly "random" infections are not random at all. Rather, they occur as the result of violations of traditional norms or the insidious effects of bewitching (Yamba 1997). To the extent that this is the case, traditional discourses call for visits to a traditional healer whose alternative treatments, not unlike those employed in the United States, enjoy an element of mystery that both increases their popularity and—potentially, at least—heightens their placebo effect.

We will see how these discourses about AIDS—particularly the first two— permeate approaches and local responses to HIV prevention. For now, we simply note how each discourse reflects a different underlying principle. Underlying the first is a belief in random chance, the product of an unintelligent exogenous force. Underlying the second and third are beliefs that the exogenous force is entirely intended—willed either by divine powers or by local witches.

The Origin of HIV and AIDS

Ontological and existential questions about AIDS in SSA are evident from these debates about AIDS' importance, divine judgment, and proximate versus ultimate causes of infection. However, other issues also affect how people understand AIDS. The first deals with views of where "this thing called AIDS" comes from. Differing beliefs about the origin of AIDS shape people's understandings of it.

The most popular answer to this question in the Western science-and-media narrative is that HIV (in its original strains) originated in Central or West-Central Africa after somehow making the species leap from chimpanzees or monkeys to humans at some point in the middle of the 20th century (Iliffe 2005).[17] Many Africans see it differently. Some agree that AIDS originated in Africa but insist that this occurred when an American or European (i.e., a white man) had sex with a monkey. This alternative narrative is an easy sell. In many African contexts, it maps onto European sexual tourism and onto widely circulating stories of African women persuaded to make their way to developed countries where, instead of marriage to a wealthy white suitor, they find themselves forced into prostitution or, at the very least, a type of private sexual enslavement to a perverted older man. During Weinreb's Kenyan fieldwork, such stories were widely discussed among young university-educated adults. Since then, coastal Kenya has become an even more popular destination for sex tourists, the majority of whom are European (UNICEF 2006).[18]

Another local (and popular) explanation is that AIDS was produced by Westerners, specifically American scientists, as a means of population control.[19] This is consistent with at least one major policy decision in SSA: the attempt to combine AIDS programs with programs run by the family planning movement. However rational this programmatic combination is from an organizational perspective, it visibly reminds people in SSA of another large-scale effort funded by the West, also focused on sex.

A Church of Christ pastor we interviewed in Malawi clearly articulated this idea that AIDS is a Western creation[20]:

> [*Do you mean AIDS was just made?*] They made it, yeah. [*Which people?*] The whites . . . the Americans, the scientists. They made that, through baboons, those big monkeys, the chimpanzee. . . . [*So . . . the AIDS patient you saw in the hospital was a deliberate move by the whites?*] Woo [no] . . . he acquired it on his own. [*Where from?*] They put it in . . . as it is now, you get AIDS through sex.

Once in a while, representatives of the (Western) scientific establishment do something stupid that both confirms and strengthens such suspicions and adds fuel to this interpretive fire. In 2002, for example, news emerged that a Ugandan clinical trial of the drug Nevirapine—which substantially reduces the odds of vertical (mother-to-child) HIV transmission—sponsored by the National Institutes of Health (NIH) had been seriously mismanaged, resulting in deaths and severe reactions that went unreported and were then covered up (Cohen 2004). Such examples of scientific misconduct are fodder for local discussions about the motives of Western science and Western scientists. They support the perception that Western interests, both political and scientific, supersede the good of black Africa and its people.

Of course, conspiracy theories are unique to neither AIDS nor Africa. They are a key motif in fictional stories about science in Africa (e.g., the 2005 Oscar-nominated film *The Constant Gardener*) and figure prominently in theories of underdevelopment and ethnographic critiques of international aid (Ferguson 1990). Alongside alternative African narratives about the origin of AIDS are alternative Western voices, some of which share certain features with African narratives. One example comes from Hooper (1999), who theorizes that AIDS emerged accidentally during the quest to perfect the polio vaccine. Others are found in the loose group of "AIDS skeptics," some of them prize-winning conventional scientists who question the link between HIV and AIDS, suggesting that it is, among other things, in the interests of "Big Pharma" to promote this relationship rather than investigate other potential causal pathways (Duesberg 1996).[21] We do not discuss these theories any further here (see Kalichman 2009 for a critical review). Our point is simply that where institutions and governments are mistrusted, as is clearly the case in SSA, alternative narratives (including conspiracy theories) readily emerge.

God, Sex, and Fertility

The final contextual factor that affects our ability to comprehend African views on AIDS considers them in relation to ideas about sex, fertility, concepts of God, and sin. At the risk of glossing over important ethnocultural and denominational distinctions and practices, we venture some general points to this end.

In SSA, the connections AIDS has to God, sex, and fertility are more than just intellectual connections. To Muslims and Christians alike, God is alive and active in the material world. God permits drought, brings rain, opens some wombs and closes others, just as in the days of the Hebrews. Indeed, the Hebrew Bible (referred to by Christians as the Old Testament) and its chronicles feel familiar to many Africans (Jenkins 2006). It is *their* story too. These books star a God who values fertility and "blesses" people with children (and some husbands with many wives). The reaping and the sowing and the begetting that are so visible in Old Testament narratives are far removed from the daily lives of most Western Christians. But these same narratives ring very close to home in agrarian societies where children are a form of wealth and fertility remains high.

African pronatalism (the valuation of fertility and childbearing) is remarkably different from what we experience in the West. Most sub-Saharan countries have not yet experienced a full demographic transition—the shift from high birth and death rates to much lower ones. And in areas where substantial reductions in fertility have been documented (total fertility rates are 2.8 in South Africa, 2.9 in Swaziland, and 3.6 in Namibia and Zimbabwe), fertility has stabilized at levels much higher than anything seen on other continents (Bongaarts 2006; Gould and Brown 1996). This implies that talk of AIDS and prevention cannot be disentangled from talk of fertility. Many scholars see the cultural predilection for high fertility as a persistent barrier to HIV prevention efforts, especially given that the standard prevention methods (abstinence and condoms) impede conception.

This does not mean that sex is enjoyed only as a way to procreate. Sex in Africa is recreational, too (Watkins 2004). But sex in Africa does tend to be more pronatalist than it is in the West. There has not been the same decoupling of sex and reproduction in long-term stable relationships that is so prevalent in Western societies. In fact, there is no culturally legitimate way to long delay or altogether avoid childbearing within a long-term relationship.[22] Likewise, even though the desired number of children continues to fall, there is no African equivalent to the developed country phenomenon where 20–30% of young women claim to want no children whatsoever.[23]

An additional difference is that marriage is more fluid—in practice if not in theory—in Africa than in the West, an issue we discuss in greater detail in Chapters 5 and 6. In spite of strong Christian and Muslim traditions, divorce is commonplace in many African countries, and it tends to be simple to enact. Though it can be hard to measure in the absence of documented legal procedures, there is considerably more serial marriage across SSA than in the West. African Christians are more biblically "literalist" than Western Christians. Since biblical stories tolerate divorce and a variety of other culturally specific sexual norms—including nonmarital sex, the existence of concubines, and widow inheritance—it should not surprise us to see religion being employed to justify serial monogamy (Smith 2004).[24]

These differences between Western and African ideas about marriage, divorce, and the extent to which fertility is valued and expected create persistent challenges to Western AIDS prevention programs. Several years ago, for example, the international community began to invest heavily in strategies that bundle HIV prevention and family planning programs together—with sex, of course, as the common denominator in matters of fertility and the risk of HIV transmission (Esacove 2010). As mentioned already, these joint programs have aroused considerable suspicion. Western interests in population control are just one source of the suspicion (Treichler 2004). Skepticism about the underlying cultural messages that these health programs intend to transmit—for example, legitimizing illicit sexual behavior and spreading new ideas about gender—represents another. We discuss these, and others, more extensively while reviewing the role of religion in HIV prevention programs in Chapter 5.

Conclusions

Understanding African responses to AIDS requires an appreciation for the supernatural, for the range of opinion about the nature and targets of Divine punishment, for alternative narratives about the origin of AIDS, and for the centrality of fertility to social life. While Africans are not uniquely mystical in seeking to identify and understand ultimate causes of disease, they are unlike most of us in the West—even the more religious United States—in terms of the nature of their religious attributions. Spiritual forces, including witchcraft, are foreign to most Westerners. But they are central to AIDS-related discourse in SSA. This sensitivity to the supernatural does not imply a rejection of Western biomedical understandings of disease. Here we stand with other scholars in our assertion that the biomedical view of what causes HIV/AIDS is readily accommodated into uniquely African understandings of ultimate causes (Feierman 1985; Ashforth 2005; Liddell et al. 2005).

In high-prevalence settings like Malawi, conversations about AIDS quickly turn into debates about theodicy. Religion is the primary lens through which perceptions of the epidemic are filtered and dominant interpretations of AIDS are constructed. As Smith (2004: 434–35) observed in Nigeria, the relationship between religion and AIDS "illustrates the inadequacy of imposing simplistic explanations and the limitations of one-dimensional intervention strategies that ignore the extent to which religion, health, sexuality, and morality intersect in people's everyday lives." Christian and Muslim narratives about AIDS are remarkably similar, suggesting either that something generically "religious" or "transcendental" underpins the interpretations we observe or perhaps hinting at the development of a shared Abrahamic religious schema that supersedes the particulars of any single tradition.

Finally, the staggering statistics about the toll of AIDS across the subcontinent masks an important reality: that AIDS in SSA is a relative problem. For some, especially those who are suffering from AIDS or caring for someone who is, AIDS is central to their day-to-day lives. For many others, however, AIDS is distant, dwarfed by more immediate concerns like poverty, work, family conflict, and other daily struggles. The unique virology of HIV—namely, that the infection usually lies dormant for 7 or 8 years before any symptoms emerge—makes the reactions to it different from reactions to other deadly diseases, and different from other problems that manifest quickly. Similarly, the low probability and randomness of transmission upon exposure can easily be read as crude empirical support for the belief that "God is punishing all of us" and not just a select few. The fact that not all who commit sexual sin get infected with HIV while untold numbers of innocents become sick and die moves questions like "why me?" to the center of the AIDS-related discourse that we, and other scholars, observe on the ground. The answers that Western science provides for this question are incomplete. In the context of an AIDS epidemic, the something *more* that remains demands explanation.

|| 4 ||

Knowledge about HIV

. . . We have received counselors from government or non-governmental organizations inviting us to a workshop like VAC (Village AIDS Committee), and whatever we get from there, we do advise our faithfuls on what transpired at the workshops. We tell them how to prevent AIDS and we tell them that AIDS has no cure. Even on how to care for someone who is suffering from the deadly disease we do advise them as advised by the Home Based Care Personnel.

—Sheikh, *Liwundi Mosque, Malawi, 2005*

What do people in sub-Saharan Africa (SSA) know about HIV? There is no single answer to this question. The informal conversations that we've had with Malawians over the years highlight that AIDS is known at some level not only by those most at risk—prime-age adults and adolescents—but also by people outside those high-risk age-groups. One of our colleagues, for example, claimed: "Everyone here knows how HIV is transmitted, even in the rural areas. My 89-year-old grandmother knows about AIDS!"[1] Another informant bemoaned the fact that "even a 4-year-old can tell you about HIV and condoms!"

What is meant by the grandma who "knows about AIDS" or the preschool age child who "can tell you about HIV and condoms"? Demographic and Health Surveys (DHS) data confirm that virtually everyone in SSA has heard of HIV, AIDS, and condoms. Africa's visual and aural landscape is filled with references to them. It is difficult, for example, to avoid AIDS-related posters in any African town that we've been in or to open an African newspaper without seeing an AIDS-related advertisement and articles. We recently plugged "AIDS posters Africa" into Google Images and got "about 508,000 results." In fact, art historians are now beginning to take note of these as a new phenomenon in African art (Ezra 2007), and ethnomusicologists are cataloging and archiving the wide variety of folk and pop songs inspired by AIDS (Barz 2005; McNeill and James 2008). Radio-based drama series feature AIDS as a central theme—part of the "social marketing" of AIDS-related issues. Drama groups act out AIDS-related plots in national tours of villages. AIDS-related "discourse" is thick and omnipresent. Talk of AIDS permeates public settings. References to AIDS are everywhere.

None of this tells us much about how much people actually know about AIDS, however, nor does it tell us if what they know is accurate. But it is precisely in relation to these more qualitative indicators of knowledge that we expect to find variation across religious groups. There are two reasons for this. The first touches on what economists call *program placement* effects. Where a dearth of resources means that AIDS information programs cannot be established everywhere, decision makers are likely to target the subpopulations they think will be most receptive to the campaign and to work in areas that are relatively easy to access. Since AIDS-related discourses were originally associated with the West and because AIDS in Africa initially affected the urban middle class more than the rural poor, it is reasonable to expect AIDS information programs to have first targeted urban, relatively educated subpopulations who were seen to be at higher risk of infection and were more open to Western discourses. This has implications for religious differences in AIDS-related knowledge since the religious characteristics of urban subpopulations are different from their rural and less educated counterparts. At least until the 1980s, highly educated individuals were more likely to associate with older Mission Protestant churches, while members of the smaller African denominations (the African Independent Churches, or AICs) tended to have comparatively low levels of education. With few exceptions (Uganda and Tanzania), Muslims in SSA typically have lower levels of education than Christians, which also may give rise to religious differences in knowledge about AIDS.

The second reason for expecting religious variation in knowledge of AIDS is related to "social networks," a standard sociological mechanism through which information, particularly new information, gets communicated. Over the last decade, a number of important studies conducted in SSA have highlighted how people's social networks affect not only their knowledge of AIDS but also their behaviors related to it (Agadjanian 2006; Helleringer and Kohler 2005; Smith and Watkins 2005). These results echo findings from prior research on family planning. Social networks spread both positive and negative information about contraception and family planning (Agadjanian 2001; Kohler, Behrman, and Watkins 2001; Valente, Watkins, Jato, Straten, and Tsitsol 1998).

It's no surprise that network effects are strong in SSA. Other informational resources (e.g., Internet and libraries) are limited, and the primary sources of new information—government agencies and nongovernmental organizations (NGOs)—are not fully trusted. This pushes people to rely on their networks— friends, confidants, and other trusted individuals—to evaluate new information. Is it accurate? What are the moral implications? Since social networks are, to differing degrees, centered around religious groups, religion occupies a central position in the relationship between networks and knowledge.

What do we mean by "networks"? There are two crucial dimensions. One is the frequency of contact with other people. The other is the level of network *homophily*, which is the extent to which people in one's network share the same characteristics. Social network theory predicts that people with better knowledge of new information—a category that, in the SSA setting, includes information about AIDS—interact with large and diverse groups of people, each of whom bridges another network. In contrast, people with the lowest levels of knowledge about some innovation—those who are the last to know—are stuck in homophilous networks in which no one (or nearly no one) has contact with people who are different from themselves. In short, at least in relation to information flows, good networks are open and have many "bridgers" (Burt 1995, 2005), while bad networks are dense and impervious.

In SSA, each of these network characteristics—frequency of contact and homophily—varies by religious tradition. Some traditions expect regular (i.e., weekly) attendance, while others also obligate members to participate in collective religious activities like Bible study or mutual assistance (we provide detailed examples of this in Chapter 9). In relation to homophily, some churches, particularly in rural areas, draw all members from the same village, and others, especially in areas where the religious marketplace is open and competitive, attract members from different villages. In towns and cities these differences can be pronounced. Some of the larger Mission Protestant and evangelical churches draw from different ethnic groups, different parts of the country, and different socioeconomic classes.

So what is known about AIDS in SSA, and how is that knowledge patterned religiously? Takyi (2003), using data from Ghana, found higher levels of AIDS-related knowledge among Christians than among Muslims or practitioners of traditional African religions and speculated that different levels of religious participation may have led to different levels of exposure to new ideas about AIDS. Our own early work in Malawi was not fully consistent with this. On one hand, like Takyi, we found evidence pointing to differences between religious traditions in levels of AIDS-related knowledge. For example, we found that informal discussions about AIDS among members are less common in Pentecostal and "Revivalist" churches than they are in Mission Protestant traditions like Anglican and Presbyterian churches. On the other hand, and contrary to what we expected, we also found that within each of these denominations, religious involvement had no bearing on an individual's likelihood of discussing AIDS with other members. In fact, this emphasis on interactions within congregations explains why Christians are different from Muslims here. African Islam tends to emphasize *private* religious practice (prayer five times a day) over collective religious life (mosque attendance). In Christian denominations, collective religious life is much more important.

DHS data allow us to look at this question across SSA in a more systematic way. Since the 1990s, the DHS has asked nationally representative samples

Table 4.1 **Typical Survey Questions about AIDS-Related Knowledge**

Questions
Have you ever heard of AIDS?
Can the risk of HIV transmission be reduced by having sex with only one faithful, uninfected partner?
Can the risk of HIV transmission be reduced by using condoms?
Can a healthy-looking person have the AIDS virus?
Can a person get HIV from mosquito bites?
Can a person get HIV by sharing a meal with someone who is infected?

Sources: Demographic and Health Surveys, MDICP.

across SSA (and elsewhere) a range of questions that allow researchers to track how much people know about HIV. Some of these questions are shown in Table 4.1. They range from whether people have heard of AIDS—a remnant from questionnaires fielded much earlier in the epidemic—to more specific questions about pathways of transmission, perceptions of infected individuals, and strategies for preventing infection. The last two questions in Table 4.1 are "trick" questions. Their aim is to identify misconceptions or incorrect beliefs.[2]

This range of questions, from most general and superficial "heard of" to more specific information about prevention methods and misconceptions, allows us to compare different levels of knowledge about AIDS across religious traditions. The most qualitatively important of these levels is what the DHS refers to as *comprehensive knowledge*. The DHS considers individuals to have comprehensive knowledge of AIDS if they:

1. correctly identify the two major ways of preventing the sexual transmission of HIV (i.e., using condoms and limiting sex to one faithful, uninfected partner);
2. reject the two most common local misconceptions about HIV transmission;
3. know that a healthy-looking person can have HIV.

Country-Level Variation in AIDS Knowledge

In Table 4.2, we calculate four levels of knowledge of HIV and AIDS using pooled data from 35 SSA countries in which DHS surveys, including related Multiple Indicator Cluster Surveys (MICS) and AIDS Indicator Surveys (AIS) have been fielded over the last decade. Our results show that there is a considerable gap between superficial and comprehensive knowledge of AIDS. While 91% of respondents claim to have heard of AIDS—and the heavy presence of AIDS-related phenomena, discussed already, makes us suspicious of any claim not to have heard of it—the numbers drop precipitously as the criteria for "knowledge" become more demanding. Across these 35 countries, only 55% of respondents correctly identify two prevention methods; one-third have no "misconceptions" whatsoever; and a mere quarter have what the DHS defines as "comprehensive knowledge."

As expected, these averages hide important religious variation. We can see this first at the national level, highlighting differences between Muslims and all others. Figure 4.1 highlights the relationship between each of the four levels of

Table 4.2 **Level of Knowledge of HIV and AIDS across SSA**

Level of Knowledge	%
Heard of AIDS	91
Knows Two Prevention Methods	55
Has No Misconceptions	33
Comprehensive Knowledge	25

Notes: Tabulations across 35 SSA countries with data from the most recent Demographic and Health Surveys, Multiple Indicator Cluster Surveys, or AIDS Indicator Surveys.

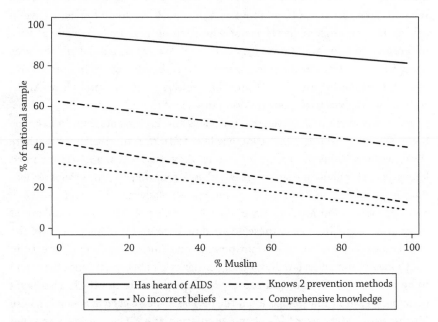

Figure 4.1 Relationship between level of AIDS knowledge and percentage Muslim
Source: DHS and related MICS and AIS Surveys (N = 35)

knowledge used in Table 4.2 and the percentage of the country's population that is Muslim. The lines are linear predictions based on bivariate regressions of the national-level data. In each case, there is a clear negative relationship: as the percentage of the country's population that is Muslim increases, the level of AIDS-related knowledge in that population falls. As one gets to the more qualitatively important parts of knowledge, where respondents know how to prevent HIV and have no misconceptions, the differences between the two religious poles become extremely pronounced. In countries with almost no Muslims, roughly 40% of the population has accurate knowledge about how HIV is transmitted (including no misconceptions). In predominantly Muslim countries, this is true of only 15% of the population.

Within-Country Variation in AIDS Knowledge

The national averages reflected in Table 4.2 and Figure 4.1 should not be overinterpreted. After all, they ignore the fact that other determinants of knowledge—in particular, the intensity of the epidemic and average education levels—also vary across countries. Studies that highlight within-country religious variation in knowledge of AIDS paint a clearer picture.

In general, results from these within-country studies are similar. As noted earlier, Takyi (2003) found that Christian women in Ghana had higher levels of knowledge about HIV than Muslims and those practicing traditional African religions. The fact that Christian women in the Ghana study tended to live in urban areas and had higher levels of education only partially explained these differences in accurate knowledge about HIV. We replicated Takyi's analyses using DHS data from 27 different countries in SSA, focusing on comprehensive AIDS knowledge. Figure 4.2 illustrates these differences in comprehensive AIDS-related knowledge by religious tradition in each of these.[3]

Results confirm that, in general, Catholics and Protestants tend to have the highest levels of comprehensive knowledge of AIDS. In the 18 countries where these two traditions are coded separately, they each win the battle for most knowledgeable population seven times and draw four times. Other groups are less knowledgeable. In only 4 of these 27 countries—Madagascar, Rwanda, Zambia, and Zimbabwe—did Muslims have more knowledge of HIV than members of other groups, and in none of these do Muslims account for more than 2% of the population. Nor are these Muslim populations "indigenous": most are from South Asian immigrant families, raising issues of comparability since they tend to be more urban, literate and educated, all of which are positively associated with more accurate knowledge about the disease. Indeed, even in Senegal, where Muslims constitute over 95% of the population and Muslim leaders engaged with government efforts to address AIDS early in the epidemic (Green 2003),

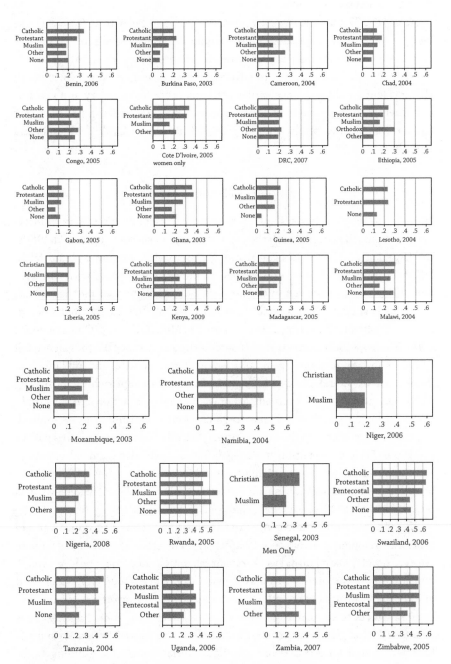

Figure 4.2 Comprehensive AIDS Knowledge by Denomination
Source: African Demographic and Health Surveys

Muslim men[4] are less likely to exhibit comprehensive knowledge about HIV than their Christian counterparts.

Across the 27 countries we examined, the only country with a relatively large indigenous Muslim population and roughly equivalent levels of knowledge across religious traditions is Uganda. This is interesting because Uganda is widely acknowledged as one of the AIDS success stories in SSA. It reduced both HIV incidence and prevalence earlier than any other SSA country and features prominently in discussions of "best practices" for AIDS-related policymakers (Green, Halperin, Nantulya, and Hogle 2006; Parkhurst 2002; Parkhurst and Lush 2004).

Co-opting Religious Leaders

The story of religious leaders' integration in the dissemination of crucial information about AIDS begins with the story of Uganda's success. In the mid-1980s, the Ugandan government began working closely with community- and faith-based organizations to deliver a clear AIDS prevention message with the acronym ABC: Abstain from sex until marriage, Be faithful to your partner, or use Condoms if abstinence and fidelity are not possible. The widely cited, though recently problematized (e.g., Murphy, Greene, Mihailovic, and Olupot-Olupot 2006; Timberg 2006), evidence of Uganda's success is that HIV prevalence fell from 15% in 1991 to about 5% in 2001 (Green 2003; Stoneburner and Low-Beer 2004). One of the take-away messages from Uganda's approach to addressing AIDS was that early government acknowledgment and action are essential.[5] A second lesson was that religious organizations constitute critical—indeed, until recently, sometimes the only—infrastructure of civil society in this part of the world. Early intervention in Senegal, for example, also included efforts to train religious leaders to disseminate crucial information about AIDS and has been credited with containing its epidemic; HIV prevalence in Senegal has remained stable at 1% since 1986 (Meda et al. 1999).

The observation that most Africans attend churches and mosques and are otherwise religiously active (see Chapter 2) translated into the belief among Western development and aid workers that religious leaders could be leveraged—much like radio programs—to disseminate knowledge about HIV widely and quickly. Public health organizations soon stepped in, kicking off a string of coordinated efforts to co-opt religious leaders as vehicles for spreading messages about HIV. This trend was evident long before the United States President's Emergency Plan for AIDS Relief (PEPFAR) initiatives started funding faith-based organizations (FBOs) to combat AIDS. A paper presented at the International AIDS Conference in 1992 described a workshop on "Islam and AIDS" with 50 participants in Sierra Leone. It concluded, "In a country where literacy rate is very low, Religious [sic] leaders can be very good AIDS educators in spreading messages and educating the general public on AIDS Prevention and Control" (Mansaray, Kosia, and Mikiu 1992). In 2005, this Malawian pastor concisely described the co-option process we heard about from many of the leaders we interviewed:

> The NAC [National AIDS Commission] people came to see me in 2001; they also visited other leaders—like chiefs—and told us that whenever more than five people gather, we should be telling them about this virus to make sure everyone understands how it spreads. And we should do this until everyone knows.

Among dozens of other (secular) multilateral health organizations and NGOs, UNAIDS, Population Services International (PSI), UNICEF, the World Health Organization, and the Global Fund have issued reports on religious leaders' untapped potential in the fight against AIDS (AHARP for the World Health Organization 2006; Lux and Greenaway 2006; Population Services International and AIDSMark 2007; Summers 2002; UNICEF 2007). A 2004 audit of the national AIDS policies of six southern African countries lists among their recommendations: "Traditional and religious leaders can improve community participation in all HIV/AIDS initiatives and increase the awareness of the HIV/AIDS epidemic at the community level" (Zungu-Dirwayi 2004: 35). They also recommended formalizing programs and curricula to educate religious leaders about HIV and to increase their involvement in combating its spread. During our fieldwork in Malawi, we attended several such workshops. Our field notes from 2007 describe part of one. We present a lengthy passage to give a sense of the materials covered, seminar participants, and general rhythm of the workshop:

> I spent the afternoon at a training workshop with a group of Reverends from at least a dozen different churches. Most of them are from villages around here but some distant villages too—they're all sleeping here while the workshop is going on. Three got rides from Mangochi and two came all the way from Zambia. There are 26 of them: 3 women and 1 toddler wandering around the meetings when he's not tied on his mother's back. The agenda for their 3-day program was posted on the door, and when I asked the guy who looked like he was in charge more about it, I got an invitation to participate. The workshop is sponsored by the Student Christian Organization of Malawi with funding from some Irish NGO. Before diving into the first topic, lots of prayer and songs. Everyone got a packet of photocopied information about AIDS. The stuff in here includes: diagrams of t-cells, a comic-like step-by-step of proper condom use, a table indicating CD-4 counts (ranging from

healthy to "at death's door"), though there are no CD-4 count machines at Balaka District Hospital, so I'm not sure how someone knows what their count is if they're not very, very sick. Comic-like drawings of how AIDS doesn't spread: people shaking hands, kissing, eating together. Also: lots of material on recommendations that HIV-positive mothers breastfeed their children exclusively for 6 months to prevent transmission to children. A picture of "mixed feeding" with a big X over it (probably was a red X before all the photocopies). The mother in the drawing is young and sitting next to an older woman (her mother). The young mother is taking her breast out of the top of her shirt to nurse the baby and the older woman is offering to give the baby a bottle. NO! Seems to be a lot of emphasis on this issue, which makes sense since this might be the only recommendation to have changed in a long time. A lot of prayer and singing between sessions. All the materials are in English, and some of the participants can't speak any English, though a few are very, very fluent. About half of the teaching is being done in Chichewa. Here are the topics for tomorrow: "Healthy Family Relationships (Mutual Faithfulness)," "Challenges Young People Face," "HIV/AIDS and Counseling," "Sex and Sexuality: Sexual Abstinence," "Youth Culture and HIV/AIDS."

Everywhere in SSA that we have looked for evidence of efforts to involve religious leaders in disseminating and promoting accurate knowledge about HIV, we have found it. This includes places such as Sudan (UNDP Sudan) and Somalia (UNDP Somalia), low-prevalence countries beset by civil war and political instability (more pressing problems). Efforts to involve religious leaders were commonplace in the epidemic's early stages—before everyone knew what AIDS was. That said, even though many religious leaders were willing to take on this role, it is clear that they did not become mouthpieces for a coherent public health message. Rather, the thousands of religious leaders trained through these workshops have combined discrete pieces of information about AIDS with a moral framework that allows them to interpret AIDS—as God's judgment, as a scourge, and sometimes simply as a disease.

This is certainly clear from our own work. Based on participant observation we conducted in 114 religious services in Malawi (Trinitapoli 2006), we know that most religious leaders frequently talk about AIDS in regular services and that the information they provide is quite accurate. But the overall consequence of the move to embrace religious leaders as disseminators of information about AIDS was this: information about AIDS circulated widely and quickly but not in the morally neutral manner the internationally sponsored workshops and curricula intended. Rather, messages went through a process of "translation"— from a supposedly amoral public health idiom to an explicitly moral-religious one. In the following chapters we provide more specific examples of how this process of moralization "works" in relation to HIV prevention.

Conclusions

Public health experts have been fond of invoking "ignorance about AIDS" as a primary reason for its spread across SSA. In line with the Health Belief Model (HBM), teaching people that HIV is a sexually transmitted disease and that it can be prevented has been a crucial component of the prevention efforts that swept the continent. Expanding knowledge about AIDS was especially important in the early years of the epidemic—when large numbers of people started dying from a mysterious wasting disease that they likely had contracted about 10 years earlier. Today, however, ignorance can hardly be blamed for the continued spread of HIV. After nearly two decades of exposure to public health campaigns, funerals, rumors, and informal conversations about all of these events, virtually everyone has heard of AIDS. In certain subpopulations, detailed knowledge about HIV is also widespread. This tends to be truer for Catholics and Protestants than for Muslims and practitioners of traditional religion. Even while some misconceptions persist, a majority of Catholics and Protestants, especially in high-prevalence countries, can spontaneously identify modes of transmission.

Religious leaders have played an important role in achieving these relatively high levels of knowledge. Early in the epidemic, in particular, religious leaders were central in spreading crucial information about AIDS among their memberships. But religious leaders were not simply mouthpieces for neutral, public health-style information and messaging. Relaying information was not their primary goal—as religious leaders it never could be. Their goal was both to educate their flocks about the basics of a new and mysterious disease and to interpret the epidemic, and the personal experience of illness, within a specific theological and cultural framework. The results of their efforts are clear: since the beginning, messages about AIDS that have spread through religious individuals and institutions have been imbued with an overtly religious tone.

Would the results have been substantially different if the public health campaigns had bypassed religious leaders altogether? Not necessarily. As we argued in Chapter 3, religion and religious thinking infuse many aspects of daily life in SSA. Even without the intentional engagement of religious leaders in the task of disseminating knowledge, we are convinced that AIDS in SSA would still be interpreted religiously and experienced in vocabularies and scripts that draw on religion.

These religious differences in levels of knowledge are important. Notwithstanding the conceptual and empirical flaws of the HBM, basic knowledge of

HIV was necessary for stimulating large-scale behavior change related to AIDS, whether in terms of prevention, the focus of Chapters 5 and 6, or stigma and care, which we address in Chapters 8 and 9. But basic knowledge is insufficient for stimulating large-scale behavior change. This observation informs our approach to the role of religion in what is arguably the world's biggest health policy intervention—the ABCs of prevention.

PART THREE

PREVENTING HIV

We now turn our attention to religious differences in how people in sub-Saharan Africa (SSA) avoid infection. We begin (Chapter 5) with an examination of the strategies promoted by public health groups. Our focus here is on the ABC campaign—the central approach to HIV prevention in SSA. In Chapter 6 we describe a different set of prevention strategies—the ones emerging as people "navigate AIDS" (Watkins 2004). These local responses are an amalgam of prevailing understandings of HIV and preexisting values about sex, marriage, and divorce. Finally, Chapter 7 examines the combination of prevention strategies promoted by religious leaders and pursued by lay members. These range from straight biomedical approaches to faith healing. In either case, our main focus is on congregations.

5

The ABCs of Prevention

The greatest medicine and the surest way [to avoid plague] is to
do penance, love God above all things, fear him, [and] keep the
commandments, completely submitting your will to them.
—Hans Folz, Nürnberg, 1482[1]

ABC—for Abstain, Be faithful, use Condoms—is the basic HIV prevention lexicon. Referring to both the behavior of individuals and to the programmatic priorities that have shaped interventions to promote these behaviors, ABC has served as the cornerstone of HIV prevention across Africa for almost 20 years.[2] Anyone living in or traveling around sub-Saharan Africa (SSA) will see and hear signs of ABC. It is the programmatic face of AIDS—on billboards, the outside walls of public buildings, the backs of T-shirts, in radio programs and sermons in churches and mosques.

The core elements of ABC have been part of HIV prevention strategies since before they became known as the ABCs. For example, beginning in 1990 Museveni's government in Uganda sponsored campaigns that emphasized two messages: "Zero grazing" (i.e., remain in your own pasture; be faithful) and "Don't forget to carry your 'coat'" (i.e., always have a condom handy). Slightly later, in Tanzania, Father Bernard Joinet, a Catholic priest and clinical psychologist, developed a series of prevention messages centered on the idea of a "Fleet of Hope." Based on the story of Noah's ark, the Fleet of Hope provided a simple metaphor: AIDS is a flood that is destroying the people around us, but you can escape the flood by jumping into one of three boats: abstinence, fidelity, or a (rubber) lifeboat.

Three underlying subtexts can be seen in each of these approaches. First, by appropriating and then playing with locally meaningful imagery these campaigns were intended "to awaken people's emotions" (Williams, Milligan, and Odemwingie 1997: 45). Second, in a nod to the idea of self-efficacy that we discussed in relation to the Health Belief Model (HBM), they were intended to help people "believe they can escape the epidemic" by changing their own behavior (Williams et al.: 45). Third, both Museveni's original "Zero grazing" and "Carry a coat" and Joinet's Fleet of Hope approaches were intentionally

created as a middle ground, a single, comprehensive approach to HIV prevention whose emphasis on abstinence and fidelity in marriage would appeal to
religious groups and whose promotion of condoms would appeal to those in
public health.

Not surprisingly, the same three subtexts are found in the phrase *ABC*. Said
to be have been created by Juan Flavier, a Filipino Minister of Health (1992–95),
ABC quickly diffused to other regions through international networks of expa-
triate advisors and World Health Organization (WHO) officials (Hardee, Gribble,
Weber, Manchester, and Wood 2008). Since, like Museveni's and Joinet's original approaches, ABC represented a compromise between public health and religious professionals, it was particularly appealing in countries that already had
pragmatic and functional partnerships between ministries of health and religious leaders. Both Uganda and Senegal fit this model (Green 2003). As Uganda
began to document dramatic declines in HIV prevalence, and as Senegal appeared
to hold off any increase in HIV prevalence whatsoever, ABC became the favored,
though unofficial, prevention strategy promoted by the U.S. Agency for International Development (USAID). All this had occurred by the end of the second
Clinton administration. Then in 2003, during George W. Bush's first administration, ABC became the official cornerstone of the United States President's Emergency Plan for AIDS Relief (PEPFAR). It was at this point that ABC became sharply
politicized, because a Congressional earmark mandated that 33% of PEPFAR
funding be devoted to the A-factor, that is, abstinence-only programs. This led to
pointed debates over the moralization of U.S. aid to Africa and speculation that
funding for HIV prevention was becoming a tool of the religious right (e.g.,
Goldberg 2007).

In this chapter we examine religious patterns in A, B, and C across SSA. Looking both at the behavior of individuals and the role of religious leaders in this
now ubiquitous approach to prevention, we argue that the overwhelming majority of Christian and Muslim leaders have taken a pragmatic approach to the
ABCs. The dominant view is quite simple: it's best to abstain and be faithful, but
condoms offer some protection to those who don't act in accordance with A and
B. We also show that religious messages about HIV prevention translate into
measurable differences in the behavior of individuals, with important consequences for the current and future shape of the epidemic.

A Is for Abstinence

In the context of a generalized HIV epidemic rooted almost wholly in sexual
transmission—as is the case in SSA—abstaining from sexual intercourse is, of
course, the most effective way to avoid infection. Somewhat surprisingly, given
the politicization of abstinence-based education in developed countries, there is

broad agreement on this in SSA. Both secular and religious groups have embraced abstinence as a cornerstone of combating the AIDS epidemic—particularly where it's most feasible—among young, unmarried adolescents. Posters and radio messages advocating abstinence garnish the landscape in both urban and rural areas, while TV programs and pop music dramatize the importance of "saying no."

Even with this broad agreement between secular and religious groups for promoting abstinence, the style and content of secular and religious abstinence campaigns vary, each one reflecting a different set of motives. Our general observation is this: global health groups fighting AIDS in Africa promote abstinence for instrumental, material reasons; religious groups, Christian or Muslim, promote abstinence as a moral issue, sometimes in addition to instrumental reasons and sometimes alone. The differences between these two general types of abstinence messages are relevant, since each appeals to a different subpopulation. Before describing and giving examples of each, we take a step back to describe the broader context in which abstinence is being promoted across SSA.

Africa's New Adolescents

Marriage in most of SSA is different from its Western counterpart. First, in contrast to most Western societies, which have had high rates of nonmarriage for centuries—bachelors and spinsters are long-established types in Western society (Hajnal 1965; Thornton 2005)—marriage in SSA has historically been universal. And it remains almost universal outside of South Africa and Botswana. Second, marriage in SSA happens earlier, occurring shortly after puberty in most settings. This, too, differs from Western societies since even in the early modern era, prior to the Enlightenment and Industrial Revolution, many European women did not marry until their late teens or early 20s (Offen 1999). Likewise, even though mean (and median) age at first marriage in SSA has increased in recent years, it is still much lower than in developed countries: it is currently around 19 for women across SSA (Bongaarts 2006) compared with 26 in the United States, 25.3 in the United Kingdom, and 31 in Germany (UNPD n.d.).

Abstinence campaigns in SSA are directed at adolescents and youth, respectively defined as people between puberty and late teens. Importantly, throughout Africa *youth* is primarily defined by the person's stage in the life course (i.e., before marriage) rather than by age (i.e., 15–24 or < 18). The rising age at marriage in SSA has opened up space in many African societies for an abbreviated version of unmarried adolescence. In fact, HIV prevalence in SSA is positively correlated with age at marriage (Bongaarts 2007) at both the aggregate and individual levels. In other words, the AIDS-belt countries with the highest ages at first marriage also have the highest national levels of HIV prevalence (e.g., South Africa, Bostwana, Namibia). This is consistent with the assertion that a longer period of nonmarital adolescent sexual activity (which typically involves a higher number of partner changes) facilitates the spread of HIV.

Local leaders, religious and traditional, promote abstinence as a direct cultural response to these transitions. It reflects the fact that, especially among women, the traditional combination of late puberty and early first marriage meant that historically there was no need for long-term premarital abstinence. Now, however, things are different. Delayed marriage in itself has created large cohorts of sexually mature but unmarried adolescents. Visit African college campuses, open African newspapers and magazines, watch African music videos, and it is evident that sexualized cultural influences are affecting popular ideas about how this stage of the life course should be experienced in SSA—just as in developed societies. Abstinence campaigns attempt to put the brakes on this process. And they do so with an idea that is new to SSA. One of the clearest signs of this is that many African languages lack a word for abstinence, forcing abstinence campaigns to develop a new vocabulary to promote this new idea and behavior.

Even with this convergence in sexualized adolescent culture, there is an important difference between Africa's "unmarried adolescents" and "youth" and their Western counterparts. Compared with the latter—juggling school and homework with part-time jobs and a host of extracurricular activities— the life course in SSA is much less predictable. The general context of deep poverty and the absence of publicly funded social safety nets (outside of South Africa and Botswana) require adolescents in SSA to assume responsibilities that far exceed what is expected from their Western counterparts at equivalent stages of life.

We see this first and foremost in levels of school enrollment. The latest UNICEF data suggest that only 33% of eligible youth in SSA are in secondary school (37 and 30% of boys and girls, respectively), with only minimal regional variation (39% in eastern/southern Africa and 29% in central/western Africa).[3] Likewise, for the minority who remain in school, interruptions are common, especially among the poor for whom tuition fees and familial responsibilities often require their attention and labor. These responsibilities can be intensive— again, in contrast to the comparatively predictable lives of school-age adolescents in developed countries. They include agricultural tasks—plowing (for men), weeding (for women), harvesting (both)—not all of which are synchronized with the academic calendar. They also include caring for younger siblings or sick family members, selling goods at local markets, maintaining the family's house and compound—mud huts, thatched roofs, and pit latrines need frequent attention—and fetching water (women), sometimes at a considerable distance. Finally, these responsibilities are generally not limited to their own households. The nature of extended family support networks demands that adolescents help out in other households too.

Types of Abstinence Campaigns

Two distinct types of abstinence campaigns target the emerging demographic of African adolescents. A poster campaign in Malawi implemented by Population Services International (PSI), a leading global health organization, neatly sums up the instrumental abstinence message: those directed at fulfillment of long-term goals. Part of the "Youth Alert!" peer education campaign (established in 2001) that stressed abstinence and personal goal setting, the poster features a young man standing outside a school while three young women—the variation in their attire and stance hints at different levels of modesty—beckon. Books in one arm, the young man holds up his other hand, simultaneously stopping the girls and waving good-bye. The poster reads: "Sex Can Wait . . . But my future can not. Abstinence is the best way to prevent HIV/AIDS, STIs and Unwanted pregnancy." A blurb at the bottom of the ad fills out the message in the young man's own voice. Notably, this blurb does not mention AIDS at all. It talks about how girlfriends compete with studies for the young man's time. The ad emphasizes that he needs to stop having sex so that he can "become what [he] wants." The central explicit idea is that abstinence is the safest way to get ahead. The key implicit idea is that people should want to get ahead.

The same message is also directed at women. An abstinence poster from South Africa, for example, portrays a young woman about to enter Secretarial College while resisting an invitation from a suitor, his wealth signaled by car and earring. "A real woman waits," the poster declares. A simpler poster from Zambia—no suitors here—simply urges girls (all dressed in their school uniforms) to abstain from sex to stay in school. "Value your lives," it commands them. Neither of these posters mentions AIDS.

A second type of instrumental message related to abstinence is less about being goal-oriented and more about being "cool." This type of message builds on sophisticated marketing techniques—segmentation and branding—that specialize in adolescents.[4] Their underlying narrative is that it's not only serious-minded, goal-oriented individuals, like those featured in the previously mentioned education-focused posters, who are into abstinence. It's also the cool people who adolescents really want to emulate—attractive models smiling and doing fun things, relatively wealthy individuals—and this provides the foundation for several official abstinence curricula.[5] "Stay strong, say no to peer pressure," says one Zambian poster with this type of message. "Not everyone is doing it, we are NOT!" declare a group of girls in another Zambian poster, this one titled "Virgin Power, Virgin Pride." "Sex is worth waiting for: Zip Up," says a Nigerian poster, picturing two couples, each hugging and smiling. The examples go on and on.[6] But the common denominator is the absence of any ideological motivation for abstinence. Its promotion is image-driven and utilitarian.

The abstinence as cool theme is also embodied in attempts to change language. The first large-scale abstinence campaign in Kenya, the 2004 Nimechill Campaign, offers a clear example. Its aim was to promote abstinence until marriage but, failing that, to at least "foster youth's self-efficacy to refuse sex and delay sexual debut" (AIDSMark 2007: 2). Its core method was to arm adolescents with the ability to resist peer and partner pressure to have sex by making abstinence cool—thus the term *nimechill*. Narrowly understood, *nimechill* is a composite of the English slang "chill"—as in to be cool—and the Swahili *nime* (the present perfect "I have"). It is simply "I'm cool." But in the absence of an existing word for "sexual abstinence" in Kiswahili, the campaign added a new verb "chill" to Kiswahili, and assigned that word a new and local meaning, *ku-chill* (to abstain). Framed in the perfect tense, *nimechill* was therefore "I've chilled; I'm abstaining." Likewise, *ni poa ku chill*—it's cool to chill/abstain—was one of the campaign's refrains (USAID and PSI 2006). "Sex? No way, *tume chill* [we're chilling]" appeared in another (afrol News 2008). Similar themes can be found in Zambia and Malawi, where the phrase "Abstinence *ili che* [is cool]" appears within many AIDS posters. *Kudziletsa*, a new Chichewa word for abstinence, was also invented as part of the new AIDS lexicon. *Kudziletsa* literally means "to restrain yourself" but is used almost exclusively with regard to sex to describe both the avoidance of sex and faithfulness. "Abstinence *ili che*" appears on posters far more frequently than *kudziletsa*, which suggests a perception—at least on the part of those designing the posters—that *ile che* delivers the abstinence message most effectively.[7]

The pro-abstinence messages in these "instrumental" posters articulate with religious messages, but they contain no religious content or even innuendo themselves. The campaigns have effectively decoupled premarital sex and morality. They promote abstinence as good on the grounds that it helps people achieve their material goals or on the grounds that it's cool. Religious messages about abstinence, whether Christian or Muslim, are different. Over and above any other reason for abstinence—which they may or may not refer to—religious messages insist that premarital sex is simply wrong. God says that one must remain abstinent until marriage.

Somewhat surprisingly, religious messages of this type are comparatively rare—at least visually. Instead, they tend to be promoted orally within the walls of religious institutions. Numerous studies have confirmed that messages of abstinence and fidelity are commonplace in religious services throughout SSA, including South Africa (Garner 2000), Mozambique (Pfeiffer 2002), Nigeria (Orubuloye, Caldwell, and Caldwell 1993), Uganda (Epstein 2007; Green 2003), and Malawi (Trinitapoli 2006; Watkins 2004). And while the intensity of such messages varies across denominations or between Christian and Muslim groups, the basic content of the messages does not. Adolescents are encouraged to "Save sex" for marriage rather than have premarital "Safe sex," because that is the right thing to do (Ebrahim and Nawab 2008).

In Malawi, we observed many of the messages you might expect to hear religious leaders preaching about abstinence from a strictly religious perspective, with an emphasis on God's law. A guest speaker at an African Independent Church (AIC) emphasized the primacy of abstinence over condoms (which we discuss in detail later in this chapter):

> Doing sex with a condom is not safe because it is not 100% safe. . . . But let me warn you: you are not safe in the eyes of God because God hates premarital sex.

We also heard more instrumental messages about abstaining to preserve health and future opportunities almost equally. A Malawian sheikh in one of our research sites bemoaned the state of the youth in his area, linking their lack of abstinence to general changes in authority structures, including those stemming from democratization:

> In our days . . . we were less sexually active. But today's youth grow very fast and mature when they are at 10 or 11 years old. With the coming of democracy they take the law in their hands. You cannot advise them. They say they are free to do or enjoy. We just watch, helplessly. They go out, get the disease, and come back to suffer and die.[8]

To summarize, there are a number of reasons that can be used to promote premarital sexual abstinence. In fact, a more or less complete list—including a religious abstinence message, though not of the hellfire and brimstone type—appears in another poster from Zambia. It urges adolescents to "finish school, fulfil [sic] your dreams, don't be a father yet, don't get STD's or AIDS, obey God's commandments, don't disappoint your parents, Be Proud! Abstinence *ili che*." Everything is covered here. The poster promises that those practicing abstinence will achieve their goals, remain healthy, please God, make their parents happy, and, to top it all off, *ili che*, will also be cool!

Interpreting Abstinence

The strength and visibility of the abstinence campaigns in SSA raises a number of questions. How are the abstinence messages understood and interpreted, in particular in societies in which adolescents' lived experience is so different from ours and in which abstinence as a concept never before merited a precise word in local languages? What effect, if any, do abstinence campaigns have? How much variation is there in both the understanding of, and response to, these abstinence campaigns in SSA? And how do all of these vary across religious groups and congregations?

Focus group data collected from young people in Ghana and Uganda shed light on the first of these questions: what youth in Africa think about abstinence and abstinence messages.[9] The focus groups produced dozens of comments that could have been lifted straight out of any health worker's script, such as "The best way is to avoid sex. Sex can wait." Or, "a boy who loves you will respect your desire to wait to have sex." While many young people emphasized the importance of heeding advice from elders to remain virgins until marriage—"obey our parents and have self-respect"—few drew directly from religious doctrine as a motivation for abstinence. Only one young woman and three young men (out of about 40) tied abstinence back to religious beliefs when discussing it as a strategy for avoiding infection. A young man from an urban area in Ghana described the path he believes young people should take: "I have heard that it is a sin to have premarital sex. So if you are ready to marry, the couple has to go to the hospital to be tested for the disease." A Ugandan man who responded to the moderator's question about the best ways of avoiding infection with the statement "Abstain and get saved!" was met with laughter and dissent. Another participant responded:

> There are people who get saved. But reverends these days, you hear that they are the ones with prostitutes. You hear they rape from their offices. These days people get saved to cover themselves . . . You put that one of being saved aside.

Young people in Ghana and Uganda also disagreed about the possibility of dating without being sexually active. While some recommended setting sexual limits with a romantic partner before getting seriously involved, others believed that a romantic relationship without sex is impossible and urged others in the group to avoid relationships altogether until they are ready to be sexually active. This advice is consistent with research showing that many young Malawian women perceive schooling and having a boyfriend as fundamentally incompatible pursuits (Poulin 2009). This, in turn, echoes the instrumental abstinence messages previously described: choose between sex now and securing a better future.

Focus groups also illuminated variations on traditional abstinence messages. We consolidated dozens of statements about ways youth can help themselves remain abstinent into five categories:

1. Choose a hobby or some way to keep busy.[10]
2. Avoid wearing tight dresses, miniskirts, and "shaking your bum."
3. Don't drink alcohol.
4. Know God first and then you can abstain, or "give your life to Jesus."
5. Substitute mutual masturbation for penetrative sex.[11]

Although it is not clear how representative these opinions are or how widely accepted they are by their peers in the focus group setting, they highlight the diversity of opinions on abstinence as a method of HIV prevention for adolescents in SSA. Likewise, although only one of these extra messages—the fourth—is overtly religious, the first three are at least secondarily so. In other words, although adolescents rarely attributed their motivation for remaining abstinent to religion, the methods or strategies that that they described as helping them remain abstinent are thoroughly consistent with messages that they hear from religious leaders: stay busy, dress and behave modestly, and stay away from alcohol. These strategies are also thoroughly consistent with the social control mechanisms many religious groups institute—more about that in Chapter 6. Likewise, they match the indirect ways religion shapes the sexual behavior of American adolescents (Regnerus 2007).

What are more effective in SSA settings, instrumental or religious messages? Later in the book we show empirically that a mix of strategies appears to be most effective. For now, we point out that what makes the religious messages particularly relevant in SSA is the fact that the purely instrumental messages—especially those focused on the choice between school and sex—are ill-suited to the actual lives of so many African teens. As we have already noted, only about a third of eligible teens in SSA attend secondary school. Among the two-thirds that don't, there are some who are taking time away from school and many more who hope to go back to school. But most won't. In all likelihood, further schooling is off the table. In our view, this reality weakens the salience of instrumental messages to their lives.

Likewise, the images associated with the "abstinence is cool" theme are completely removed from the realities of everyday life for most African adolescents: a mixed crowd in a bar, women with spaghetti-string tops, or preteens sitting on a tidy bed with a snuggly toy all capture small urban pockets of African adolescents. They are a world away from the daily realities that most African adolescents experience.[12]

In contrast to these instrumental messages, religious messages are not limited to a particular demographic. Our analysis of the MRP sermon data revealed approximately equal focus on the youth and married persons, on men and women. Religious leaders make universal moral claims, focusing on the essential moral value of abstinence rather than on its instrumental value. And they don't shy away from describing the strategies that are worth adopting to achieve that moral goal. This may make religiously based abstinence messages more tenable and also more effective in terms of behavior change.

Religious Variation in Abstinence

Measuring actual abstinence is, of course, quite difficult—much as many researchers would like to, we don't follow adolescents around with notebooks and cameras, faithfully recording every sexual interaction. Rather, we rely almost solely on adolescents' own reports of their sexual activity. These reports are most commonly gathered during face-to-face survey interviews. Somewhat less frequently, they are collected in self-administered questionnaires, which the respondents fill out either on paper or a computer. Both formats are plagued by error (generally underreporting for women and overreporting for men), and there is conflicting evidence about which methods generate the most valid data, at least in SSA settings (Mensch, Hewett, and Erulkar 2003; Poulin 2010).

Notwithstanding these methodological issues, available survey data do tell us something (though certainly not everything) about the sexual behavior of individuals.[13] Simple tabulations of data from adolescents in Uganda, Ghana, Malawi, and Burkina Faso—from a Guttmacher Institute (AGI) survey—are presented in Table 5.1. They show relatively high absolute levels of abstinence among adolescents in Africa, ranging from a high of 85% in Ghana to 64% and 68% in Malawi and Uganda, respectively. In contrast, reported abstinence is substantially lower (52%) among high school students in the United States.

Although there are no meaningful differences in reported sexual activity by religious affiliation, more detailed analyses do illuminate a pathway by which religion influences abstinence. It works through religiosity. After controlling for individuals' age, education, and wealth, those who attend religious services regularly (at least once a week) are twice as likely to report being abstinent as those who attend infrequently (less than once a month). Additional analyses suggest that the relationship between religious involvement and sexual activity among young people is primarily due to religious differences in attitudes about acceptable sexual behavior. While 47% of those who attend infrequently believe it is okay for a couple to have sex before marriage if they love one another, only 35% of those who attend regularly report the same. Controlling for this particular belief eliminates significant differences in sexual activity across religious groups and levels of religiosity. In other words, religion appears to shape adolescents'

Table 5.1 **Reported Abstinence among Unmarried Adolescents**

Country	%	Source
Burkina Faso	74	AGI
Ghana	85	AGI
Malawi	64	MDICP
Malawi	65	AGI
Uganda	68	AGI
United States[a]	52	CDC

[a] High school students only.

sexual behavior by influencing their beliefs about what behavior is acceptable and under what conditions.

These results are consistent with a study of 5,000 Zambian adolescents. It, too, found that members of religiously conservative groups become sexually active at later ages, likely reducing their chances of contracting HIV (Agha, Hutchinson, and Kusanthan 2006).[14]

Analysis of our own data from Malawian adolescents reveals more about this mechanism. After controlling for all individual-level sociodemographic characteristics, we find some significant differences across religious groups—in contrast to the AGI data. Muslim adolescents, in particular, are considerably less likely to report remaining abstinent than their Catholic, Mission Protestant, or AIC counterparts. Importantly, Malawian adolescents who attend religious services every week are nearly twice as likely as those who attend only rarely to report abstaining from sex. And attending congregations in which AIDS is discussed on a regular basis—and in which there are frequent messages about AIDS—is strongly related to abstaining (Trinitapoli 2009).

Summarizing A

In Africa, as in the rest of the world, many unmarried adolescents are having sex, despite the fact that this runs contrary to the teachings of their religion. Parents and religious leaders concerned with the sanctity of sex—holy and acceptable only within marriage—may see the sexual activity of young people in their own churches and mosques as a failure to effectively transmit values of chastity, discipline, and purity to the next generation. But religious involvement does have the unintended consequence of *delaying* the onset of sexual activity. This is completely consistent with research on adolescent sexuality in the United States, where religious adolescents are also less likely to be sexually active than their less religious counterparts even if they also become sexually active before marriage (Regnerus 2007). A recent study of married young adults in the United States revealed that only about 11% wait until marriage to become sexually active, with an additional 22% having sex before marriage but only with their future spouse (Uecker 2008). In other words, religious teachings about abstinence delay "sexual debut" even if they rarely succeed in what some would consider their primary aim, which is to save sex for marriage. This is true in the United States, and we can see that it is also true in Africa.

Delaying the onset of sexual activity may not sound like much. But as already noted, in SSA HIV prevalence is higher in countries where marriage occurs at later ages (Bongaarts 2007). The most plausible explanation for this is that a longer average period of nonmarital sexual activity facilitates the spread of HIV in a population. For this reason, delayed sexual activity has a cumulative effect that epidemiologists have identified as a potentially important point of intervention. In analyzing the decline in HIV prevalence in Uganda, for example, Edward Green (2003) links the observed delay in sexual activity among adolescents and the timing of Uganda's turnaround. Green attributes the substantial declines in HIV prevalence in Uganda to the country's massive ABC campaign and emphasizes that the greatest decline occurred among the youngest age groups, in which people started having sex at later ages. To the extent that religious teachings about abstinence are responsible for delaying the onset of sexual activity for young people—alone or in combination with a more goal-oriented instrumentalism—they can have important consequences for curbing the spread of HIV in a particular country or district, even though they might not dramatically reduce the risk of infection for a given individual.

We revisit the abstinence issue in the next chapter in the context of discussions about organic responses to AIDS. For now, however, we move on to the next letter in the AIDS prevention lexicon.

B Is for Being Faithful

"B" stands for "Be Faithful."[15] Like abstinence messages, messages about faithfulness in Africa abound. They have also been one of the central foci of AIDS-prevention programs across the region (Green 2003; Stammers 2005). Perhaps most famous is Uganda's promotion of "zero grazing" from 1987 to 1992 (Epstein 2005; Hardee et al. 2008). Here, a faithfulness policy was framed in terms that would resonate in a socially conservative, agricultural society. Remember: two-thirds of today's sub-Saharan African population lives in rural areas, so they could easily understand it and easily talk about it.

On purely conceptual grounds, "Be faithful" is an appealing policy in SSA contexts. The main reason is that, unlike in Western societies, marriage in SSA is almost universal. That is, although the proportions vary across and within countries, almost all African adults outside South Africa and Botswana marry at some point in their lives. They also tend to stay married, remarrying following divorce or the death of a spouse. By definition, then, were all people to remain abstinent before marriage and faithful within it, the spread of HIV—at least the sexually transmitted variety that drives the African epidemic—would be contained.

In the real world, of course, this is impossible. In fact, one thing that distinguishes the African AIDS epidemic from its counterparts in Asia and the United States is the high proportion of new infections occurring within marriages or long-term partnerships, whether from one's spouse or from extramarital relations (Bongaarts 2007; Clark 2004). Fidelity, it seems, is a problem in SSA. There is clearly considerable extramarital sex in some areas in SSA. This is true even if the proportion of men reporting extramarital partnerships is quite variable—it ranges from very low in Ethiopia (1%) and Rwanda (5%) to over one-quarter of men in

Liberia and Lesotho. And this is also the case despite the fact that public attitudes about extramarital sex in SSA are quite conservative; remember that abstinence among unmarried adolescents is higher in SSA than in the United States.

High rates of male labor migration have been touted as the most important structural characteristic affecting fidelity (Chirwa 1997; Epstein 2007; Wolffers, Fernandez, Verghis, and Vink 2002). The relative absence of work opportunities in rural areas—especially for those with some education—encourages labor migration to urban areas or to other rural areas in which there is large-scale (industrial) farming, such as tea and coffee plantations in Kenya, tobacco in Malawi. This movement is highest for prime-age adults, that is, people between their late teens and late 30s. It also tends to be higher for men than for women, even if rural wives are joining their husbands in cities more than they once did (Jolly and Reeves 2005). Labor migration physically divides spouses, long-term partners, and casual partners. Our analysis of Demographic and Health Surveys (DHS) data from 26 countries showed that between 19% (Mozambique and Ethiopia) and 53% (Lesotho) of married men spent *at least one month* away from home (i.e., away from their wives) during the past year, and these numbers are even higher when unmarried men are included.

Much has been written about labor migration in the context of AIDS, particularly about the migration of men to South African mines from other southern African countries, since long-term living in all-male hostels is seen to directly affect the spread of HIV. Epstein (2002: 90) describes it as follows:

> The long absences from home, the tedious, dangerous work, the drab anomie of life in all-male miners' hostels, the gangs of prostitutes clinging to the chain link fences around the mines—are all believed to contribute to miners' higher risk of HIV infection.

HIV infection doesn't end with these men, however. On their cyclical returns home, they carry the virus back to waiting wives. Indeed, Epstein argues that this is the primary reason HIV prevalence is as high, if not higher, in rural areas of Botswana, Lesotho, and southern Mozambique than in urban areas or migrant-receiving regions in general (see Bouare 2007).[16]

Men are not the only ones bringing AIDS into the home. Though often portrayed as little more than victims of men's sexual misadventures, women, including those left behind by migrant spouses, are also sexual agents. They have sexual desires, and they sometimes act on them. Their relative poverty, combined with the fact that sex is more openly transactional in SSA than in Western societies, makes it is easy to understand why women in SSA might look for a regular extramarital partner who can provide sex, companionship, and a little material support. That this is a widespread phenomenon can be seen in the high levels of HIV *serodiscordance* among marital couples, that is, where one partner is HIV positive and the other is negative. In 4 of 10 countries studied by Bishop and Foreit (2010)—Cameroon, Côte d'Ivoire, Kenya, and Swaziland—there are more serodiscordant couples where the woman is HIV positive than where her husband is. This is a clear sign that the women were infected by a partner other than their husbands, even if we cannot say whether that occurred before or during the current marriage. Indeed in Zambia, the authors estimate that at least 70% of HIV-positive individuals who were currently married or cohabiting "had to have acquired their infection from someone other than their current marital partner" (Bishop and Foreit: 2).

This brings us to another important factor that underlies frequent extramarital relations in SSA, but that doesn't appear in the public health literature: boredom. This is a much more profound type of boredom than the one referred to by the aforementioned Ghanaian informant ("when you are bored, you tend to look for bitches"). It refers to the dull repetition of much of daily life. Most people's daily lives are severely circumscribed by the lack of ready cash and, in agricultural areas, the unending demands of subsistence living—long days fetching water, prepping food, walking long distances, planting, weeding, harvesting. All these tasks mean that outside small pockets of the middle class and wealthy, people in Africa have few choices about what to do, what to wear, what to eat, where to go, and so on. Likewise, home provides few options for leisure: only a minority of people have TVs, books, or magazines, even if they have the time to engage in leisure—during less intensive agricultural seasons, men typically have more leisure (Whitehead 1999). It is not difficult to imagine how an extramarital affair in this environment might add pleasure and intrigue to an otherwise tedious existence. Flirting and sex are fun (remember?). They don't cost anything. And if nothing else, flirting with a variety of people—some of whom might go on to become sex partners—is one way to spice up a daily life which offers excruciatingly little variation.

Related, though not specific to SSA, is the fact that men and women, married and unmarried, regularly experience predictable and unpredictable attractions to one another. Researchers tend to ignore this obvious fact in studies of sexual behavior and disease transmission—attraction and lust are hard to model. But our male informants and evidence from the ethnographic journals collected in Malawi for over a decade leave no room for doubt. Men notice and appreciate the beautiful women around them, even while aware of the dangers of AIDS. The journals document dozens of conversations between male friends that go something like this. After describing that "all the girls that he sees look very beautiful," he explains further:

> . . . These days, there are more beautiful girls than it was in the past . . . Those girls are like bait, just the same as a fisherman does when he wants to hook fish. He first of all puts bait at his hook so that fish should be attracted with the bait without knowing that it will be hooked.

Along these same lines, religious leaders frequently equate beautiful women with temptation directly from the devil. This can happen at any time. One imam playfully described the threat of recently bathed women attending the mosque, urging the men who attend to go straight home after prayers lest they be tempted. Others preach about Satan's plot to destroy families by sending beautiful women as temptation for men; spiritually disciplined men might have the strength to resist, but weak men will perish, taking their families along with them. The following is an excerpt from a sermon that we observed in a "strict" Baptist congregation in southern Malawi. It is typical in the sense that it highlights the slippery slope down which people—in this case, men—can slide, away from faithfulness and into temptation:

> He first gave an example of the sin of lust and adultery. Today the devil might bring to you a beautiful woman. You see her and smile at her. Tomorrow he will bring her to you again. By the next day she comes to you, something starts moving in you. The devil then starts asking you questions: "What about her?" "What do you feel?" "Go after her." At this point in time you have your conscience right, you can even tell the devil that "No. Get away from me. I am married and I'm happy with my wife." At this point the devil will run away from you, but if you just nourish his questions, you create an internal conflict. He will advance by telling you, "I know you're married, but how do you compare her to your wife?" With time you begin to accept the devil's lies. You will confess that the girl is more beautiful than your wife. The devil will keep on bringing this lady into your life until you're defeated and fall into sin. Once you sleep with that girl that marks the beginning of your ending. But if you could say no just the moment you first saw that girl, the devil could run away from you.

We can't say for certain why any given person engages in extramarital relationships, in SSA or anywhere else in the world. But we do know that it happens. We now seek to document variation in this phenomenon according to key dimensions of religion—by tradition, individual-level religiosity, and the broader religious context.

Religious Variation in Faithfulness

All of the world's major religions forbid extramarital sex for married persons. And research from across the globe suggests that both religion and religiosity influence the sexual behavior of married adults. Studies of married adults in the United States, for example, show that those who attend religious services regularly are less likely to report an extramarital sexual partner than those who do not (e.g., Burdette, Ellison, Sherkat, and Gore 2007). Likewise, members of religiously distinctive groups (e.g., Pentecostals in Brazil, Zionists in Zimbabwe) report faithfulness to a greater extent than others in their communities (Gregson, Zhuwau, Anderson, and Chandiwana 1999; Hill, Cleland, and Ali 2004).

DHS data from men in 27 countries (Figure 5.1) allow us to examine whether the proportion of married men reporting an extramarital partner varies across major religious groups. While we observe significant differences in many of the countries from which we have estimates, there is no obvious pattern to these patterns. In other words, among the three major traditions, no single group is consistently more or less likely to report extramarital partners. This is not surprising. Since all religious traditions unequivocally object to sex outside marriage, it is nearly impossible to hypothesize about expected differences in any particular place. There is no evidence that Islamic teachings about sex and family life are different in Gabon—where Muslims constitute a majority and Muslim

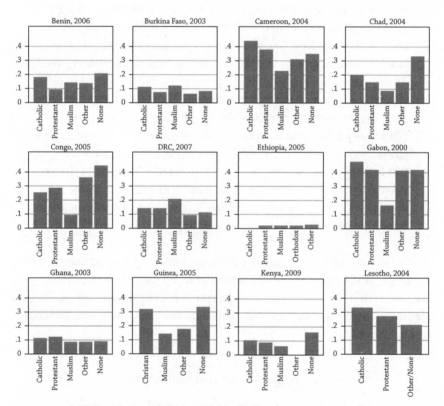

Figure 5.1 Proportion of Married Men Reporting at Least One Extramarital Partner During the Past 12 Months by Denomination

Note: We exclude Cote D'Ivoire, where data were collected only from women, from these analyses.

Source: African Demographic and Health Surveys

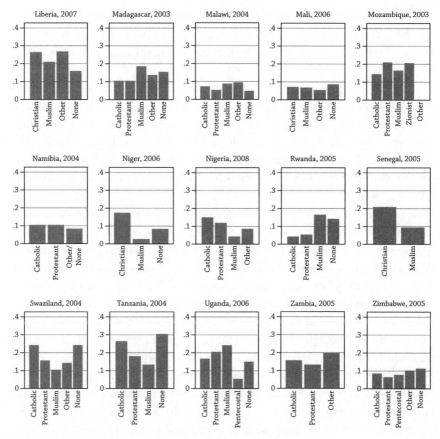

Figure 5.1 (continued)

men are less likely than their Christian counterparts to have an extramarital partner—than in Uganda, where extramarital partners are most prevalent among Muslim men. These findings—or lack thereof—move us to ask different questions about how religion shapes the discourse on faithfulness. Namely, we focus on how religiosity, as opposed to mere affiliation, illuminates differences at a local rather than a national level.

Religion shapes how people think about fidelity, temptation, and risk. People in SSA are simultaneously vigilant to the risks posed by their spouses and optimistically trusting—or at least resigned to trusting them, often interpreting this tension through a religious lens. Davis, a 26-year-old Malawian man who regularly attends a Presbyterian church told us this when asked how worried he is about AIDS:

> We worry, because you really can't know what your partner is doing. But we trust each other. But trusting each other can also be a bad thing. The one who betrayed Jesus Christ [Judas] was eating together with

him! It's the same for us. If Jesus was betrayed by a man who ate with
him, then couldn't my wife betray me? Could I betray her? I am very
doubtful that I could betray my wife. But maybe she could betray me.

Likening the possibility of infection by an unfaithful spouse to Judas' be-
trayal of Jesus is a telling metaphor for the AIDS epidemic in Africa today. Davis
acknowledges his own concern about infection while admitting his main source
of worry is his own partner—someone he should be able to trust.[17] In an environment much crueler than the one that we experience in developed countries,
the possibility of infection by an unfaithful spouse is just another in a long list
of injustices.

Analyses of our Malawi data provide ample evidence that religion influences
the sexual behavior of married persons. A reported recent extramarital partner
(during the past year) was no more or less prevalent among polygamous men
(compared with men with only one wife), educated men (compared with those
with no schooling), or wealthy men (compared with the poor). However, net of
a host of other controls, men affiliated with Mission Protestant and Pentecostal
congregations were less likely than Catholics to report an extramarital partner.
We also found Muslims—here a combined sample of women and men—to be
most likely to report extramarital partners. But across denominations, the religiously involved, as measured by frequent attendance at religious services, were
half as likely as those who attended services infrequently to report having had
an extramarital partner during the past year (Trinitapoli and Regnerus 2006).[18]

Why is this the case? How exactly does religion shape sexual behavior? Garner's (2000) study of sexual behavior in Kwazulu Natal Province, South Africa,
documented a similar pattern of lower levels of extramarital and premarital sex
among Pentecostals compared with members of other religious groups. He suggests four mechanisms through which religion can influence individuals:

1. Indoctrination: Religious organizations instruct members about sexual
   behavior, directly shaping the behavior of their members.
2. Subjective religious experiences: Song, ritual, and nearness to God foster
   internal motivation to follow a particular teaching or practice.
3. Exclusionary practices: Religious congregations preemptively exclude persons not conforming to their beliefs and kick out members who deviate from
   their teachings.
4. Socialization: Members are embedded in a network that provides support,
   surveillance, and social control.

Our detailed data on the religious landscape of Malawi allow us to empirically
assess which of these four suggested mechanisms has the greatest explanatory
power. Using data from married men and women in 2004, we looked not only at

individuals' own religious beliefs and practices but also at the characteristics of the congregation they attend.

First, our analyses[19] showed that attending a religious congregation in which AIDS and sexual behavior are discussed frequently is unrelated to the reported sexual behavior of married persons. However, men and women who attend congregations in which the leader reports actively monitoring the sexual conduct of members are 68% more likely to report faithfulness to their partner (Trinitapoli 2009: Table 4).[20] To eliminate the possibility that unfaithful people who were associated with a strict church had left or been kicked out, what social scientists call a *selection effect*, we controlled for whether individuals had changed congregations during the past five years and found no relationship. In other words, voluntary or involuntary religious switching—Garner's (2000) exclusionary practices—is not the primary force behind the religion–faithfulness connection. Likewise, there was no relationship between reported faithfulness and other messages reported by the religious leader having to do with AIDS or sexual morality (in fact there appeared to be opposite relationship, though it was not statistically significant). The observed religion–faithfulness pattern was not, in other words, the product of a substantial internal reorientation consistent with Garner's first "indoctrination" mechanism. Finally, we found only a weak effect of personal religiosity, an indicator of subjective religious experiences, on reported faithfulness.

In fact, of the four mechanisms Garner (2000) identified as driving the relationship between religion and faithfulness, the most important in our Malawian sample was old-style social control, active vigilance on the part of the leader, albeit strengthened by a level of personal religiosity. In contrast, internal motivation to follow religious teachings on sexual behavior and practice marital fidelity had no measurable effect.

Vigilance on the part of the leader is not the only thing that matters for the faithfulness of members. Using the same multilevel approach we used to measure HIV prevalence in Chapter 2, we examined the relationship between a host of village- and individual-level factors and the likelihood that married respondents report having an extramarital sexual partner during the past year.[21] Consistent with expectations from our previous discussion of sex ratios and labor migration, in villages where men outnumber women, both women and men are more likely to report extramarital partners. But the religion findings are particularly intriguing. As with other analyses of faithfulness, more religious women are less likely to report having had any extramarital sex. But village-level religiosity has the opposite effect for women. Where the average level of religiosity is high, women are *more likely* than those in less religious contexts to report an extramarital sexual partner. This relationship is shown in the bottom three lines of Figure 5.2. Village-level religiosity does not constrain the sexual behavior of women. In fact, highly religious villages[22] provide a context in which significantly (though not substantially) more extramarital sex occurs.

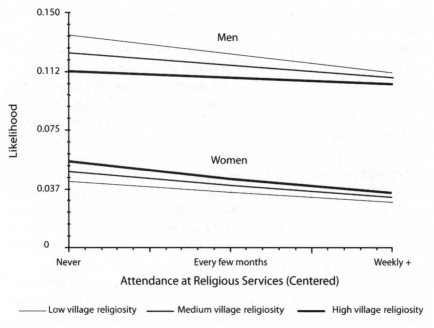

Figure 5.2 Likelihood of Reporting an Extramarital Partner by Village and Individual-Level Religiosity

As we saw in relation to the effects of village-level religiosity on HIV status, religious context shapes the sexual behavior of men quite differently. First, the intercepts for each line are different from one another—both visibly and statistically—demonstrating that just residing in a religious village lowers men's odds of reporting an extramarital partner. Second, the negative gradient of each line shows that the most religious men are the least likely to report such a partner and that this is true across religious contexts. Third, and important for thinking clearly about religious context, the magnitude of these negative gradients differs by village-level religiosity. In less religious villages, the impact of individual religiosity is greater. Here, religious distinctiveness seems to matter most. In highly religious villages, highly religious men are also the least likely to report an extramarital partner. In these same villages, however, the difference between the sexual behavior of highly religious men and that of their less religious counterparts is minimal. Pulling these analyses together with our village-level HIV prevalence findings from Chapter 2 suggests that high levels of village religiosity constrain the sexual behavior of men, independent of their own religiosity. Arguably it is these most religious villages that offer "protection" from HIV infection for women.

These results map neatly onto the denominational differences identified in previous literature. For the religious congregations in which members' sexual behavior is policed tend to be nested within the sexually conservative denominations that seroprevalence studies have shown—on the whole—to be associated with lower HIV prevalence. But this is not always the case. What our analysis confirms is that the primary pathway from religion to marital faithfulness is through an extrinsic mechanism, social control. This is not specific to any particular religious tradition. It also operates independently of personal beliefs about sexual morality.

C Is for Condoms

We say that the most important thing is to abstain because if you abstain, you avoid everything. For those who cannot abstain it is better to use condoms. The Bible has no verse that says, "Do not use condoms."
—Akiki, *17 years old, Uganda, 2004*

This gadget called the condom . . . is causing the spread of AIDS in this country.
—Lucy Kibaki, *Kenya's "First Lady," 2006*

Religious groups have generated broad consensus around abstinence and fidelity, the A and B of primary AIDS prevention methods. "C" is a different story. There is considerable disagreement about both the desirability and acceptability of condoms, and this is found both within and across religious traditions. Further complicating matters, attitudes toward condoms are only loosely correlated with their actual use, making the relationship between religion and condoms even thornier.

The official Catholic position on condoms is well-known. The Church's categorical opposition to condom use—along with all forms of modern contraception—has been front and center in debates about the role of religion in HIV prevention in Africa. Hostility toward condoms by religious leaders from other traditions has also been noted. During her time in Uganda, for example, Helen Epstein (2005) witnessed a pastor set fire to a supply of free condoms intended for college students, proclaiming, "I burn these condoms in the name of Jesus!" Likewise, Mozambican archbishop Francisco Chimoio's allegations that European countries are deliberately manufacturing condoms infected with HIV to decimate African populations received considerable media attention in 2007 (AIDS Lunacy 2007; Shock at Archbishop Condom Claim 2007). More recently, the opposition of some Islamic leaders to condoms has also been noted (Moszynski 2008).

Cases like these have been broadly publicized in the West. The contrast between forces of light (e.g., African or international aid workers promoting condom use) and forces of darkness (e.g., an African priest burning condoms and promoting abstinence) makes for a good story. One represents the Africa that we'd like to see. The other fits deeply held beliefs about Africa as a place filled with superstitious nonsense. In other words, stories of priests standing in

the way of progress can be easily cast in ways that fit Western readers' predispo-
sitions about both Africa and religion (i.e., both are backward). The condom
issue in SSA, therefore, underscores bigger representational questions about
how we write about people unlike ourselves.[23]

The popular media are not alone in playing with such unhelpful caricatures.
Some scholars build on similar stories, asserting that religion and religious beliefs
are a (if not *the*) barrier to HIV prevention in SSA (Pisani 1999; Preston-Whyte
1999; Rankin, Lindgren, Rankin, and Ng'oma 2005). This is particularly true of
those who believe that condoms are the solution to the AIDS problem and that
religious opposition to condoms is the primary barrier to their widespread use.

There are at least three problems with this negative view. First, it ignores the
fact that religious leaders were among the first in SSA to legitimize the use of condoms. Second, it ignores the considerable differences in opinions about, and use
of, condoms that one finds *within* denominations. Third, it assumes that the official position of a church or religious group on condoms—whether for or against—
is reflected in popular attitudes to condoms or, more importantly, their use.

As already noted, pastors setting fire to condoms or Chimoio-like allegations
about condoms being laced with HIV as part of a plot to depopulate Africa make
for good news stories in the West. But for every religious leader who is vocally
and visibly anti-condom, many more seem to have championed condom-based
prevention methods. This goes back at least as far as the late 1980s. Early in this
chapter, for example, we talked about Father Bernard Joinet, founder of the
"Fleet of Hope" in Tanzania. Joinet was a Catholic priest. His aim was to develop
a prevention approach that was consistent with his own (mainstream) religious
beliefs. This included the use of condoms. Another notable example is Ugandan
Bishop Karuma of the Anglican Church, one of the first religious leaders to explicitly link the B and C messages, saying, "If you are foolish enough to have sex
outside, don't be stupid enough not to use a condom" (cited in Hardee et al. 2008:
11). Echoing him were Muslim leaders in Uganda who, beginning in the late
1980s, endorsed condoms as what Badri (2007:15) later referred to as "the lesser
of two evils." This endorsement made condoms a core component of the Islamic
Approach to HIV/AIDS (IAA) developed by the Islamic Medical Association of
Uganda (IMAU) in 1989.

Even the Catholic Church, the most visible target of criticism over the condom issue, harbors many dissenting voices in the tradition of Joinet. In 2006,
for example, Cardinal Carlo Maria Martini caused a stir when he called the use of
condoms for HIV prevention "a lesser evil" (Cardinal Backs Limited Condom Use
2006). A recent editorial in the *Lancet* reported that 65 of 100 Catholic priests
polled in the United Kingdom agreed that it was morally acceptable to promote
condom use to curb the spread of HIV (*Lancet* Editorial 2006). Perhaps most surprising, *congregational distribution* of condoms has been documented in Catholic
parishes across South Africa—at least when authorities aren't looking (Timberg

2006)—mirroring cases in Pentecostal, Salvation Army, and Presbyterian churches in Malawi (Gama 2003).[24]

This broader body of evidence demonstrates that, as a whole, religious groups have cultivated a more balanced position vis-à-vis condoms than is often attributed to them. We characterize this position as the *unenthusiastic acceptance of condoms*: a pragmatic, humane, but somewhat distasteful solution to the imperfections of the human character. In the words of Anglican bishop S. Tilewa Johnson of The Gambia: "We are aware that we live in a world where not everybody is holy and for some people abstinence or one partner is not a viable proposition, therefore, the only sensible and responsible line of action is a use of condoms" (Colombant 2005: para. 3). Likewise, Badri's keynote lecture to the third International Muslim Leaders Consultation on HIV/AIDS in Addis Ababa in 2007 criticized the anticondom positions of some Muslim scholars as "immoderate" and went on to say:

> . . . No strategy is able to purge society from promiscuity and fornication. An Islamic strategy should therefore find solutions to deal with such expected sexual adventures. It is in this situation that an Islamic approach should endorse the use of condoms as the lesser of the two evils. (Badri 2007: 14–15)

From a non-Western perspective, this unenthusiastic acceptance of condoms represents a pragmatic midpoint between the two extremes. Badri (2007: 15) describes this midpoint well:

> One [extreme] regards condoms as the major line of defense against HIV infection and sometimes behaves as if it is the only form of protection. To these the answer to better prevention is more and more condoms. The other considers any advocacy for its use an open invitation to promiscuity . . . We must reject the first extreme of condoms . . . condoms . . . and more condoms since it is based on the philosophy and mores of the Western sexual revolution . . . However we should also reject the absolute "No" to condoms. Even if we do our best to advocate abstinence and being faithful to spouses, we would fail with many young people. No society can succeed in completely stopping its people from engaging in sex outside marriage.

Badri's positions are almost identical to those of mainstream Christian groups— as a mental exercise, substitute "Christian," "Catholic," "Anglican" or some other denominational identity wherever Badri mentions "Islamic." Like his Christian counterparts, Badri's refusal to decouple sex and morality, as we discussed earlier in relation to instrumental abstinence posters, makes it impossible for him to uncritically embrace condoms. But that does not stop him or others in competing religious traditions from treating condoms as a useful last resort.

Does this unenthusiastic acceptance of condoms as a last resort imply a demotion from its equal footing in the early ABC campaigns? To some extent, yes, as can be seen by comparing early versions of Joinet's Fleet of Hope to later adaptations. While early Tanzanian versions show three equally sized wooden boats linked by planks, later adaptations have two wooden boats—abstinence and fidelity—and a smaller rubber lifeboat associated with condoms. In the same vein, some Ugandan adaptations of the Fleet of Hope feature a single boat labeled *Abstinence and Fidelity*, while people using condoms bob about in the water wearing lifejackets (Hardee et al. 2008: 9). The message of both adaptations is clear: condoms are riskier than abstinence or faithfulness. They are for those who have already slipped up, but they are better than nothing: they still offer some protection.

Muslim and Christian leaders of the churches and mosques we observed in rural Malawi between 2004 and 2005 echoed this pragmatic though unenthusiastic position on condoms. An imam who leads the largest mosque in his district explained:

> Abstinence is the best way of prevention against the disease. Also God has told us not to come near adultery. But the fact is that man cannot live without sinning. In the cases where abstinence fails, one can use condoms so that he should not get the disease.

A Church of Christ pastor put his pragmatism in particularly stark terms:

> There is too much ignorance on the part of the youth to take heed [abstain], because they have not reached a point of self-conviction where they completely adhere to the word of God. In this case, the youth need to be assisted in the other way around [condoms]—otherwise just encouraging *kudziletsa* [abstinence] might result in the death of the believing community.

In other words, condoms are OK if for no other reason than to preserve the life of the congregation. He continued, ". . . If all the members are dead, I will be the leader of what?"

This unenthusiastic acceptance of condoms is not only a religious thing. It represents a consensus position among African leaders and opinion makers in general. A good indicator of this can be seen in the comparative coverage given to Pope Benedict XVI's deliberations about AIDS and condoms by American and African newspapers. Leading American and British newspapers opened with headlines like, "Pope says No to Condoms." In other words, they emphasized the condom and public health angle. Coverage in African newspapers, in contrast—the *Daily Times* in Kenya and the *Nation* in Malawi are examples—highlighted the Pope's remarks about the importance of "friendship with those who suffer," mentioning the issue of condoms only briefly at the end.[25] Broadly interpreted, this difference in media coverage suggests that promotion of condoms is more important in the West than in SSA. The (at least partial) demoralization of sex in the West makes it difficult to emphasize A and B without coming across as an unenlightened conservative. C has, therefore, become a cornerstone of the rubric Western scholars use to evaluate the effectiveness of AIDS-prevention programs and, by extension, the practitioners of those programs. But condoms are less important in Africa. Since A and B are the preferred prevention strategies, debates about condoms are sidelined. Indeed, condoms are typically seen as the most foreign aspect of the fight against AIDS. They are a product of the "sexually liberal" West.[26]

Framed in terms of sexual morality, A and B are widely considered to be the preferred prevention strategies across SSA. Many African leaders, from the national to local level, view condoms as an intervention that undermines efforts to promote abstinence and faithfulness, which both religious leaders and the population as a whole see as the most effective prevention strategies. This is the alternative reading of Lucy Kibaki's comments at the start of this section as well as those associated with others. Janet Museveni, for example, Uganda's first lady, has launched similar critiques of condoms.[27]

Religious Variation in Attitudes to Condoms and Condom Use

So much for broad declarative statements about the acceptability or desirability of condoms: How much religious variation is there in attitudes to condoms and in actual condom use? To answer this properly we need to distinguish:

1. Attitudes to condoms, as voiced by three different types of social actors, each of whom represents a discrete analytic level:
   a. International/national leaders of the religious denomination
   b. Local religious leaders, that is, leaders of individual churches and mosques
   c. Individuals, that is, regular laypeople
2. Reported condom use, again, by regular people

Ultimately, only the second point is directly relevant for HIV transmission. But tensions between attitudes at the three levels are illuminating and, as we show, relevant for understanding prevention.

First, despite massive public health campaigns promoting their use, condom use remains low across the subcontinent. We know this because (1) this is what people tell survey researchers, and (2) the fervor of condom promotion leads people to exaggerate their condom use, not underreport it.

Just as we did with AIDS-related knowledge and faithfulness, we examined religious differences in condom use across all countries in SSA in which DHS data have been collected. Figure 5.3 illustrates religious differences in condom use the last time respondents had sex—using only those who have had sex in the past year. Because the DHS data reveal low levels of condom use across Africa, with men reporting higher levels of use than women, we focus only on men here. A number of important patterns and nonpatterns emerge from these data. Taken together, they illustrate the limitations of using official religious doctrines to infer religious differences on the ground. First, despite the well-known official prohibitions against all forms of modern birth control (especially condoms), African Catholics are *no less likely* than Protestants (e.g., Presbyterians have no

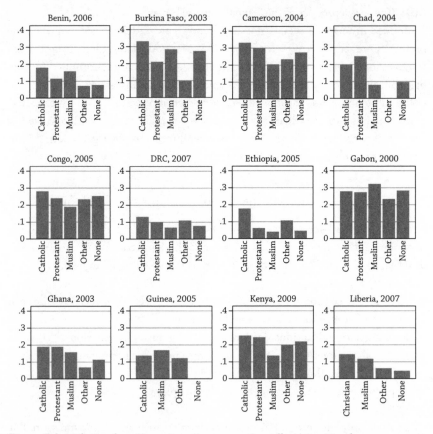

Figure 5.3 Male Condom Use at Last Sex among Sexually Active Men by Denomination

Note: We exclude four countries from these analyses: Cote D'Ivoire, where data on condom were collected only from women; Swaziland, where data on men's condom use are missing; Lesotho, where data on men's condom use appear to have been miscoded; and Mali, with insufficient religious diversity to make valid comparisons between groups.

Source: African Demographic and Health Surveys

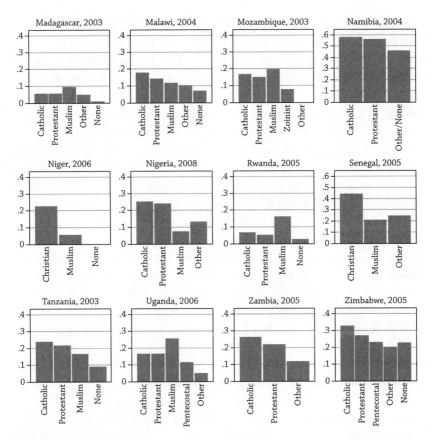

Figure 5.3 (*continued*)

Note: The scales of the graphs from Namibia and Senegal, where reported condom use is comparatively high, are different from all others.

such prohibition) to report using condoms in any African country. This is true even in Namibia, the only country in which reported condom use among sexually active men could be described as high. Second, with some exceptions, primarily in East Africa (Mozambique, Madagascar, and Uganda) or with very small or largely non-African Muslim populations (Rwanda, Gabon), condom use tends to be lowest among Muslims, even though they are not subject to any prohibitions from mainstream Islamic authorities (Badri 1997/2000; Musallam 1983). Third, there is no consistent condom use pattern across the religiously unaffiliated: nowhere do they have the highest levels of condom use, but in several countries they do have the lowest. This, too, suggests that there is no outright religious hostility toward condoms that suppresses their use. If there were, we would observe higher levels of condom use among the religiously unaffiliated.

The gap between official religious doctrine and the actual sexual behavior of lay members in SSA should not surprise anyone. The convergence of Catholic and non-Catholic fertility in the United States points to the limited relevance of Catholic doctrine on birth control for the behavior of most practitioners (Mosher, Williams, and Johnson 1992). So, too, does the fact that predominantly Catholic countries like Italy and Spain have some of the lowest fertility rates in the world. There is no good reason that people in Africa should, on average, be any more susceptible to official church rulings on condoms than their European and American counterparts are on contraceptive use in general.

The same argument can be used in relation to our parallel finding of low condom use among Muslims. Although contraceptive use is broadly permitted by almost all Islamic legal authorities (Musallam 1983) and contraceptive prevalence is high in some Muslim countries (notably Iran and Tunisia), contraceptive prevalence in Muslim populations in general is almost always lower than in neighboring non-Muslim populations (Morgan, Stash, Smith, and Mason 2002). Most Muslim legal authorities agree that condoms are permissible, and the IAA endorses them. Yet condom use is considerably lower among this group. This gap between official messages and actual behavior begs a different explanation. In the case of contraception generally, Obermeyer (1992) linked that difference to cultural conflicts between Islam and the West. We suspect that the same phenomenon is driving the patterns we observe with regard to condoms. Mainstream Islamic authorities may permit their use and may even teach that, under certain circumstances, condom use is obligatory (Badri 1997/2000). But in general, the contemporary geopolitical tensions referred to in Chapter 1 clarify why the popular associations between condoms and all things Western make them especially undesirable to African Muslims.

In summary, then, official prohibitions against, or endorsements of, condoms may or may not influence whether lay Africans concerned about HIV infection actually use them. An official denominational message is merely one of multiple influences on the decision to use condoms. Official religious messages compete with other factors, many of which have nothing to do with religion. For example, condoms are seldom used in longer-term relationships, including marriage. Rather, they are seen as specific to extramarital relations. The strong pronatalism we discussed in Chapter 3 also contributes to the low levels of condom use observed across SSA. Yet another stems from a strong preference for sex without condoms (see Tavory and Swidler 2009) that may or may not be particular to SSA. In our own work, we have heard endless complaints about condom use from both men and women: "it's like eating a sweet with the wrapper on" and "you wouldn't eat a banana without peeling it."[28]

In addition to their formal teachings and messages about AIDS, churches and mosques provide fertile ground for informal communication about HIV, and we believe that it is these informal interactions that are most relevant to the question of condom use by members. Studies on the content of religious services in Mozambique (Agadjanian and Menjívar 2008; Pfeiffer 2004) and Malawi (Trinitapoli 2006) have shown that local religious leaders almost never speak about condoms directly from the pulpit. How, then, might the position of the religious leader be reflected in the behavior of members? While mentioning condoms directly in a mixed (age and sex) setting like a religious service may be taboo, condoms (and other forms of contraception) appear to be more of a topic for discussion at group meetings, which are frequently sex-segregated (Yeatman and Trinitapoli 2007). Evidence from Malawi also shows that while religious leaders seldom speak directly about condoms, almost 30% claim to have privately advised members to use them (Trinitapoli 2009).

Data from the MDICP presented in Table 5.2 also reveal denominational variation in individual attitudes toward the acceptability of condoms. Results here are surprising. They show that Muslims are significantly more likely than members of any other group to say that it is acceptable[29] for a married couple to use condoms for HIV prevention (53%), New Mission Protestants are the least accepting of condoms (28%), and Catholics, Pentecostals, and Mission Protestants (e.g., Anglicans and Presbyterians) fall somewhere in the middle (37–39%). Here we see again how large the gap between reported attitudes and behavior can be. Reported condom use[30] shows very different denominational patterns. While attitudes toward condom use vary along religious lines, denominational differences in condom use are minimal. Mission Protestants report marginally higher condom use, but the differences are tiny and not statistically significant. Likewise, Muslims, though much more likely to view condoms as acceptable, are at the bottom of this tightly clustered group in terms of actual condom use.

Two potential sources of religious differences in condom use remain. First, there is the issue of variation within denominations—for example, differences

Table 5.2 **Denominational Differences in Attitudes to Condoms and Condom Use in Malawi, 2004**

	Condom Acceptability (%)	*Condom Use (%)*
No Religion	32	21
Catholic	39	20
Mission Protestant	28	25
Pentecostal	37	23
African Independent Church	32	24
Muslim	53	19
New Mission Protestant	28	23
N	3101	2997

Source: MDICP-3.

across all the Catholic churches in our sample and differences within the group of mosques from which we have data. Do differences in local religious leaders' attitudes to condoms, in particular in their willingness to countenance or promote condoms as a back-up, translate into actual differences in their use among the laity? In systematically observing religious services across rural Malawi, we documented a range of positions on condoms. Sometimes condoms were explicitly prohibited by religious leaders. Other leaders had relaxed prohibitions on condom use and were encouraging members who cannot abstain to use a condom to avoid contracting HIV (Trinitapoli 2006). Here there is a measurable effect of religion on condom use. Specifically, sexually active Malawians who attend congregations in which the leader thinks that condoms are acceptable are nearly 50% more likely to report having used condoms themselves (Trinitapoli 2009).

Second, a number of studies have shown that religious individuals who are sexually active are less likely to use condoms when they do have sex (Agha, Hutchinson, and Kusanthan 2006; Nicholas and Durrheim 1995). This finding is consistent with research on religion and sexual behavior among adolescents in the United States (Bearman and Brückner 2001; Ku, Sonenstein, and Pleck 1992). On the other hand, this pattern is inconsistent. For example, a recent study of black South Africans found the expected negative relationship between religiosity and sexual activity (i.e., more religious, less sex) but no association between religiosity and condom use (Burgard and Lee-Rife 2009). This is similar to what our research in Malawi reveals. Net of their own reported risk behaviors, sociodemographic characteristics, religious affiliation, and attitudes about condoms, those who attend religious services frequently are neither more nor less likely to report using condoms. Likewise, there is no difference between the attitudes of the most religious individuals—those who attend religious services frequently and participate in Bible studies or choir groups—and those who attend infrequently or not at all.

Conclusions

A couple of key results emerge from this chapter. First, there is broad consensus across all religious groups about the role that abstinence and fidelity can play in preventing the further spread of HIV. There is also broad consensus about condoms—a pragmatic but unenthusiastic acceptance of their use. Second, and importantly, these official views do not explain much variation in ABC behavior. Thus, even where official doctrine officially prohibits or permits condom use, there is no direct relationship between that official position and the reported behavior of individuals. Indeed, what one's own pastor or imam does matters far more than the official position of a higher-level denominational leader. The next chapter takes this emphasis on the importance of local leaders several steps further, as we talk about other local approaches people use to supplement the official AIDS lexicon.

Beyond ABC: Local Prevention Strategies

And some holding it best to live temperately, and to avoid excesses of all kinds, made parties, and shut themselves up from the rest of the world; eating and drinking moderately of the best, and diverting themselves with music, and such entertainments as they might have within doors; never listening to anything from without, to make them uneasy. Others maintained free living to be a better preservative, and would baulk no passion or appetite they wished to gratify, drinking and reveling incessantly from tavern to tavern, or in private houses . . . A third sort of people chose a method between these two; not yet confining themselves to rules of diet like the former, and yet avoiding the intemperance of the latter; but eating and drinking what their appetites required, they walked everywhere with odours and nosegays to smell to . . . Others of a more cruel disposition, as perhaps the more safe to themselves, declared that the only remedy was to avoid it: persuaded, therefore, of this, and taking care for themselves only, men and women in great numbers left the city, their houses, relations, and effects, and fled into the country: as if the wrath of God had been restrained to visit those only within the walls of the city . . . Divided as they were, neither did all die nor all escape; but falling sick indifferently, as well those of one as of another opinion.

—Bocaccio, *The Decameron, p.xxi–xxii.*[1]

Three decades into the epidemic it is clear that, in their attempts to avoid infection, many people in sub-Saharan Africa (SSA) employ prevention strategies that are not an official part of ABC. These strategies can be characterized in a number of ways. They are local and unorthodox—they arise in spite of the fact that no transnational network of nongovernmental organizations (NGOs) or state institutions promotes them. They are organic, emerging naturally as people "navigate AIDS" on their own (Watkins 2004), making assessments about the things that constitute "risk" and what they can reasonably do to avoid those things. They are also popular: many people use them.

In general, these local prevention strategies are oriented toward leading a lower-risk sex life. They work in one of two ways. The first is by limiting the person to less risky partners by promoting partner reduction, more careful partner selection, or the termination of risky relationships. The second is by limiting behaviors that are believed to lead to risky sex, in particular drunkenness.

In this chapter we describe these local prevention strategies and discuss their relationship to religion. A few general themes emerge from this description. First, many of these strategies evoke the extrinsic social control mechanisms mentioned toward the end of the last chapter. They depend on, and draw their strength from, social surveillance. Second, religion influences the risk of HIV infection over and above offering a concrete set of guidelines about the acceptability of different types of sexual behavior. Third, the promotion of local non-ABC strategies and combinations of strategies cuts across denominations. In other words, there is more variation in local prevention efforts within denominations than across them. This is consistent with the patterns we noted in relation to the ABCs.

There are at least two non-ABC prevention strategies that we do not address here as local ones. The first is the use of protective charms, amulets, or talismans. Although such charms have historically been widely used throughout Africa to protect wearers from other dangers—for example, from malaria (Maslove, Mnyusiwalla, Mills, McGowan, Attaran, and Wilson 2009), risk of pregnancy (Kalipeni and Zulu 1993), or injury in battle (Robinson 2004)—there is limited evidence that such methods are used to help protect wearers from HIV infection.[2] This stands in contrast to the prominent role of traditional medicine in the *treatment* of AIDS, especially in the pre-antiretroviral therapy (ART) era. (We return to this point in Chapter 7). The second non-ABC strategy is male circumcision. Although it clearly falls outside of ABC and although it has been replicated in several rigorous clinical trials (Auvert, Taaljard, Lagarde, Sobngwi-Tambekou, Sitta, and Puren 2005; Williams et al. 2006), male circumcision for HIV prevention did not grow locally and organically. Rather, its increasingly mainstream position rests on findings from formal epidemiological studies and, after some initial reticence, directives from the international health organizations.

Early Marriage: Prevention or Risk?

> If someone is 18 years old, he should have a wife because that's the age that the prophet had a wife. So that person should get married so as to avoid temptation.
> —Jawara, *imam, Senegal*

The extent to which early marriage helps prevent HIV has generated heated debate over the last decade. Those who argue that early marriage is protective build on the A and B in the ABC strategy. Their argument sounds feasible. If two people abstain until marriage, and they are then fully faithful within marriage, they will never be (sexually) exposed to HIV.

Naysayers don't deny the effects that early marriage can have on prevention in theory. They simply dismiss the underlying A and B assumptions as unrealistic, pointing to the fact that people in the real world often have both extramarital partners and premarital partners. This is particularly true of men, since men tend to become sexually active earlier and marry later: "spousal age difference" in SSA is roughly 5 years between a husband and a first wife and greater still in marriages between a man and his later wives (in polygamous marriages). As a result, naysayers argue that pushing a young woman into marriage early may unwittingly increase her risk of HIV infection since it generally means marrying someone older and more sexually experienced. And because sex within marriage is almost always "unprotected"—there is virtually no condom use within marriage, though other forms of contraception are increasingly common—early marriage may raise the risk of HIV infection, especially for women (Clark, Bruce, and Dude 2006).

Not surprisingly, the debate over (early) marriage as prevention has not yet been settled empirically. Measuring the *actual* effect of early marriage on the likelihood of infection is difficult. Ideally, researchers would prospectively follow a large sample of adolescents from their mid-teens into their early 20s, collecting survey data on sexual behavior, sex partners, and marriage and also biomarker data on HIV status. While we know of two ongoing research projects that are doing exactly this,[3] to date no study has provided an unambiguous answer to this question. Furthermore, the bits and pieces of evidence that can be used to either support or reject the argument are not easily generalized to settings with different levels of, for example, premarital and extramarital sex, relative ages at marriage, and sexually transmitted infection (STI) prevalence.

People's attitudes on the ground are consistent with this empirical ambiguity. In our Malawi data, for example, we asked adolescent women and men whether they thought that marriage could help them avoid AIDS. A little more than half of the respondents—57% of women and 53% of men—thought so; most of the rest thought not. Divided opinions were also evident from the focus group data from unmarried adolescents in Ghana (see Chapter 5, section on "Interpreting Abstinence"). On one hand, some adolescent boys and most adolescent girls in those data talked about marriage as a risk. Seeing condoms as an unrealistic part of married life, they believe that they could be more easily infected by an unfaithful spouse than by an unfaithful boyfriend or girlfriend, with whom they could insist on using condoms (Hearst and Chen 2004; Shelton 2006).[4] On the other hand, some young people value abstinence and view early marriage as an effective strategy for avoiding infection, though *only under certain conditions*. For example, one young Ghanaian man who advocated for abstinence put it this way:

> If you can't abstain, choose a girl and marry. But before you marry this girl try to study her moves. Don't just marry. Since testing is not easy, you can learn about the girls from villagers who know girls' moves and characters.

This is, in most contexts, a reasonable suggestion. Rather than simple-mindedly promoting early marriage as a universally safe venue for sexual activity in the era of AIDS, the informant merely asserts that the safety marriage can provide is contingent on both partners being both negative to begin with and faithful to one another in the future. The point of careful partner selection raises other questions about how one can know about a person's sexual history—and their likely future sexual behavior. Here the informant suggests relying, in a village setting at least, on the oldest and least formal mechanism of social control: gossip.

Gossip provides an entry point for thinking about how the relationship between religion and AIDS works through the early marriage mechanism. Religious congregations and leaders play a central role in the transition to marriage for young Africans. When the Ghanaian man quoted before referred to the importance of "studying her moves" to determine whether a woman is marriage material, he was referring both to direct observation and to reliance on local knowledge (i.e., gossip) about a romantic interest's sexual and health history. These are the two primary methods for developing confidence that a love interest might make a good and safe sexual and marital partner.

This mechanism was described to us at length by a lay leader of one Catholic parish in a particularly remote area of Malawi. In the context of talking about the importance of marriage—and careful partner selection—for avoiding infection, he declared: "We advise the youth to choose a well-behaved girl or boy, and when they want to marry they should let the mediators know so that they can do a background check on the particular person." An Assemblies of God pastor in one of our Malawian research sites takes a particularly hands-on approach in managing marriage prospects for young adults in his congregation. He matchmakes from his tightly knit pool of born-again young adults, making exceptions in cases only where he can verify the religious and health status of a member's romantic interest.

In this sense, local gossip can be thought of as a functional substitute for current *and prospective* HIV testing. Getting confirmation that a potential partner is currently HIV negative is important. But knowing the character of a potential partner—his or her likelihood of remaining faithful and of being a good provider—is essential for evaluating the chances of remaining negative. Of

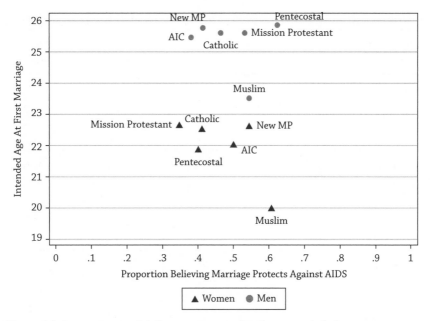

Figure 6.1 Denominational differences in attitudes about – and ideal age at - marriage
  Source: MDICP, 2004 (N=13)

course, these tests of character cannot be determined clinically. They can be inferred only from people's behavior and social characteristics.

Empirically, we find little evidence of denominational differences in attitudes about marriage for risk reduction. Figure 6.1 presents ecological associations between the belief that a person can avoid AIDS by getting married and the desired age at marriage for men and women across denominations.[5] Among Christian men, there are no denominational differences in ideal age of marriage, but Muslim men aspire to marry at earlier ages. Muslim women are similar in having a much lower ideal age at marriage than women belonging to various Christian denominations; they are also more likely to see marriage as a protective institution. Overall, however, we find no clear associations between the prevalence of the belief that marriage protects and the ideal, or intention, of marrying early.

To test for differences in *actual* age at marriage across denominations we use Demographic and Health Surveys (DHS) data from Swaziland, Zimbabwe, and Malawi. These are the only high HIV prevalence countries with data available to distinguish between a sufficient number of denominations. Table 6.1 shows that across all three countries, Muslims have lower than average ages at marriage, and so do those who self-identify as "Traditional" (Swaziland and Botswana) and Zionists (identifiable only in Swaziland). In contrast, Mission Protestants, Pentecostals (Swaziland),

Table 6.1 **Age at First Marriage for Women Married in the Last 10 Years**

Religious Affiliation	Swaziland 2006	Zimbabwe 2005–2006	Malawi 2004
Protestant	23.5	20.0	—
Anglican	—	—	18.2
Church of Central Africa, Presbyterian	—	—	18.9
Roman Catholic	24.1	19.7	18.0
Pentecostal	23.9	19.6	—
Seventh Day Adventist/Baptist	—	—	18.2
Apostolic Sect	23.7	18.7	—
Charismatic	24.1	—	—
Zionist	21.3	—	—
Other Christian	—	19.5	17.6
Muslim	20.0	18.1	17.7
Traditional	22.0	17.3	—
Other	24.5	18.0	20.3
None	23.1	18.8	18.3

Source: Demographic and Health Surveys.

and Charismatics (Swaziland) have higher than average ages, as do Catholics in Swaziland and Zimbabwe.

Does this early marriage strategy work? We don't know for certain and must await the results of ongoing studies that have been set up to examine this specific question. But we do know that the majority of our Malawian informants think that, under certain conditions, marriage is protective. They believe that their sexually inexperienced peers who marry young are less likely to become infected than their counterparts who remain single or who marry—in the case of women, in particular—much older partners. To the extent that this is true and that religious leaders encourage early marriage of this type, they may well be reducing the spread of HIV. Of course, this is a difficult message to incorporate into a public health campaign. But that fact doesn't invalidate early marriage as a prevention strategy. Indeed, the very fact that it is not part of an official public health campaign may make it more culturally appealing and effective.

ABC and D: Divorce

Religious leaders may play an even more salient role when it comes to regulating divorce. Divorce rates in Malawi have risen sharply since AIDS became visible, and some evidence suggests that this is true in other AIDS-belt countries as well.[6] In Malawi, the rise in divorce is not exclusively a "secular" phenomenon. That is, it is not merely driven by changes in the ideology of family formation or by growing individualism. Rather, the increasing frequency of divorce also appears to be linked to AIDS, making it look like divorce is being used as a way to avoid HIV infection within marriage (Reniers 2003, 2008).

One indicator of this change comes from evidence that the association between suspected infidelity and divorce in Malawi has been increasing by 5% a year (Reniers 2008). Although there is evidence that adultery has decreased over time, where it still happens, it is followed more often by divorce, and this is true both for men and for women. Together, these facts suggest that individuals are ever more willing and able to sanction their spouses' sexual indiscretions—a violation of the "B" in ABC—with divorce.

Another indicator is the fact that, for both lay Malawians and religious leaders, infidelity is by far the most acceptable reason for an individual to divorce a spouse. We know this because we directly asked rural Malawians a series of questions about the acceptability of a woman leaving her husband under a variety of circumstances. Infidelity consistently came out on top. Like-wise, our interviews with religious leaders show that the majority tolerates divorce under such circumstances. "If she catches him, the Bible allows it," said one, emphasizing the need to catch an adulterous spouse "red-handed." Beyond merely tolerating divorce, some religious leaders virtually mandate divorce in the case of infidelity, saying things like: "She should leave him; he can kill her," or "Yes, she must [leave him] if he is moving around with other women care-lessly. Nowadays it is dangerous." Interviews with Muslim clerics in Senegal reveal very similar messages. "In the Koran, if there is a *maladie*, it is permitted to end the marriage. . . . because that can get transmitted and reach the family." Just as we saw with condoms (Chapter 5), divorce is widely described as the lesser of two evils.[7]

Among religious leaders, less divorce-friendly voices can also be heard em-phasizing the sanctity of marriage over and above the risk to individual parties, even for serodiscordant couples. One Senegalese imam, for example, described his advice to serodiscordant couples: "Don't reject your conjoint. Help. Abstain from sex or use condoms. Ask lots of prayer and pardon so that health comes back. Do all so that the family still remains, especially for the kids. Divorce only makes it harder." But in both our formal data and informal conversations with people in the field, the voices categorically opposing divorce are a distinct minority.

Predictably, there are denominational differences in the ability to use divorce as an anti-HIV strategy. However, the direction of some of these differences did surprise us. The first notable point is the substantial difference we observe between official denominational (doctrinal) positions and the stated position of local religious leaders. This can be seen in column 1 of Table 6.2. We asked 187 religious leaders whether they thought that divorce was acceptable under a variety of circumstances. We then counted those who opposed divorce under all circumstances as truly opposing divorce. Overall, the denominational extremes are what we expected: Catholic leaders were least accepting of divorce, and Muslim leaders most accepting. However, not only did a third of the Catholic leaders think that divorce was acceptable in certain circumstances—a position that is contrary to official Church teaching—but also between 20% (New Mission Protestant) and 30% (Mission Protestant) of other Christian leaders also considered divorce to be completely unacceptable. This, too, strikes us as odd since even if Protestants have historically discouraged divorce, official denominational positions have never outlawed it.

A second important point is the substantial difference between the stated position of local religious leaders (column 1) and the divorce history of individuals who belong to those denominations. The latter—specifically, the percentage of ever-married Malawi Diffusion and Ideational Change Project (MDICP) respondents who had ever divorced—are given in columns 2 and 3 for MDICP women and men, respectively. It is immediately apparent that there is much less interdenominational variation in actual divorce than in religious leaders' views of divorce. Overall, Muslim women and men are most likely to have divorced at

Table 6.2 **Religious Acceptability of Divorce and Actual Divorce in Malawi**

| | | *Percent Ever Divorced* | |
	Religious Leaders Claim Divorce Is Never Acceptable (%)	*Women*	*Men*
Catholic	66.7	28.0	43.2
Mission Protestant	30.0	26.7	33.5
Pentecostal	25.0	22.5	34.2
African Independent Church	23.7	36.0	39.3
Muslim	0.0	44.0	44.9
New Mission Protestant	20.6	30.1	32.1
N	187	1520	1050

Source: MDICP-3, 2004 and MRP, 2005.

some point (44.0 and 44.9%, respectively). But among men in particular, almost the same percentage of Catholics and African Independent Church (AIC) members divorced at some point in their lives. Overall, the Pentecostals have the lowest levels of divorce—far less than the Catholics—even though relatively few of their leaders categorically oppose it.

We estimated these relationships in more robust ways, and the mean differences between denominations remained.[8] In particular, Pentecostals were the least likely and Muslims the most likely to ever have been divorced. But there was absolutely no relationship between a religious leader's opposition of divorce and actual divorce patterns in his (almost always a "his") congregation. In contrast, divorce was negatively associated with religious attendance (i.e., the more frequent the attendance, the less likely the divorce) and positively associated with the extent to which people attend congregations where they discuss AIDS frequently.

So is divorce a successful strategy for avoiding HIV? Again, we think that it may be. But we also suspect that it's most likely to be used as a strategy when other prevention strategies are not working. This may account for the somewhat strange Pentecostal position: even though Pentecostal religious leaders are relatively unlikely to claim that divorce is always unacceptable, Pentecostals themselves experience considerably less divorce. It is as if they *don't need to use* the divorce strategy as much as their counterparts in other denominations.

We also suspect that this is a gendered strategy. Although in theory both men and women can use divorce to end a marriage, in practice women are often disadvantaged. For example, the official position of Sunni Islam (dominant in most of SSA) permits only male-initiated divorce.[9] Women are supposed to use their male kin or Islamic leaders to persuade a husband to grant a divorce. Even in Christian denominations, where legal barriers to women's divorce are not explicit, men are typically better positioned to get a divorce. Religious leaders who are opposed to divorce for any reason (even suspicion of infidelity or HIV infection) discourage or even prohibit it entirely, and their authority may have an especially strong impact on women.

On the other hand, involvement in a religious community that takes a neutral stance on divorce or would support a wife's decision to leave her husband might have the opposite effect. Religious leaders who teach that divorce is biblically justified in cases of infidelity may actually empower women to leave an unfaithful spouse, as might congregations with a history of providing instrumental support to members going through periods of hardship for all sorts of reasons. Having a social safety net in her religious congregation may enable a woman who wants to end a marriage she believes is putting her at risk of HIV to actually do so. Congregation-based support might be especially critical in patrilocal cultures, where returning to one's natal family after the end of a marriage tends to be more difficult.

Transactional Sex

A third local, non-ABC strategy focuses on transactional sex. This topic is disquieting for Westerners since Western cultures have long idealized romantic love as inconsistent with overt economic exchanges or other types of utilitarian ends (in many classics of Western literature the choice between two potential partners, one representing love and the other more sensible economic or utilitarian ends, lies at the core of the plot). At the very least, unromantic utilitarian considerations, especially those having to do with money, sully the purity of true love; at most, they give such relationships a sheen of prostitution.

As in the rest of the world, romantic love is important in Africa (Hunter 2010; Poulin 2009).[10] One wouldn't think so from much of the academic literature on AIDS and sexual relationships in SSA. Aside from long-standing inquiries into the role of prostitution in spreading HIV, a growing body of research has focused on the prevalence of informal types of sex-for-money exchanges among women who do not self-identify as commercial sex workers or prostitutes (Caldwell, Caldwell, and Quiggin 1989; Hunter 2002; Luke 2006; Poulin 2009; Wojcicki 2002). New estimates suggest that sizable proportions of young adults exchange sex for money or gifts; estimates for the year preceding data collection range from 2% of women in Burkina Faso to 25% of Zambian men (Chatterji, Murray, London, and Anglewicz 2005). The evidence for, consequences of, and the meaning of transactional sex are hotly contested topics among AIDS researchers (see Hunter 2010; Swidler and Watkins 2007). We interpret findings about the widespread accompaniment of nonmarital sex by money and gifts as evidence of a light commodification of sex, not dissimilar to what we observe among our students and friends in the United States. But statements that transactional sex is "driving the AIDS epidemic" are plentiful and have inspired debates about the "right" relationship between sex and money—debates we see playing out both among researchers and on the ground.[11]

Scholars have identified two distinct types of transactional sex in Africa. The first, sometimes referred to as "survival sex," has historically received the most attention in the AIDS literature. Rooted in gender paradigms, it deals with sex as a commodity that women—sometimes adolescent men—"sell" as a last resort since they have no other way to provide for themselves. In the United States, survival sex is commonly associated with homeless youth (Greene, Ennett, and Ringwalt 1999). In SSA, it typically refers to younger women who may have a physical home but lack resources for essentials like food and soap, whether for themselves, their children, or other dependents. Survival sex is driven by deep physical privation and need. It is a last resort. It therefore differs from commercial prostitution, which also involves women (and men) who are not living on the brink of starvation or deprivation.

The other type of transactional sex is not about "need" in this narrow material sense. Rather, it describes women (primarily) who want to acquire certain types of material goods. To some extent, these goods are more important symbolically than in terms of cost; they are a material expression of a potential partner's desire and, subsequently, commitment (Hunter 2010). They are part of the courtship ritual. Based on their quasi-ethnographic data, for example, Swidler and Watkins (2007: 3) summarize the initiation of a typical romantic relationship in Malawi this way:

> The courtship, sometimes brief, begins with words of flattery from the man, perhaps along with a soda or a packet of cookies, and the sexual encounter is typically followed by a more substantial gift (a bar of soap, money to buy a piece of clothing). These gifts are not negotiated as a price but are framed by the man and received by the woman as an expression of "love."[12]

Discussions of transactional sex in the AIDS literature tend to ignore the more romantic side of gifting. Instead, they focus on sugar daddies or "3-C boyfriends," that is, male partners who provide cash, cars, and cell phones (Pisani 2009). Here, transactional sex is also referred to as *consumption sex* (Leclerc-Madlala 2003) and is linked to the fact that African societies, notwithstanding the general poverty, are becoming increasingly materialistic (Hunter 2002). In other words, increasing consumer choice and consumer impulses are raising the bar on certain types of social transactions, including sex. Indeed, this may be one of the main reasons for the positive relationship between wealth and HIV prevalence across SSA. Since poor men have little disposable cash to spend on gifts, transactional sex gives the wealthy access to more sexual partners.

Given that *survival sex* stems from deep need, risk of HIV infection through survival sex can be minimized, at least in theory, simply by providing resources and meeting those needs. Religion, in the form of faith-based assistance or aid that we describe in detail in Chapter 9, comes into play here. It provides a safety net that frees people from the need to sell sex to meet basic needs.

The relationship between religion and consumption sex is quite different. This has less to do with material support than with what are commonly referred to as *values*. For example, in responding to a moderator's question about the best ways to avoid STIs and AIDS, members of a focus group in Uganda nodded in agreement with the woman who advised, "Don't look at materialistic things our parents can't afford. Be satisfied with what you have."[13] This is a clear reference to consumption sex. The nodding heads of other people in the group show that it is also a phenomenon with which they are deeply familiar: desiring things leads young women to pursue sexual relationships that bring both material and emotional support but also put them at risk for contracting HIV. This is obvious to many young women in Africa. Indeed, in Chapter 5 we touched on this very phenomenon when describing the instrumental posters directed at younger women: ignore the temptations posed by wealthy suitors; stay in school.

Religious warnings against greed or against becoming a "material girl" demand the same type of abstinence, albeit for different reasons. They encourage people to focus on otherworldly rewards. These messages are common in religious services. During our observations in Malawi, for example, a Presbyterian preacher elaborated on the infamous scripture passage about the love of money being the root of all evil, saying, "Girls give sex in search of money, and boys break others' houses to steal and find money." While visiting a Baptist church, we heard another pastor warn his members of the dangers of excess. The story was about a wealthy man who was greedy not only for money but also for women: "He wanted all women to be his." The man married six beautiful women and built a house where they could all live together, but his greed was insatiable and he still chased after other women. Eventually, the man brought AIDS into the family, and they all lost their lives. A Catholic priest similarly warned his members:

> Men, once they have money, think that they can ask anyone for sex. And men who have these small groceries [stores], they have just a little bit of money, but so many women are so poor that they think these men have lots of money. So they exchange soap for sex. Or money for sex. They are looking for some support.

In the context of the AIDS epidemic, these types of religious messages about materialism and consumption are exceedingly relevant. They aim to dull the desire to want—or want to give—material goods in exchange for sex. By emphasizing the fundamentally sacred nature of sexual relationships, these messages stand in opposition to the increasing commodification of sex. A slow courtship involving some gifting is one thing. Consumption sex with a wealthy man is another thing entirely.

Alcohol Consumption

A fourth local strategy for preventing HIV addresses alcohol consumption. This is a qualitatively different strategy than those we have described to this point. Rather than directly limiting people's exposure to risky sexual partners, the focus on alcohol is one step removed: it builds on the assumption that drinking is a slippery slope that leads to risky sex.

The consumption of alcohol is high in many SSA societies, both of traditional locally distilled spirits or beers and Western-style equivalents. Alcohol consumption is not, as some have thought, limited to community or religious rituals. Rather, in many areas there is a long history of private drinking and drunkenness that predates the colonial era (Willis 2002). As evidence, taxes on regulated types of alcohol—mainly Western-style beer—are a primary source of income for many African governments (Bird and Wallace 2003; Bryceson 2002).

In rural areas, drinking occurs in compounds—usually organized around a local woman who brews the best local beer. In urban areas and the trading centers of small market towns, drinking occurs in bars and drinking dens— South African *shebeens*, Rwandan *cabarets*, Malawian *bottlestores*—where the female beer sellers or bargirls can make additional money selling sex.

In recent years, the scale of drinking in SSA and its public health consequences have been moving into the public eye. Alcohol-related mortality is the primary motivation. Across Africa the local media regularly report stories about groups of people harmed by bad batches of homebrewed spirits—attractive since they are much cheaper than the regulated alternatives sold in stores that use Western formulas. Once in a while these bad batches kill a shocking number of people: 80 people in western Uganda in April 2010 from a single batch of *waragi* ("banana gin") and more than 200 people in Machakos, Kenya, in two *changa'a* incidents in 1998 and 2000. In all cases the homebrew had been laced with industrial alcohol or methanol.

Yet the greater visibility of high alcohol consumption in the public health literature stems from more than just mortality. It also affects other indicators of public good: high rates of fetal alcohol syndrome—according to some, the highest in the world (May et al. 2005; Viljoen et al. 2005)—are found in South African towns. SSA's high death rates from road traffic accidents have also been linked to alcohol, as have the high rates of crime, STIs, even civil unrest and genocide (Hatzfeld 2007).

Not surprisingly, AIDS has begun to play a major role in spotlighting Africa's alcohol-related problems. A series of studies from Rakai, Uganda, has shed important light on the relationship between alcohol use and HIV infection. Researchers followed more than 16,000 men and women for nearly a decade, testing them for HIV at various points in time. Compared with those who reported not ever drinking, individuals reporting that they consume alcohol also reported behaviors that would elevate their risk for contracting HIV: more sexual partners in the past year, more extramarital partners, and inconsistent condom use. Even controlling for these behavioral factors, individuals who consume alcohol before having sex were more likely to be infected with HIV (Zablotska et al. 2006). Similarly, alcohol consumption before sex was often associated with sexual coercion and intimate partner violence, both of which are established risk factors for HIV. Again, even controlling for these two factors, the consumption of alcohol was associated with more new infections. Likewise, researchers in Zimbabwe reported not only that visits to bars are one of the few predictors of infections (a rate twice as high as for those who do not visit bars) but also that attitudes toward drinking matter. In particular, women who said they did *not* believe that beer drinking is an essential form of relaxation for men were significantly less likely to be infected with HIV during the period they were followed (Lopman et al. 2008).[14]

These established relationships in the scientific literature are also reflected in popular opinion. The association between alcohol and perceived risk of AIDS stems, in part, from the associations between beer and bargirls, between drunkenness and other undesirable behaviors (e.g., partner violence). Importantly, however, this association as recounted on the ground long predates the more recent public health campaigns against alcohol. For example, the Malawian journals (that local informants began writing for the MDICP in 2000) feature dozens of stories where drinking and womanizing or drinking and nonuse of condoms, the immediate proof of which could be seen in an ensuing pregnancy, go hand in hand. Alcohol, in the words of one South African poster we found, "invites risky sex."

Over the last few years, the increasing visibility of drinking as a problem has given rise to two very different types of official policy responses in Africa. The first can be seen in calls to legalize different types of homebrew to regulate it. This is an attractive option for many governments given the importance of alcohol-generated tax revenues. A different type of policy is aimed at encouraging more responsible drinking or discouraging drinking altogether. Both strategies aim to reduce the risky behaviors commonly associated with drinking. At the softer end of this campaign is the call to drink in a more responsible, measured way. For example, a South African poster featuring Pollen Ndlanya, a South African football (soccer) star, appeared around the 2009 FIFA Federations Cup. It begins with the slogan "Champions drink responsibly" and then goes into the risks that can stem from irresponsible drinking (car accidents, unplanned pregnancy, HIV infection).[15]

The more radical approach in the same vein is to discourage drinking altogether. This is being tried in Botswana. In November 2008, the new prime minister, Ian Khama, introduced a 30% levy on alcohol (and also reduced operating hours of bars and bottle stores) with the aim of reducing alcohol consumption "to reduce crime, road accidents and the spread of HIV, the virus that causes AIDS" (Balise 2008). Thus far, Botswana is the only country in SSA to have pursued an explicit antidrinking policy, and its impact remains unknown.

Like the on-the-ground connections between drunkenness and AIDS, religious responses to the alcohol–AIDS relationship also predate drinking's appearance on the radar of public health officials and, consequently, their official policies. Religious groups exhibit marked differences on this topic, both in their attitudes about drinking and the expression of their positions. The Muslim prohibition against alcohol, in particular, is well-known. And even if many Muslims in Africa still drink some alcohol (Akyeampong 1996a), the general prohibition lowers alcohol consumption in Muslim areas.[16] Indeed, Gray (2004) suggests that this may partially explain the generally lower HIV prevalence in countries with large Muslim populations; it represents one less risk factor to which these populations are exposed.

Not only Muslims are anti-alcohol, however. Some Christian groups sound equally abstemious. In fact, the antidrinking strains found within certain denominations of African Protestantism arrived with the early missionaries. In the 1915 edition of the *Missionary Review of the World*, for example, a missionary in the Basuto area of southern Africa describes visiting a prison in which 18 of the 21 prisoners had committed crimes (6 for assault, 12 for livestock theft) under the influence of alcohol. "Alcohol is the black's worst enemy," he declared (Pierson 1922: 151).[17] Another missionary, this one from Nyasaland (present-day Malawi), described beer "as the greatest enemy of the economic and moral welfare of the Nyasa natives" (Pierson: 151).

Some of these abstemious attitudes are reflected in views given by our informants. Aside from stories about beer-drinking womanizers, one of the journals also contains a more feel-good story about a man who falls in love with a woman and asks her to marry him. She agrees, but only on the condition that he gives up alcohol. He does so, and some years later he tells his old friends that he is happy that he did so, not only because of his marriage but also because giving up drinking has left him with more money in his pocket.

More generally, in both our interviews with religious leaders and in the ethnographic journals, alcohol is referred to in uniformly negative ways. At the milder end are Catholics, who simply warn about excess: alcohol is not inherently wrong, but "overdrinking" is. As we move toward smaller Protestant churches, the language becomes more critical. A pastor in the Africa Continent church urges members to pray for "those who drink beer." A Baptist leader draws a ring around "drinking beer, adultery, pride." All are difficult to stop because "you're gripped by the devil and you have no power over your actions." An Assemblies of God pastor warns a drunkard that the "devil will get him sooner." And a pastor in the Zambezi Evangelical church takes some pride in the fact that his uncompromising anti-alcohol stance costs him members: "Our church detests beer drinking. We are losing many members because I stand by the Word of God." These accounts are consistent with the alcohol stance of Pentecostals in Malawi described by Dijk (2002). In all of these accounts, the consumption of alcohol is treated as an indicator of a certain type of person. Someone who drinks is seen to be at higher risk of a number of things. HIV is one of them.

Does this attitude to alcohol affect actual behavior across religious groups? The evidence is mixed. On one hand, there are indications that visiting bars varies substantially by denomination. This can be seen in Table 6.3. It shows the percentage of men in the MDICP sample who report having visited a bar in the

Table 6.3 **Percent of Rural Malawian Men That Have Been to a Bar in the Last Month**

	%
No Religion	34.6
Catholic	36.8
Mission Protestant	21.6
Pentecostal	30.6
African Independent Church	35.1
Muslim	7.8
New Mission Protestant	17.5
N	1467

Source: MDICP-3, 2004.

last month. The mean of 24% hides considerable variation across three main clusters. A high cluster, ranging from 31 to 37%, includes Catholics, AICs, Pentecostals, and those with no religion.[18] A middle cluster, around 20%, includes Mission and New Mission Protestants, the latter being lower. And the low cluster, with 8%, consists only of Muslims. This, alone, offers suggestive evidence that Muslims and then Mission or New Mission Protestants are less likely to become infected through the alcohol route than members of other groups.

On the other hand, for all the anti-alcohol positions staked by certain denominations, we see only a few signs of active policing of drinking by religious leaders. In only one church—a small African Independent denomination—did the religious leader talk about what he does when he hears that a church member got drunk. "We go to his home and ask his problem. We tell him that as you know we don't allow beer drinking so why are you doing this?" If the person insists on drinking, he is "removed" from the church.

Some religious leaders use more veiled threats, however. For example, when asked why his mosque does not have problems like adultery or drunkenness, one sheikh suggested that it is fear of punishment. In particular, people are scared that they won't be able to receive his support, including his willingness to officiate a religious ritual (e.g., a funeral) at the person's compound. In general, though, threats and overt policing of this type are less common than the simple effort to persuade members to give up drinking that we observed in dozens of churches and mosques throughout Malawi. Moreover, information about a person's drinking habits is an important component of the local knowledge used to assess the quality of that person. Along the lines already suggested, this can be for purposes of marriage (in relation to choosing a well-behaved spouse) or the legitimate right to divorce (a beer-drinking husband is easier to get rid of).

Conclusion

Religion is relevant for HIV prevention in ways that extend beyond A, B, and C. This chapter has presented evidence that religion shapes attitudes to sex and sexual behavior, marriage, divorce, consumption and interpersonal gifting, and the use of alcohol. All of these affect HIV transmission. Policymakers have almost completely overlooked these local prevention strategies. This is not surprising, since these local strategies are difficult, if not impossible, to promote programmatically (imagine the "Leave Your Sleazy Spouse Now" public health campaign). Yet despite the fact that they can't be institutionalized, the non-ABC strategies described here are critically important for prevention. They represent how people living in the midst of AIDS actually navigate it (Watkins 2004). Most do not commit to a celibate life or to consistent condom use. Instead, people modify their sexual behavior to reduce—though not completely eliminate—their risk. These modifications involve sets of decisions that rest on perceptions of who will be a safe partner, a continuous reevaluation of that assessment, and decisions about behaviors that could lead down a high-risk road. Many of these decisions are informed by religion. Religious leaders have the capacity to either legitimize different types of prevention strategies or delegitimize them; this is true both of ABC and local, non-ABC mechanisms used to curb the spread of AIDS. As one of the key institutions responsible for generating these attitudes, religion regulates local prevention strategies. From the leaders of local churches and mosques down to the laity's social networks, messages and activities associated with religion fill an important discursive space.

Institutionalized Religious Strategies

On the vast and frightful theatre of our sufferings we had not to seek the prelate. He was always wherever the greatest peril was to be found. His zeal knew no other measure than the wants and miseries of his flock. His firmness was never once shaken by the various forms by which death surrounded him.

—Anonymous[1], *1720*

When someone has died, men have to dig graves. I go and find them digging because this is a chance to preach to the men there. And it becomes a blessing—it allows people to hear the Word of God.

—Pastor of Chopi Christian Church, *Malawi, 2004*

Chapters 4, 5, and 6 show that religion affects HIV prevention in multiple ways. Religious affiliation and practice are associated with levels of AIDS-related knowledge, the ABCs of prevention, and the management of other local prevention strategies related to partner selection, divorce, transactional sex, and alcohol consumption. Though most of the evidence is focused on individuals—laypeople—there are at least hints that local religious leaders and organizations also play an important, though frequently underspecified, role in prevention. The central questions we address in this chapter are as follows:

How much variation is there in the religious leaders' and institutions' engagement with AIDS or the intensity with which they preach about AIDS?

To what extent are these levels of engagement consistent with central doctrines of their tradition?

What types of strategies are associated with the lowest—and highest—HIV prevalence?

What role, if any, does traditional medicine play among members of different denominations?

Different Organizations, Different Strategies

The data we collected from religious leaders in Malawi are unique in that they allow us to make comparisons across 187 different congregations, representing several distinct religious traditions. Just as we did with individuals, we categorized all of the congregations in our sample into six broader denominational blocs using the typology detailed in Chapter 2, summarized here in Table 7.1. As noted in Appendix G, these 187 communities range in size, level of organization, wealth, transnational connections, training of religious leaders, and so on. They also approach AIDS in varied ways.

We identify four distinct types of engagement with AIDS; each of these is associated with a different approach to preventing infection. Specifically, engagement with AIDS can have:

1. A *moral dimension* where religious leaders preach about sexual morality and AIDS on a regular basis (almost every week). This also covers prevention strategies like early marriage and consumption-driven transactional sex.
2. A *biomedical dimension* where religious leaders promote HIV testing and condoms for prevention, largely in step with secular public-health recommendations.
3. A *faith healing dimension* where religious leaders or congregations offer miraculous healing (or the hope of it) for illness. In rare cases, this includes healing for AIDS explicitly, but most of the time it refers to healing in a more general way, such as the laying on of hands to address unspecified maladies.
4. A *pragmatic dimension* where religious leaders advise members to divorce a spouse who is putting them at risk for infection.

Table 7.1 **Overview of Rural Malawian Religious Congregations by Denomination**

	N	%
Catholic	21	11
Mission Protestant	40	21
Pentecostal	32	17
African Independent Church	38	20
Muslim	22	11
New Mission Protestant	34	18

Source: MRP, 2005.

The relative prevalence of each of these prevention strategies across the 187 Malawian congregations can be seen in Table 7.2. Moral messages about HIV are ubiquitous (72%). Faith healing is also relatively common (41%). Pragmatic solutions such as divorce (32%) are somewhat less so, but all in all, the smallest proportion of leaders (23%) embrace and promote biomedical prevention strategies.

There is an equally important message in Table 7.2, however. As implied by the fact that the percentage column sums to 164%, religious leaders and congregations are not restricted to one prevention strategy alone. To address the problem of AIDS in their congregations and communities, religious leaders often combine different strategies. We follow suit. Rather than thinking about each strategy in isolation, we consider the relative prevalence and effectiveness of these different *combinations*. For example, moral teaching about sexual behavior combined with practical (biomedical) advice on condoms and testing might be very different from moral teachings alone. The same can be said about a "faith-only" approach that combines moral teachings on AIDS with miracles and healings.

We analyzed these combinations using an established technique called qualitative comparative analysis (QCA; Longest and Vaisey 2008; Ragin 2000). The approach is simple: we labeled each congregation according to the presence or absence of each of the four prevention strategies. For example, where there was a moral dimension to the congregation's prevention strategy, the congregation was coded as M. Where the moral dimension was absent, it was coded m. We did the same for the other three dimensions of engagement with AIDS prevention: F represents the presence of a faith-healing dimension, and f its absence; D the presence of the pragmatic prevention strategy discussed in Chapter 6 (divorce), and d its absence; and B and b the presence or absence, respectively, of biomedical prevention strategies. A congregation that is characterized by all of these

Table 7.2 **Prevalence of HIV Prevention Strategies in Malawian Congregations**

	N	%
Moral	135	72
Biomedical	43	22
Faith Healing	73	40
Divorce	60	32

Note: N = 187.
Source: MRP, 2005

factors—a rare combination—would be labeled MFDB, and a congregation whose leader offers healing but does not talk about AIDS from a moral perspective or promote biomedical or local prevention strategies would be mFdb.

Table 7.3 shows the prevalence of the 16 possible combinations of these four strategies. We refer to each one as an *approach*. Several patterns are worth noting. First, in a large majority (77%) of congregations, religious leaders report addressing AIDS in some way; that is, there is at least one approach. Second, even with this high number, very few congregations are associated with all four strategies; only 3% of the total are coded MFDB. Rather than trying everything, congregations approach prevention selectively. The most common approach (characterizing 21% of congregations) is Mfdb. These leaders address AIDS in moral terms by preaching and teaching about it regularly, but they do nothing else. The second most prevalent approach is a combination of moral teachings

Table 7.3 **A QCA Categorization of Approaches to HIV Prevention in Malawian Congregations**

Approach	N	%
Mfdb	40	21
MFdb	32	17
mfdb	23	12
MfDb	17	9
mFdb	14	7
MfDB	14	7
MFDb	12	6
MFdB	8	4
MfdB	7	4
MFDB	5	3
mFDB	3	2
mFDb	3	2
mfDB	3	2
mfDb	3	2
mfdB	3	2

Note: N = 187.
Source: MRP, 2005.

and faith healing (MFdb). A total of 7% of congregations take a "healing-only" approach—these are the mFdb congregations, while an equal number of congregations do everything but faith healing (MfDB). Only 1 of the 16 theoretically possible approaches does not actually occur in our data: mFdB (faith healing with biomedical).

As we would expect, the specific combination of strategies varies substantially across religious traditions. This can be seen in Figure 7.1.[2] First, Mfdb, the most popular strategy overall, is the modal approach in only one group, but there it absolutely dominates. Almost 60% of New Mission Protestant congregations are characterized this way. Although this approach is also relatively common in Catholic and African Independent Church (AIC) congregations, it does not exceed 15% of congregations in these or any other group. Moreover, in some—specifically, in the Muslim and Pentecostal traditions—it accounts for less than 5% of congregations.

The second most popular combination of strategies is MFdb (i.e., faith healing combined with moral messages). This is the modal combination in Mission Protestant congregations.[3] At first glance, the frequency of a faith-healing strategy here is surprising; these are typically associated with Pentecostals and not with Anglicans or Presbyterians. But remember that we are talking about the MFdb and MFDb combinations here. Faith healing alone (mFdb) is most popular among Pentecostals, and it hardly exists in the other traditions.

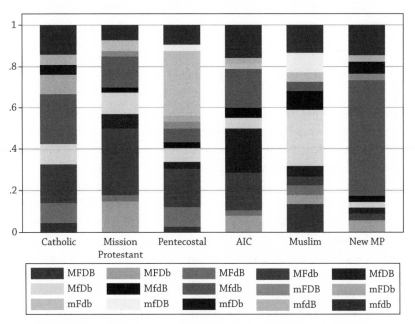

Figure 7.1 AIDS strategy of congregations in Malawi by denomination
Source: MRP, 2005

Going back to the MFdb combination, this is also relatively common in Catholic, Pentecostal, and AIC congregations, and it is very uncommon in Muslim and New Mission Protestant congregations.

Finally, the complete toolkit or the "we-try-everything" approach (MFDB) is largely a Muslim strategy, though the combination of moral and pragmatic (i.e., divorce) strategies is the most common approach for Muslims. In general, Muslim leaders exhibit greater flexibility on teachings on family life than, for example, New Mission Protestant congregations. Together with the evidence about divorce presented in the last chapter, we consider this as evidence that divorce is a *legitimate* prevention strategy that is becoming increasingly common, particularly within Malawian Islam.

Although there are differences across these six religious traditions, we observe considerable variation within them, too. Given that our construction of broad categories allows for considerable heterogeneity within traditions, we expected much of this diversity. The Mission Protestant, AIC, and Pentecostal categories, for example, include a highly variable array of denominations within them. But we also find considerable variation within the categories that are, formally at least, more unitary. Catholic congregations, for example, exhibit an array of strategies, with almost 15% of Catholic churches supporting a pragmatic separation or divorce policy, either by itself or in combination with healing. Likewise, there is no single dominant strategy associated with Muslim leaders. In fact, the only bloc in which a majority of the congregations are associated with a single strategy is the New Mission Protestants, where almost 60% report an Mfdb strategy.

Effects on HIV Prevalence

It is one thing to describe these strategies and to show how they vary across congregations. It is more complicated to determine whether these strategies work. The ideal scientific approach would be to field an experiment in which we randomly assign individuals to congregations where different strategies are present. We would then follow these individuals over time to measure and compare the effects of their congregational context on their behavior and HIV status. For obvious reasons, conducting an experiment of this type is impossible. We therefore do the next best thing, which is to use biomarker data from the Malawi Diffusion and Ideational Change Project (MDICP) to answer the following question: across 164 congregations in our sample, how do the 16 possible combinations of prevention strategies described in Table 7.3 covary with HIV?[4]

Results of this analysis, shown in Table 7.4, are consistent with others that we have already discussed previously. First, congregational HIV prevalence does vary by religious tradition. It ranges from 5% (New Mission Protestant, Catholic, Muslims) to 9% (Pentecostal) and is highest in small congregations, from which we have relatively few observations of HIV status. Second, and more important, HIV prevalence is more variable when examined by congregational strategy than by denomination. In particular, prevalence is highest—in excess of 9%—in congregations where faith healing is present (i.e., mFdb, MFdb, MFDb). This suggests one of two possibilities. Either people who know or suspect that they are HIV positive are joining these congregations with the hope that they will be healed, or HIV prevalence is higher because the emphasis on faith healing is a less effective strategy.[5]

The configuration of prevention activities in low-prevalence categories is also telling. First, the congregations that do nothing about AIDS—mfdb congregations—have low prevalence (4%). We suspect a reversal of the causal mechanism here. That is, it is unlikely that they are silent on AIDS because of denial. Rather, they might be doing nothing because AIDS is really not a significant problem in their community—at least relative to other problems they face (see Chapter 3). For

Table 7.4 **Congregational HIV Prevalence by Prevention Approach**

Approach	N	% HIV+
Mfdb	38	0.06
MFdb	27	0.09
mfdb	21	0.04
MfDb	15	0.07
mFdb	11	0.18
MfDB	13	0.02
MFDb	12	0.09
MFdB	8	0.07
MfdB	5	0.04
MFDB	3	0.03
mFDB	3	0.09
mFDb	3	0.08
mfDB	3	0.08
mfDb	3	0.08
mfdB	3	0.23

Note: N = 168.
Source: MDICP-3, 2004 and MRP, 2005.

example, the leader of a Jehovah's Witness characterized as mfdb knew a lot about AIDS and talked extensively about how the epidemic has changed his community. His congregation, however, seemed insulated: "From the time I joined in 1995 I had never seen somebody who died because of AIDS. No! And the way this religion is, it happens that five or seven years pass without hearing that a child or somebody has died." This is in stark contrast to the impression of a leader of a large high-prevalence congregation in the same district. He talked about how fatigued he was from officiating at multiple funerals each month. Likewise, while elaborating on his view that end times are near, the lay leader of another large church—a Catholic outpost parish where we estimated HIV prevalence to be 16%—described the burden of funeral responsibilities this way:

> . . . When I was in standard 2 [second grade] I never knew what a funeral was all about. Funerals were rare back then. When there was a funeral it was like a special occasion. But now they [funerals] are like a song. When you are on your way to the grave you hear that there's another funeral, and another one.

It is, of course, important to be cautious about interpreting ecological associations like the ones we are describing here. Yet the high levels of congruence between multiple types of data (qualitative vs. survey data) collected at different levels (i.e., biomarker data from individuals vs. religious leaders' perception of the mortality burden) give us confidence that these congregation-level associations are tapping into very real patterns on the ground.

The other two low-prevalence approaches share two strategies: M and B. The combination of moral underpinnings with biomedical advice (openness to condoms, promoting HIV testing) corresponds with lower-than-average prevalence— as low as 2% among the 13 congregations that also promote divorce as a strategy for avoiding HIV. One particularly illustrative congregation from this category (MfDB) centers on our 2005 interview with the leader of an AIC congregation in Central Malawi.[6] After introductions and pleasantries, the interviewer asked about the topic of the respondent's last sermon. The respondent answered that the sermon was not only about sexual morality but also about his profound sense of responsibility for this issue: "We church people have all rights to preach about the reducing of immoral sexuality." He went on to describe how in the past year he has presided over the funerals of five adult members, two of whom he suspected had died of AIDS. He also described how, that very week, "we will go to the hospital all of us for blood testing."[7] In fact, this was the source of his optimism about the future of his congregation amidst the AIDS problem: he promoted AIDS prevention using a variety of strategies, preaching about sexual morality, distributing condoms, and leading a campaign for testing. He was also pleased with the results of his efforts. One was fewer funerals, and the other was the positive response he gets from members regarding his leadership on the AIDS issue.

> When I have brought [the information], my members show happiness. And that tells me that my counseling information is working. If they were showing me that they were not happy, I would have known that they did not understand. What I do is this: after talking about AIDS, I ask the choir to sing one chorus which also talks about AIDS. We also do dramas that concern such issues! My members show that they have started believing what I am saying.

Almost all congregations are engaged in some sort of prevention strategy, although only some of them would be recognized as such by public health authorities. Two observations stand out as particularly worthy of additional exploration. First, prevalence among members of congregations that take the two-pronged moral + biomedical approach is significantly lower than the national (and subregional) averages in our three Malawian field sites. This suggests that these congregations are relatively "protected" from the epidemic. Second, the fact that congregations that use a faith-healing strategy exhibit higher levels of HIV prevalence begs further questions about the role and nature of faith healing vis-à-vis AIDS in sub-Saharan Africa (SSA). It is to these two combinations of strategies that we now turn our attention.

The Moral + Biomedical Approach: Protective or Selective?

The two-pronged moral + biomedical prevention strategy is present in 18% ($N = 34$) of the congregations in our Malawi sample.[8] To better understand the commonalities between congregations that embrace these strategies, we examined these 34 congregations in more depth using the qualitative data we collected from their religious leaders and laywomen members. In particular we wanted to identify which of two possible causes of the association between M + B congregations and low HIV prevalence is the most likely one. Is prevalence low in M + B congregations because the people who belong to them are less likely to have *become* infected? Or is it because these congregations don't allow people they know or suspect are HIV positive to join, and they kick out existing members who have been diagnosed with or are suspected to have HIV? In other words, is M + B truly a protective thing, or is a selection process driving these results?

In an effort to identify the selection process, we coded all of our sermon reports and in-depth interview transcripts for *scandals, church discipline*, and *excommunication*. We came across dozens of stories, ranging from light gossip about work, school, and relationships (all roughly equivalent to the kind of gossip we would hear hanging around any American congregation) to stranger-than-fiction human drama. Overall, however, we found almost no evidence of excommunication in any of the 187 congregations. Two stories, broadly representative of disciplinary procedures commonly enacted in Malawian churches and mosques, illustrate this point.

The first example concerns Matthews, a young reverend whose AIC congregation was visited (unannounced) by one of our research assistants one Sunday in 2004. The service was being led by a church elder because Matthews, a married man, was, for lack of a better metaphor, standing trial for having impregnated a choir girl. Most services that we or one of our research assistants visited had a joyful tone: there was praise music and general effervescence. This one did not. Our research assistant characterized it as "somber." Matthews sat quietly in the front. The message went like this:

> When we sin we must repent and this shows that you have returned to your God. As I said, our behaviour is monitored not only by others but also by the people around us. [Matthews] is asked to repent because he has sinned. Our church should not condone these actions. What he has done is adultery. He is going to have a baby outside wedlock. He has been asked to repent at the reverend at Chagunda [his denominational superior]. He can only return to the pulpit after his repentance. The major sin that will prevent us from meeting our Lord is adultery. You should all avoid it. Nowadays, you will get AIDS as a certificate to your actions. We are old and we have kept the church intact. Your childish acts will break the church. Matthews should behave like an adult and a reverend. This matter is discussed because he is the reverend of the church. Since Jesus loved us we also show our love to the reverend to repent to God. When you go home avoid this evil practice not only because you can get AIDS from it but also because it is a commandment from God. Hallelujah! Amen. Go in peace and God be with you all.

Given the series of sex scandals that have rocked Western churches over the last decade, in particular the Catholic Church, it does not shock or even surprise us that we came across the case of a pastor who had impregnated a choir girl. What stands out in this story—which was also recounted to us by laywomen in the congregation and by a second observer—is that the Reverend Matthews wasn't fired. Rather, this congregation chose to emphasize not only moral and behavioral discipline but also forgiveness, even for a pretty serious offense committed by a pastor.

The same discipline-and-forgiveness approach was observed at several other congregations in which adultery was discovered. All these others involved lay-people and followed a very similar formula: the member received a suspension—sometimes for a set amount of time and sometimes until the member was "ready" to repent. Upon having completed the suspension, confessed, and earnestly repented (this often had to be done outside the congregation itself, which required additional effort in terms of travel and expense), the member was welcomed back. Of course, not all members complete the steps required to return as a full-fledged member. But according to our interview data, most do.

The second example, also related to adultery, was recounted to us by the pastor of a Church of Christ congregation and by one of our lay respondents. In her words:

> There is a certain friend of ours whose husband married a second wife. So after marrying another woman, he was suspended because accord-ing to the rules of our church, they do not allow polygamy. So her hus-band is already on suspension with his second wife. But this friend of ours [the first wife], who was still in the church, burned the house of the second wife at night. Meaning she wanted to burn the second wife and husband! She wanted to kill the second wife and her husband. But with God's power they came out alive . . . They suspended this woman, saying that what she did was against the church rules. She came to repent. Right now she has started coming to church. But up to now the man is still on suspension.

Admittedly, this story is extreme. But it tells us something about religious con-gregations as places in which forgiveness is there for the taking—forgiveness not only for illicit polygamy and adultery but also for even graver offenses like arson and attempted murder.

These two stories suggest that the relatively low levels of HIV prevalence found in M + B congregations are not the result—at least not primarily—of selection and "serosorting." That leaves one alternative explanation: this partic-ular combination of AIDS-related messaging actually influences the behavior of members (and those around them) in such a way that they minimize their risk of infection. There is indirect evidence that this is the case. In particular, although 12% of religious leaders pursuing some other combination of strategies had ever attended a formal workshop focused on AIDS-related education or issues, propor-tionally twice as many (25%) M + B leaders had. This suggests that coordinated efforts to engage religious leaders may, indeed, have facilitated the pragmatic openness to biomedical solutions (e.g., condoms when necessary, testing if pos-sible) that characterizes this group. That said, it is clear from Table 7.3 that the protective value of the M + B combination does not stem from B alone. In only three of the congregations (out of 187) do leaders promote B in isolation (mfdB), and in these three, HIV prevalence is highly variable (5%, 15%, and 50%). The most effective prevention approaches filter AIDS-related messages through a moral lens. Measured objectively, the moralizing approach to prevention is, indeed, relevant to epidemiological patterns.

Traditional Medicine and Faith Healing

Inasmuch as they point to the protective potential of the moral + biomedical prevention approach, the QCA analyses suggest that faith-healing congregations do the exact opposite. They feature higher levels of HIV prevalence. Before describing some of these faith healing patterns in greater detail, we sketch the overall healing milieu in which people solve—or attempt to solve—their health problems.

We begin with themes alluded to earlier (see Chapter 3). In particular, narrow biomedical discourses about AIDS are often seen to be incomplete in Africa. The tendency to distinguish proximate and "real" causes of infection (respectively, the how and why of HIV transmission), combined with the limited biomedical infrastructure, has massive implications for how illness is experienced in Africa. This includes AIDS. Many people living with HIV and AIDS (PLWHA) in SSA, for example, understand that antiretroviral therapies (ART) can help them hold AIDS at bay. Yet as shown in Figure 7.2, even now, after several years of "scaling up" the distribution of ART in sub-Saharan Africa, only two high-prevalence countries— Botswana and Namibia—have universal or virtually universal distribution to people with advanced HIV. Most countries fall far short of this high standard, providing ART to between 20 and 50% of people who need it.[9]

This is part of a more general problem plaguing the provision of health care in SSA. Clinics and hospitals typically suffer from a severe shortage of trained medical personnel; tragically, many Anglophone African countries train large numbers of nurses at public expense but lose them to medical systems abroad or to higher-paying sectors locally (Ahmad 2005; Mullan 2005). These problems are especially severe in rural areas, where two-thirds of the SSA population still lives and to which the urban sick often retreat in search of support and care from members of their extended family. In Malawi, for example, when we began this research project, 65% of all nursing positions in Malawi were unfilled, with rural areas (where 85% of Malawi's population reside) being particularly hard hit: only 5% of working nurses practiced in rural areas (GoM 2005). Indeed, throughout SSA, clinics and hospitals tend to have long waiting lines, and patients who do receive a diagnosis have only a small likelihood of accessing the drugs they need. Even where clinics stock ART, distributing them is no trivial matter: it requires the establishment and maintenance of intensive registration and bureaucratic

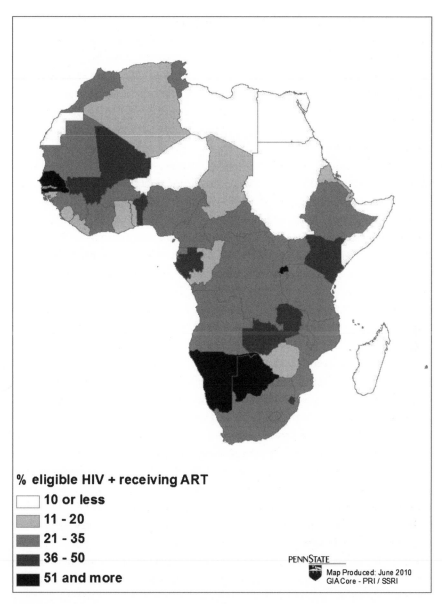

Figure 7.2 Percentage of persons with advanced HIV receiving antiretroviral therapy, using WHO/UNAIDS methodology

systems within clinics. It also demands that HIV-positive patients return to the clinic every couple of months to receive their refills.

Under these conditions, it is no surprise that many people turn to alternative sources of healing—traditional healers, religious leaders, and God in prayer— even if they are simultaneously receiving some measure of biomedical care. This combination of systems of healing is exceedingly common throughout SSA

(Manglos and Trinitapoli 2011; Meyer-Weitz, Reddy, Weijts, van den Borne, and Kok 1998) and has been so since long before the emergence of AIDS (Comaroff 1980; Feierman 1985; Morris 1986).[10] AIDS has simply cast a brighter light on these long-standing patterns while simultaneously highlighting the structural inadequacies of African health-care systems. As journalist Rachel Swarns (2002) writes, "Where clinics run short of even the most basic medicines, it is easier to believe in a miracle worker than in the possibility that the government might provide AIDS drugs."

Even if the medical systems were better, however, we suspect that many Africans would continue to use religious and traditional approaches to healing. The latter have other advantages. We have already mentioned one of these: they better match culturally embedded distinctions between proximate and ultimate causes of illness. Another is that their demands on patients are much more flexible than those associated with the unending and tightly time-specific ART regimen. Yet another advantage of these alternative sources of healing is that they are more financially accessible than Western-style clinics. Accessing God through prayer is completely free. Healing provided by religious leaders is officially unaccompanied by any fee, though tithes—which members are expected to give—can be thought of as a type of insurance premium. Traditional healers are, in this respect, a little different. Almost all charge for their services, and some charge a lot. So those who choose the traditional healing option can incur considerable expense, sometimes exceeding the cost of visits to a local clinic (Liddell, Barrett, and Bwdawell 2005). On the other hand, traditional healers remain more accessible because they tend to accept payments in cash or kind, which allows families to work out arrangements that approximate what Westerners would identify as a payment plan—making payments in produce or livestock—something that clinics are ill-equipped to do. This is particularly true of the most traditional healers (outside whose compounds one usually finds long lines of people).

While the names and various methods may vary from country to country (e.g., soothsayers in Ghana, herbalists and diviners in Botswana, or doctors of spirits in Malawi) the template is similar: old traditions, "potions," herbal remedies, and bone fragments are tools for restoring good health.[11] Blood frequently remains a powerful symbol surrounding health and illness, and bloodletting is not an uncommon recommendation by traditional healers, sometimes at the behest of parents or grandparents intent on safeguarding their children (Ingstad 1990).[12]

The relationship between traditional healers and different religious groups, and the particular methods that traditional healers employ, has relevance for AIDS. From our Malawi Religion Project data, we learned that most Christian and Muslim leaders tolerate potions but not amulets, ritual cutting but not "traditional" practices (like widow cleansing) that involve sex, and herbalists but not divination or witchcraft. For this reason, most religious leaders forbid the use of blood, bones, and especially human remains; all of these materials are associated with witchcraft.[13] Overall, this tension between, on one hand, the consensus views about different types of traditional healing among religious leaders of different stripes and, on the other, the continued use of such methods among laypeople illustrates that indigenous representations of illness are resilient. They have not yet been completely overhauled by new ways of understanding illness associated with Christianity, newer streams of orthodox Islam, or Western biomedicine. Instead, here as in other areas, syncretism reigns. New ways of understanding illness or, as in the case of AIDS, new illnesses have been *incorporated* into preexisting ontologies (Liddell et al. 2005).

This is not to say that levels of syncretism—here, the acceptability of traditional medicine and other cultural practices—do not vary across religious groups. They do. This can be seen in Table 7.5, which displays the percent of religious leaders in Malawi who advise their members to go see a traditional healer, sorted by religious group. Roman Catholic leaders, most of whom are not ordained priests—an increasingly rare commodity everywhere, not just in Malawi—are most likely to advise their flock to see a traditional healer, at 60%. Muslims and New Mission Protestant leaders come in a close second; in fact, there is no statistically significant difference between them and the Catholics. In contrast, Pentecostal leaders are least likely to suggest such a visit (just over one in five have done so), followed by Mission Protestants at 30%. What is perhaps the most surprising is the fact that AIC leaders, who in much of the literature on religion in Africa are closely associated with valuing traditional African ways, are among the least likely to suggest visiting a traditional healer. At 38%, they are closer to the Pentecostal anti-traditional healer position than to the more syncretic Catholic one.

Table 7.5 **Malawian Religious Leaders, by Tradition, Who Advise Members to See a Healer**

Religious Tradition	%
Catholic	60.0
Mission Protestant	30.0
Pentecostal	21.9
African Independent Church	37.8
Muslim	54.6
New Mission Protestant	52.9

Note: N = 185.
Source: MRP, 2005.

Overall, our analyses of MDICP data on questions about healing, divination, and witchcraft are consistent with much of the existing qualitative and ethnographic work on this topic (e.g., Ashforth 2005; Middleton and Winter [1963] 2004; Morris 1986). A sizable minority engages in these practices: in 2004, 17% reported having consulted a diviner in the past year and 29% having visited an herbalist during past year. But importantly, this widespread engagement with other forms of healing does not imply a rejection of germ theory or of biomedical prevention strategies. When asked if they knew how to protect themselves against AIDS, only a fraction of 1% said either that "God can protect," that "traditional medicine can protect," or that "charms" could protect against HIV. A slightly larger number (2%) mentioned "prayer" as a prevention strategy, though it is unclear whether prayer protects in a direct way (miraculously preventing infection upon exposure) or indirectly (protection from making decisions that could lead to infection). At any rate, these numbers are miniscule compared with mentions of the prevention strategies on the public health radar: avoid many partners (7%), avoid blood transfusions (13%), use condoms (24%), be faithful (25%), advise your partner (26%); and "abstain" (65%).[14] Finally, the MDICP data provide some evidence that engagement in these strategies is relevant to AIDS. Generally speaking, people who consult diviners and wear amulets tend to be more worried about AIDS than people who don't do these things, and those who attend congregations where faith healing plays a major role report being less worried about the disease (Manglos and Trinitapoli 2011).

To situate this discussion of faith healing more generally, we begin with a single clarifying fact. Faith healing attracts poor villagers and urban professionals alike. Stephen Gyimah (2007: 925), for example, notes that in urban Ghana many Pentecostals first report illnesses to "'healing camps' and are often kept there until the situation gravely deteriorates, when they are then rushed to the hospital." In contrast, in locales where little more than faith, prayer, and "holy water" are available, believing in their power is hardly an irrational act. After all, biblical texts admonish the people of God to anoint the sick with oil, to fast, and to pray. This theme emerges in Rachel Swarns's (2002) account. Writing about South Africa, a nation much closer to the cutting edge of biomedical technology and ability than, say, Malawi or Tanzania, she contrasts people's limited tolerance for Western medicine with the extraordinary confidence that they place in faith healers. "God is greater than pills. God is greater than the condom," insists one believer whose husband is infected with HIV. Unable to afford antiretroviral drugs, she and her husband reportedly turn to prayer, refusing the HIV counselors' entreaties to use condoms to avoid transmission to the wife.

In consonance with the peaks and valleys of the immune system disorder that is HIV and AIDS, plenty thrive and no doubt benefit psychically from the hope that communication with a personal God engenders. Swarns (2002) describes how some parishioners have died in spite of the emphasis on faith healing but that the ultimate cause of their death—so the local faith healer claims—was their own pursuit of traditional healing, which angered God. This suspicion of traditional healing is consistent with the patterns observed in Table 7.5. It suggests some inclination among Pentecostals in particular to break with their traditional approach to healing, without fully embracing a biomedical approach.

Don't get us wrong. As other social scientists have noted (Smith 2004b), very, very few congregations offer "cures" for HIV, including Pentecostals (e.g., not one leader from our sample of 187 Malawian congregations claimed to have such powers). They merely articulate a deeply held theological principle that an omnipotent God can heal any illness; the fact that this is seldom observed plays directly into the interpretations of AIDS as divine punishment we discussed in Chapter 3.[15]

This approach to faith healing—articulating it as a matter of principle even if there's little direct evidence that it works—is exemplified in this quote from a New Mission Protestant leader in Northern Malawi. In discussing how he engages with HIV-positive members, he frames faith healing as being primarily about offering hope and encouragement to the infected:

> Mainly, we discuss the goodness of the words of God and give them courage; we also discuss the ways of helping these sick people. We give hope that God can heal and He is the Healer. We want them to trust God so that they should not lose hope.

Messages of faith healing, in other words, offer hope and psychological comfort to individuals living with a death sentence. And while this was particularly true in the pre-ART era, it still holds true today. We return to this religious emphasis on offering "cheer" and "hope" to sick individuals at greater length in the following chapter.

Conclusion

Here, as in previous chapters, the available evidence shows that, although there are some important denominational differences in approaches to HIV prevention, these differences are secondary to the set of prevention strategies congregational leaders promote. As evidence that these configurations matter, we have shown that both ABC and non-ABC prevention strategies correspond to actual HIV prevalence within local religious congregations. The inclusion of faith healing in a congregation's overall set of approaches appears to be the central tipping point in this relationship. HIV prevalence is highest in churches that emphasize only faith healing and lowest in those that have no faith healing whatsoever, irrespective of whether they emphasize other approaches. In contrast, being in a community that combines regular moral messages about AIDS with openness to public health strategies (testing and condom use) provides the best protection. While we cannot fully control for the impact that HIV infection prior to joining has on these differences, our own formal analyses of denominational switching suggest that self-selection (here, congregation switching) is not driving these observed differences. (We address religious switching in greater detail in Chapter 10).

The centrality of faith healing is somewhat surprising. Consistent with findings from the anthropological literature on health beliefs and disease etiology, our qualitative data suggest that faith healing vis-à-vis AIDS does not represent a competing health care system. Rather, even where relying on faith healing is more of a Pentecostal thing, it is deeply rooted in biblical and monotheistic notions of God as healer. This is why some notion of faith healing can be found in the prevention approaches practiced across all six religious traditions in Malawi. Yet empirically, the presence of faith healing is positively correlated with HIV prevalence. This is true where faith healing is the only strategy practiced and where it is integrated into a more diverse set of strategies. It also seems to be the case whether the faith healing is intended to cure a person physically or simply comfort them psychically. We now expand on this difference between cure and comfort, turning our attention to the care of those affected by HIV.

PART FOUR

RESPONDING

Our attention thus far has been devoted to the effects of religion on the interpretation, knowledge, and prevention of AIDS. We now turn to the final means by which religion affects AIDS—the attempt to mitigate its effects, both on those who are infected by the virus and on those who share their lives: family members, friends, and neighbors.

In certain ways, this is the most profound dimension of the religion–AIDS relationship. Increasing knowledge and preventing infection are standard public health goals. But mitigating the effects of AIDS takes us into more general territory. It forces us to deal with how family, friends, neighbors, and communities respond to a person's actual sickness, impending death, and the needs of surviving dependents. It also forces us to differentiate between those who are directly infected by the virus and those whose lives are affected indirectly, though no less deeply. Press coverage over the last decade has introduced us to a host of characters from these dramas: the surviving spouse and children, stigmatized to varying degrees by community members; the emaciated but stoic grandmother, whose tiny hut is home to 10 grandchildren bequeathed by her own deceased children; the aunts and uncles who, in the best cases, generously provide their orphaned nieces and nephews with school fees (while struggling to provide for their own children, too) and, in the worst cases, heartlessly rob them of their deceased parents' wealth. Check the archives of any first-rate newspaper or Google "AIDS photo essay Africa," and you'll find heartrending stories and pictures that feature these characters.

What is the role of religion in all this? Beyond general agreement that organized religion is one of the key institutions in generating responses to the AIDS epidemic in sub-Saharan Africa (SSA), the academic literature provides no clear answer to this question. Some believe that

Christian and Islamic religious organizations are barriers to a more effective and just response to AIDS. Common references here are to the role of religion in perpetuating AIDS-related stigma and failing to contest discrimination, in each case linking back to religious groups' presumed sexual conservatism (Ahiante 2003; Atatah 2004; Moonze 2003; World Bank 1997). The sustaining logic underlying this line of argument is simple: if religion treats nonmarital sexual behavior as immoral conduct, then sexual behavior that makes people vulnerable to HIV can be interpreted as a moral transgression, which will distance HIV-positive individuals from organized religion, in turn deepening stigmatization. Note that this view is sometimes shared by church leaders. Several years ago, for example, Cape Town's Anglican Archbishop Njongonkulu Ndungane suggested that churches have contributed to AIDS-related stigma. He consequently identified fighting such stigma as one of his top priorities for the church in South Africa (Gross 2005; Ndungane 2004). Though writing earlier, Alonzo and Reynolds (1995) had already taken this argument further. They suggested that organized religion may not only reinforce stigma. It may also offer little comfort to the infected. The reason: social support to the sick and dying from these institutions requires that the sick and dying "accept the perspective of the condemners" (Alonzo and Reynolds: 311).

There are more positive voices, however. They see organized religion as an effective tool for combating AIDS-related stigma and discrimination. These voices point to the fact that the Bible and Koran, the primary texts of Christianity and Islam, do not easily lend themselves to justifying poor treatment of the sick, orphans, or widows. Likewise, they refer to the countless examples of congregations and religious nongovernmental organizations (NGOs) actively combating stigma (e.g., Gatheru 2002; Komakech 2003), providing care and support to people living with HIV/AIDS, or being key players in preventive education in spite of the limited funds at their disposal (Liebowitz 2002; Pfeiffer 2002). To these types of voices we add our own. As we described in Chapter 3 ("Interpreting the AIDS Epidemic"), typical religious responses in both Christianity and Islam in SSA involve narratives about God's judgment on sexually immoral society. However, they do not typically isolate individuals in assigning blame. We see the inability to distinguish between general moral claims and judgment on individuals as largely responsible for generating and propagating misconceptions about the role of organized religion in structuring responses to AIDS. It conveys the impression that the *average* religious congregation fosters discrimination to a greater extent than nonreligious organizations and that religious individuals are more likely to discriminate against an HIV-positive individual than their less religious counterparts.

Empirical evidence has not yet been pulled together into a systematic analysis of either of these two positions regarding organized religion and the mitigation of AIDS across Africa. Our key aim here is to rectify that omission. We examine variation in AIDS-related stigma (Chapter 8) and patterns of social support for the sick and orphans (Chapter 9) across denominations and levels of religiosity. These are, in our view, the most important aspects of AIDS mitigation. Choosing these outcomes forces us to tap into two different types of data. Those addressing stigma are primarily attitudinal, and those addressing care are primarily behavioral. Each has its strengths. Together, they are more than the sum of their parts. They provide a broad picture of the ways the effects of AIDS in SSA are mitigated, if at all, by religion.

|| 8 ||

Stigma

Even nowadays we have some people who laugh and discriminate [against] the AIDS suffering people. We need to show love
to them and give them support and care. Amen!
        —Women's prayer service, *Catholic Church, Malawi, 2004*

No social scientific study of stigma and discrimination gets far without making
reference to Erving Goffman. In his seminal work, Goffman (1963) describes
stigma as "an attribute that is deeply discrediting," one that diminishes the
bearer "from a whole and usual person to a tainted, discounted one." As Herek,
Widaman, and Capitanio (2005) note, stigma is different from prejudice and
discrimination. Prejudice is a negative attitude (an evaluation or a judgment)
toward a member of a social group. It resides in the mind of the individual. Discrimination adds the element of *action*, referring to the differential treatment of
individuals according to their membership in a particular group (Link and Phelan
2001). Stigma adds yet another element to these two. In contrast to prejudice, it
resides in the structure of social relations within a society. And in contrast to
discrimination, it contains a distinct aesthetic or moral message. Stigma may
imply differential treatment, but it is really about demarcating the boundaries
between different sorts of people in terms of their desirability. Stigmatized
people are undesirable, usually because they are seen to lack a crucial moral
quality. This makes them impure or wrong.

From the perspective of HIV prevention, stigma is dangerous since it pushes
those infected with HIV to hide their condition, including from spouses or
other sexual partners. In this way, stigma is thought to contribute directly to
the spread of HIV. But stigma has other undesirable and counterproductive
consequences. If stigma reduces the likelihood that a person will use counseling
and testing services, the pathway to lifesaving antiretroviral therapies (ART),
stigma is indirectly reducing access to the most effective drug-related therapies.
In summary—and bluntly—stigma facilitates the spread of AIDS and condemns
infected persons to an earlier death.

In the context of AIDS-ridden sub-Saharan Africa (SSA), discrimination can take a variety of forms. One form is practical in nature—it is primarily concerned with prospects for employment or social mobility. This type of discrimination can exist in the absence of stigma. One of the recurrent public policy debates in some high HIV prevalence countries in SSA concerns whether cash-strapped governments ought to give university scholarships to gifted individuals who are also HIV positive (see, e.g., Kisting 2010). Likewise, one can imagine a situation where a bank manager who knows (or speculates) that a particular client is infected with HIV rejects that client's application for a long-term loan to build or expand his business. In each of these cases, the debate can be framed in relation to narrow utilitarian concerns—HIV-positive individuals are risky investments because of their shorter life spans and not primarily because of stigma.

Stigma-laden discrimination, in contrast, concerns patterns of social contact and social exclusion. Some manifestations of this type of stigma are easily measured, and we consider them empirically here. For example, these deal with how much tolerance people have for sharing social space with people living with HIV and AIDS (PLWHA), doing business with them, or having them teach our kids. If we think of stigma as a continuum, the mundane end is an infected person's sense that they are becoming the subject of gossip: it might not be pleasant, but it is not deeply damaging. But as we move toward the other end of the continuum, things get more serious (making mere gossip look that much more attractive). Imagine, for example, a person being ostracized by people who were once friends or explicitly shunned and kicked out of organizations and groups. Or imagine the most extreme case: being abandoned by one's family and left to die alone.

Stories about extreme stigma, including shunning, can be found in press coverage of AIDS and its effects in SSA. Many of these stories make references to religion in some form or to "traditional practices" that—this being darkest Africa—are implicitly linked to, or legitimated by, religion (e.g., Ayikukwei et al. 2007; Lafraniere 2005a, 2005b). But how widespread are the actual occurrences? Do religious leaders and religious organizations contribute to perpetuating different types of AIDS-related stigma, either actively, such as by preaching messages that community members should shun PLWHA, or passively, such as by being silent about the mistreatment of PLWHA?

In our view, there is very scant evidence that religious leaders are perpetuating AIDS-related stigma, either actively or passively. Portrayals of religious leaders and religious organizations as purveyors of stigma abound, and they remind us of the debates about condoms we reviewed in Chapter 5. They reflect a tendency to spotlight loud, high-profile, atypical religious leaders rather than the quiet, low-key, and compassionate majority. This is an old criticism of journalistic coverage—its tendency to privilege colorful characters and a good story over the more mundane matter of responsibly representing average effects.

Our review of the evidence suggests that, overall, religious organizations do more to dampen stigma in SSA than to perpetuate it. This happens in two ways. The first is found in religious messages related to the notion of *love* (Klaits 2010). The second follows from the religious imperative to care for the sick and for their dependents. These mechanisms are especially important in rural areas, where institutions of the state are the least visible and effective, making religious congregations the most important nonfamilial organization in the area. Religious leaders are among the most important local players; they set the tone for local discourse and action and also coordinate these efforts in practical terms. In day-to-day life this means that religious organizations play a leading role as providers of instrumental, spiritual, and social support for PLWHA and for the orphans and widow(er)s left behind when an HIV-positive person dies.

This stigma-reducing effect of religion can be framed in relation to theories that emerged from research on racial and ethnic tensions in the United States during the Civil Rights era, in particular to what formally became known as the contact hypothesis (Allport 1979). This hypothesis asserts that, given reasonable conditions, interpersonal contact between members of different groups reduces prejudice and, consequently, stigma and discrimination. The hypothesis has been tested empirically in a number of settings, through experiments designed to facilitate positive intergroup contact as the "treatment" and then follow-up in both the short- and long-term to determine whether and to what extent personal relationships with "others" foster more tolerant attitudes. But even before it was formally molded into a social scientific hypothesis, its underlying principle was well-known. Social contact breeds acceptance. The lack of social contact generates and then perpetuates stereotypes and stigma.[1]

Variation in Stigma

Applied to AIDS, the contact hypothesis suggests that people who have lost close friends, family members, or even acquaintances to the disease are more likely to have developed compassion for those suffering with the disease and less likely to "discredit" them or treat them as a "tainted, discounted" person. Contact with infected persons may also reduce the fear and misconceptions that, as shown in Chapter 5 ("The ABCs of Prevention"), still exist—even though virtually every adult in SSA knows something about AIDS. The simple act of learning that HIV cannot be transmitted by sharing a meal, for example, forges social contact and reduces stigma.

Ironically, the contact hypothesis suggests that the very nature of a generalized epidemic is a barrier to stigma, in the case of AIDS at least. A generalized epidemic gives rise to so much contact between both sick and symptom-free PLWHA and people who are (or think themselves to be) HIV negative that significant levels of stigma cannot persist. Proximity in caregiving and burials reveals something we hear from our respondents all the time: "She was just like me" and "He didn't do anything I haven't done."

The contact hypothesis is very simple to test empirically. We do so in two stages: first at a cross-national and cross-community ecological level; and second with a focus on individuals.

Ecological Level

We examine the association between national-level HIV prevalence and two indicators of stigma commonly used in survey research on AIDS. Results of this initial exploration can be seen in Figure 8.1. The first panel combines UNAIDS HIV prevalence estimates for 11 countries with data from the World Values Survey (WVS). The WVS asked the following question: "On this list are various groups of people. Could you please mention any that you would not like to have as neighbors?" On the list were drug addicts, people who have AIDS, and members of various ethnic and religious groups. As predicted by the contact hypothesis, the relationship between HIV prevalence and the proportion of people who said they would not want an HIV-positive person as a neighbor is negative.

A similar approach is used in Panel 2 of Figure 8.1, this time aggregating Demographic and Health Survey (DHS) data on whether the respondent would buy

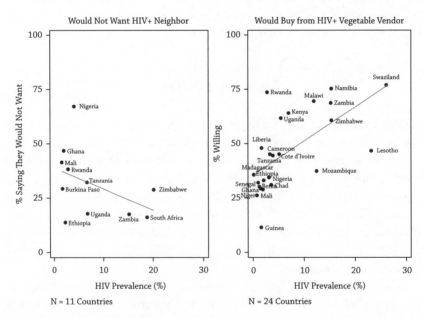

Figure 8.1 Ecological Relationship between HIV Prevalence and Stigma
Source: UNAIDS 2007, African World Values Surveys, African Demographic and Health Surveys

vegetables from a HIV-positive vendor for each country and combining these with the most recent UNAIDS prevalence estimates. Here the sample of countries is larger, and the relationship is positive and quite strong, with willingness to interact with a positive vegetable vendor rising as HIV prevalence goes up.

Both of these results are consistent with the contact hypothesis. But as we described in Chapter 2, HIV prevalence varies greatly within countries. This makes us cautious about generalizing from national prevalence estimates. For example, imagine two people living in Malawi. One lives in a village that has never experienced an HIV death. The other lives in a village where both HIV prevalence and AIDS-related mortality are high. To more accurately tap into these contextual differences, we examine data from smaller units: cluster-level data from the DHS in the 16 countries that collected HIV biomarker data and at least one stigma question.[2]

Each DHS country has between 54 and 540 clusters, and HIV prevalence within these clusters ranges from 0 to 66% of their populations.[3] Combining all clusters from the 17 countries together (N = 6584), we find a very strong and positive relationship between local cluster-specific HIV prevalence and the willingness to buy vegetables from a HIV-positive vendor. When we split the clusters between high- and low-prevalence countries, however, two interesting and important findings emerge. First, the stigma "floor" in high-prevalence countries

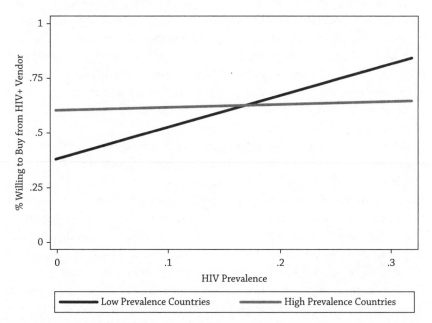

Figure 8.2 Cluster-Level Relationship between Prevalence of HIV and Stigma in High and Low Prevalence Countries

Source: Demographic and Health Surveys, 17 countries, 6584 clusters

is much higher than in low-prevalence countries. That is, in high-prevalence countries one finds that even in low-prevalence clusters more than 50% of individuals express willingness to buy vegetables from an HIV-positive vendor. In low-prevalence countries, in contrast, the relationship between cluster-specific HIV prevalence and nonstigmatized views is much stronger. There, one is much more likely to find stigmatized views in low-prevalence clusters. In other words, within countries where HIV is "rare," HIV prevalence at the very local level shapes how people think about PLWHA. Given that investments by governments and nongovernmental organizations (NGOs) in messages that combat stigma tend to be relatively equal within countries, this finding is most likely the product of social exposure to HIV. In other words, exposure to PLWHA or interaction with them erodes negative attitudes about them and, consequently, reduces stigma and discrimination. In the case of AIDS, familiarity breeds compassion and empathy rather than contempt and fear.

Individual Level

Moving from the ecological level to the microlevel, we turn to our Malawi data, in which we asked those participating in the Malawi Diffusion and Ideational Change Project (MDICP) to try to put themselves in the shoes of someone with HIV. "Imagine what would happen to you if you were HIV positive. Do you think that some people would act as though it is your fault that you have AIDS? Do you think that you would stop socializing with some people because of their reactions to your having AIDS?" While 60% of respondents thought they would be faulted for having been infected, less than 30% believed that the reactions to their HIV status would result in less socialization. In other words, Malawians are substantially more concerned about what people would *think* about them than about how they would be treated. In 2004, a full 65% said that most people in their village are comfortable around a person who has AIDS.

Survey data on what people think the people around them think also add some value to our efforts to provide an empirically grounded view of how people treat PLWHA. While individuals may be unlikely to admit their own biases to an interviewer, they give pretty accurate information on the social climate of their villages, compounds, and social circles when they tell us about what *other people* believe. For example, we asked MDICP respondents about their level of agreement with the following statement: "People in your village feel that those who are movious [a local term for promiscuous] and got AIDS through sex have gotten what they deserve." Then we asked the same question about religious leaders in their own villages: "How do religious leaders view people who have gotten AIDS through sex?" While over half (57%) of the respondents reported that others in their village would make this assessment (i.e., treat movious people who got AIDS as having gotten what they deserve), only a

Table 8.1 **Perceived Comeuppance in Rural Malawi**

Level of Agreement with the Following Statement
"People/Religious leaders in your village feel that those who are movious and got AIDS through sex have gotten what they deserve."

	People	*Religious Leaders*
Strongly Disagree	12%	17%
Disagree	31%	42%
Agree	44%	33%
Strongly Agree	13%	8%
N	3128	3038

Source: MDICP-3, 2004.

minority of respondents (41%) agreed that religious leaders feel this way. In other words, lay survey respondents perceive the religious leaders around them to be considerably less damning in their attitudes toward people with HIV than their neighbors in general.

Religious Variation in Stigma

How do these types of stigma vary cross religious groups? The graphs in Figure 8.3 address this question. Using DHS data from 27 countries in SSA, they compare respondents' declared willingness to buy vegetables from an HIV-positive vendor—our indicator of comfort with PLWHA—across major religious groups.

A number of noteworthy results emerge from these comparisons. The first concerns the differences between, on one hand, members of the "Abrahamic" religions (i.e., Christianity and Islam) and, on the other, those with no religion or who self-identify as "other." Those claiming no religion whatsoever, albeit a small group in most countries in SSA, are the least comfortable with PLWHA (observed in 14 of the 19 cases where "none" was a response option in the survey). Those who identify their religion as "other" are also substantially less comfortable with PLWHA than any type of Christian (20 of 24 cases where the country's data have both codes) and marginally less comfortable than Muslims (12 of 20 cases). In general, then, stigma is lower among those affiliated with Abrahamic religions than among those who affiliate with traditional religions or have no religion.

The second noteworthy result concerns Christian–Muslim differences. Comfort with PLWHA is significantly lower among Muslims than among any type of Christian bloc in these data. Of the 16 countries with substantial Muslim

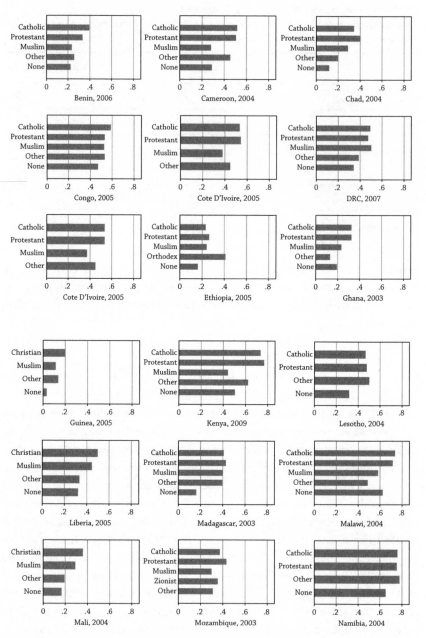

Figure 8.3 Willingness to buy Vegetables from an HIV+ Vendor by Denomination

Note: DHS data from Burkina Faso does not contain any measure of stigma and was excluded from these analyses.

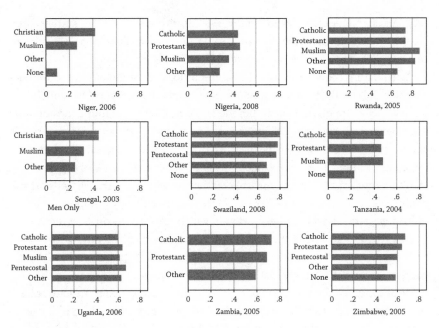

Figure 8.3 (continued)

populations, this pattern holds true in all but two countries. One is Uganda, where early sensitization campaigns targeted wide swathes of the population, and religious leaders, including Muslims, were involved in educating the public about HIV (discussed in Chapter 4). The other is Tanzania.

Finally, we observe only minor and inconsistent denominational differences between different Christian blocs. For example, in eight countries Catholics are reportedly more willing than Protestants to buy vegetables from an HIV-positive vendor; in another eight countries, Protestants are more willing than Catholics; and in five countries Catholics and Protestants are equally likely (in the remainder, the data do not distinguish between Catholics and Protestants).

These comparisons are instructive. As noted in earlier analyses, however, identity and affiliation constitute only one component—and not necessarily the most important one—of the way that "religion" writ large can influence behavior. Its broader effects are embedded in attitudes and practices that vary *within* denominations and across congregations.

To see how, if at all, stigma varies along these more complex religious parameters, we return to the MDICP data. In line with the DHS, the MDICP asked respondents if they would purchase fresh fruit from a vendor they knew to be HIV positive; approximately 24% said no. Respondents were also asked if a *female* teacher who has HIV, but not AIDS, should be allowed to continue teaching—here, too, approximately 24% said no.[4] We constructed a series of multivariate regression models that allow us to examine how response patterns on each of these two variables vary across a range of respondent characteristics, including religious characteristics. Although the two questions are only moderately correlated with one another (the Pearson correlation coefficient is 0.55), similar patterns apply to both teachers and vegetable vendors.

Aside from replicating the Muslim–Catholic denominational difference observed in the DHS data, a number of important results are evident in the models.[5] (See Appendix I for full models). First, having an abundance of what sociologists call "conversation partners"—people with whom respondents talk about religion and AIDS—is positively associated with expressing support for infected teachers. This is consistent with the idea that new, less stigmatized views emerge as part of ongoing conversations in which certain religious organizations play a part. Second, and from our perspective the most important point, individuals who attend a congregation in which the leader expresses a discriminatory attitude toward PLWHA—that is, saying the movious have gotten what they deserve—are less likely to express supportive attitudes for PLWHA. Of course, we cannot formally distinguish whether the leader is shaping the attitudes of congregation members or reflecting them. But we don't need to resolve that problem (i.e., establishing causal direction) here. It's sufficient for us to demonstrate that attitudes about PLWHA are clustered religiously. As in analyses conducted in Chapter 7, "clustered religiously" refers to variation at the congregation level rather than patterns by denomination or identity.

Finally, a noneffect in these analyses is also noteworthy. There is no observed relationship between religiosity—in this case measured by the frequency of church or mosque attendance—and an individual's perception of PLWHA. In other words, it doesn't matter how frequently individuals go to church. What matters is the conversational network they find themselves in and the tone of the religious leader's messages about PLWHA.

Muslim Exceptionalism? A View from Senegal

Both the DHS and MDICP data show that, in general, Muslims across Africa are less accepting of PLWHAs than Protestants or Catholics. Does this result reflect the views reported by Muslim leaders across the continent? To get a handle on this question we analyzed transcripts from a series of interviews about AIDS conducted with 84 imams in Senegal.[6] With regard to the African AIDS epidemic, Senegal is a special case. A largely Muslim country, it is one of the only SSA countries in which HIV prevalence is less than 1%. Its government is credited with having been one of the most proactive in relation to AIDS, among other things by co-opting religious leaders early in its interventions. But even in Senegal, as seen in Figure 8.3, Muslims in general appear to have more stigmatized views of PLWHAs than their Christian counterparts.[7] This makes Senegal an interesting case for determining whether these more stigmatizing attitudes Muslims hold reflect messages received from their imams or whether they stem from other sources.

For the imams themselves, it doesn't seem to be the lack of contact with people who are HIV positive. Even in this low-prevalence country, most imams reported having counseled members they knew to be HIV positive. Imams' opinions about how they and their communities have dealt, and should deal, with AIDS revealed broad consensus. Many spoke about their efforts to dispel faulty beliefs about transmission. They saw, or at least articulated, it as their responsibility to combat misinformation and stigma in the community.

We did, however, identify differences between the imams in their views on the existence and level of stigmatization of PLWHA in their communities. Most did not perceive it to be a problem, talking about how people with AIDS were still, in the words of one, "surrounded by family and not rejected by the population." One imam reported:

> If they are stigmatized, I don't know about it. In our neighborhood, one was a man and one was a woman. Everyone thought that they caught the disease [*maladie*]. But the two people lived with their family. Nobody stigmatized them. They lived well. But both of them died.[8]

Other imams, in contrast, reported that stigmatization is indeed a problem, evoking the themes of social exclusion in their description of stigma as the desire to "flee when they see that you are infected," to not "share a bowl with you if you have HIV," or the "reflex to not shake hands with someone who has HIV." These imams also described the negative consequences of such behavior as leading to the social isolation of PLWHA. This is the real danger, one imam suggested: "It's not the *maladie* that kills; it's the isolation that kills. You can live with HIV and live a long time and they will watch others without die before them." Indeed, this focus on the dangers of isolation was not restricted to the interviews. We heard this message in Malawi in the sermons we observed, in informal conversations with friends and colleagues, and in songs about bringing cheer to sick friends. These messages about the dangers of isolation have two distinct audiences: healthy individuals are urged to generously provide assistance; and HIV-positive individuals are encouraged to disclose their status and seek help, from congregation members in particular. "If they isolate themselves, they will still have their *maladie*. Better if people know and can help," said one imam.

One can hear at least an echo of the contact hypothesis in these comments. For by condemning those who refuse to share social space with people infected with HIV, these Senegalese imams seek to foster social relationships between PLWHA and the broader community. In the words of one, "Working with someone doesn't make you infected by HIV. Eating with someone doesn't make you infected. A good Muslim should not react like that."

So why are levels of AIDS-related stigma greater among Senegalese Muslims than Senegalese Christians? In the absence of direct information from a sample of Senegalese pastors, it is impossible for us to say for sure, but the Senegal data contain at least two hints. First, the divided opinions about whether there is stigma in their communities derives, at least in part, from the lack of a standardized definition of stigma. At least one of the imams sets the bar in this debate relatively high. There is no stigma, he appears to suggest, where HIV-positive individuals are still living with their family. Yet another imam talks much more generally about stigma: about fleeing social contact or even avoiding shaking hands, a key interaction ritual across SSA societies whose absence would definitely be interpreted as a social slight.

The second hint comes from responses to questions about how imams themselves interact with HIV-positive members. Almost all emphasized the importance of discretion and confidentiality in their counseling. Yet some went further, being reluctant to discuss particulars of any case in their interviews. For example, typical responses to the question, "Do you know personally anyone living with HIV?" were: "If I do, I don't say it," or "Yes, but I can't really discuss it with you." These responses are contrasted with the answers of imams we interviewed in high-prevalence Muslim areas of Malawi. There, in response to the same question, several imams began to list all the HIV-positive women in the mosque by name, and one began pointing us in the direction of each of their homes. On one hand, it is hard to imagine that stigma is not a problem in places where even talking about counseling remains such a sensitive issue. But we also see substantial variation in how religious leaders interpret confidentiality as a part of their professional code. The boundary between stigma that silences discussions about AIDS and a professional code of confidentiality (much like what we, in the West, expect from our religious leaders, therapists, and physicians) is, indeed, a blurry one.

Summary

Across Africa, PLWHA use religious leaders as resources. For example, data from HIV-positive women in the Democratic Republic of Congo show that after getting over the initial shock of an HIV-positive diagnosis many women told interviewers that the first person to whom they disclosed their status was their pastor. They gave three key reasons: he (almost always a "he") could be trusted to be discrete; he would pray for her; and he could both give her the necessary courage to disclose her status to others—namely, a partner—and be present to calm the partner and counsel the couple (Maman, Cathcart, Burkhardt, Omba, and Behets 2009).

Going to a pastor who is liable to condemn and stigmatize you as an infected sinner is completely irrational. That is not to say that it never happens—it probably does, but we found no evidence that this happens with any frequency. This makes sense. In a diverse religious marketplace, like the one that exists across most areas in SSA, HIV-positive individuals will disclose their status first, if not exclusively, to the most forgiving and empathetic individuals they know. If pastors and other religious leaders truly were as uncharitable, mean-spirited, and consumed with fire and brimstone as they are sometimes made out to be, then the Congolese women in this study would have named some other figure as their go-to person. Likewise, there would be evidence that HIV-positive individuals distance themselves from religious leaders and religious life. This is not the case.

Instead, the picture that emerges from the data on the relationship between religion and stigma is consistent with the picture given by Maman and colleagues (2009). Religious leaders are perceived to be less stigmatizing than "people" in general. More religious people report less stigmatizing views than their less religious counterparts. Christians tend to stigmatize less than Muslims, and Muslims tend to stigmatize less than traditionalists and those with no religion. These are important results. They point to substantial differences between religions even while showing that more institutionalized religions feature less stigmatizing attitudes among their members. We now turn our attention to one of the main sources of these religious differences in stigma: social support networks.

9

Safety Nets

Do not doubt that God is seated at your bedside, and that He is there to gather up your tears and sighs, to heal your wounds, to fortify your heart.

—Binet, 1617[1]

To those who have helped the poor, the hungry, and the oppressed, God makes a promise. Then your light shall break forth like morning. . . . And your righteousness shall go before you. The glory of the Lord shall be your rear guard. Then you shall call and the Lord will answer. You shall cry and He will say, "Here I am." That is from Isaiah 58: 8–9. Amen.

—Prayer, *Seventh Day Adventist church, Malawi, 2004*

AIDS puts heavy demands on social support systems. From the time that people living with HIV and AIDS (PLWHA) become symptomatic and sick until their deaths they need support in a number of ways: practical assistance managing themselves and their households, securing and preparing food, and caring for the dependents, particularly children, in their charge.

In developed countries, these types of support are offset by the taxpayer. Publicly funded health systems pay for or subsidize antiretroviral therapies (ART), and social security systems provide financial assistance to those who are too sick to work. This leaves local nongovernmental organizations (NGOs) and support groups with the task of providing peripheral goods and services such as companionship, counseling, and legal assistance. In poor developing countries in sub-Saharan Africa (SSA), things are different. With some important and partial exceptions (South Africa, Botswana, and Lesotho), most African states do not have the health infrastructure, public safety nets, and social security systems that characterize wealthy countries. So although free ART are now being distributed widely across SSA through government programs, all other types of support come from somewhere else.

In developing countries in general, this "elsewhere" is primarily the extended family. This is certainly true in sub-Saharan Africa. Individuals tend to be deeply embedded in family-centered exchange networks. Resources and assistance are commonly given to and received from first-order relatives like parents, children, and siblings; second-order relatives (i.e., uncles, aunts, and cousins) also play important roles (Weinreb 2002). When one node in the family network fails, substitutions occur. For example, instead of drawing upon assistance from a brother, a sick individual may draw upon an uncle or distant cousin. In this way, networks reconfigure and perpetuate reciprocal and cyclical forms of exchange (Weinreb 2006). When assistance through these familial mechanisms fails—it can happen, though rarely does—people appeal to nonfamilial sources. Friends are a potential source; friendships can become close enough to turn into what family sociologists call *fictive kin*. In the absence of either of these family- or friend-based support networks, the most broadly available source of support is from religious organizations.

Herein lies one of the key differences between religious organizations in wealthy countries and their counterparts—sometimes the same denomination—in developing countries: their central role as providers of social support. There are, of course, church-based shelters and soup kitchens that provide for a wide variety of needs in developed countries, often to people who are homeless, mentally ill, or living off the grid. But in general, over the course of the last 150 years, developed states have committed themselves to providing all citizens with a social safety net that covers basic needs such as food, essential health services, a modicum of education, and a pension for the elderly. These are the main elements of modern "welfare systems" in all developed countries.[2]

The new states that began to emerge in SSA during the late 1950s did not embed the same commitments to their citizens in law. Consequently, the only functional substitutes to the state with regard to social security are the same ones that existed in pre-Victorian Europe: family, community, church (these latter two are often linked together), and NGOs, the modern equivalent of Victorian charities. Even with the proliferation of NGOs in SSA over the last two decades (see Chapter 1), for the vast majority of people in SSA this boils down to family and religious congregation.

Providing social support is an ancient tradition within both Christianity and Islam. Both inherited norms of charity and forms of tithing from Judaism that were intended, among other things, to support the neediest, irrespective of their familial connection (Wilson 1997). There are clear signs of this in the message of the social prophets (i.e., Isaiah, Hosea, Amos, Micah), in particular in their repeated reminders that orphans and widows should receive adequate care and support. Arguably, however, nonfamilial care reached its apogee within Christianity. Historical studies suggest that care was one of the main reasons for the great success of Christianity in Gaul during the Plague of Justinian (6th century) and then again in areas of Mexico during the series of virgin epidemics that followed the *conquistadores*. Christian leaders, unlike local shamans and polytheist counterparts, were seen to remain in the vicinity of the plague to care for those who were suffering (Reff 2005). Likewise, the earliest extant designs of monasteries included hospitals where the sick and dying could be tended (Stark 1996).

These long-standing traditions were replicated by Christian missionaries in SSA. The mission hospital tradition in SSA has both theological and practical roots. Motivated by Christian ideas about love, charity, and healing, clinics and hospitals were an instrument for outreach and a tool for winning converts (Isichei 1995). The earliest missions always included medical facilities that provided not only care for the sick but also, in many cases, training for local nurses (Frazer 1914; Krapf 1860; Pavitt 1989). Indeed, mission-based clinics and hospitals are still common across Africa. This is the context in which we consider the relationship between religion and AIDS mitigation: providing care both for the sick and for orphans.

Visiting the Sick

The emphasis that many religious leaders put on not isolating PLWHA (described in Chapter 8) is part of a larger set of activities that centers on visiting the sick. In rural areas of SSA, the common practice of "visiting" absent members serves a few purposes. First and foremost, it allows people to check in on absent members to see if they are ill and to assist them with daily tasks like hauling water and firewood, sweeping, and bringing food (normally maize) and other supplies (e.g., soap). When necessary, visitors also help with other regular tasks such as fixing roofs and smearing the house.[3] In doing so, another aim of these visits is also fulfilled: to provide more general moral support. Our Malawian informants refer to this as *cheer*. In Botswana, friends and relatives visit the sick to *give love* (Klaits 2010).

One can reasonably ask what makes this a religious thing. An equivalent practice in the United States, bringing meals to a sick friend and their family, is not normally considered religious behavior. It is simply a nice thing to do. In our Malawian research sites, however, visiting the sick is both organized and interpreted religiously, in particular where the recipient is not a member of one's own extended family. The practice is organized within congregations as a religious activity (Trinitapoli 2006). Granted, not all those who are sick have HIV or an AIDS-related illness. However, recent studies have provided evidence that the sheer magnitude of AIDS-related illnesses has prompted individuals to organize within their religious congregations to provide both material and psychological support for PLWHA (Agadjanian and Sen 2007; Klaits 2010; Pfeiffer 2004; Trinitapoli 2006).[4]

Based on 15 years of ethnographic fieldwork focused on a single evangelical congregation in urban Gaborone, Klaits (2010) argues that the heavy burden of

AIDS-related morbidity and mortality has pushed caregiving relationships to the center of discourses about Christian love and morality in this context. Klaits highlights the centrality of congregational life to organizing the provision of care for the sick and consolation for the bereaved. Local interpretations of illness, suffering, death, and grief all hinge on imperatives to "sustain love in the time of AIDS" (Klaits: 283). Among the healthy, Christian practice has become synonymous with caregiving, as exemplified by this closing statement from a pastor at a young person's burial: "Our work here is done. Now let us return, for we must not neglect the sick" (Klaits: 214).

The data we collected by observing religious services in Malawi paint a picture of how visits to the sick are generally organized within congregations. In one Presbyterian congregation we visited, this job was managed by the chairlady, who delivered her weekly report on all the sick members each Sunday immediately following the sermon. Her report was followed by the collection of a special offering. We subsequently learned that this combination of report–offering was very common in Christian churches across traditions. We also learned that in some congregations members leave for the sick person's household immediately after circulating the plate, singing songs as they travel together. They stay at the house to pray and provide assistance. In another congregation the list making and offering taking looked similar, but the visiting was conducted several days later by a committee that brought gifts (maize and sugar) for the household. In most cases, the visiting seemed to be handled by women; this was subsequently confirmed by our survey data and documented in another study of faith-based care conducted in Mozambique (Agadjanian and Sen 2007). However, in some cases, mixed-sex groups went to visit a sick member, particularly when visits were conducted immediately after services with the intention of bringing cheer though songs and prayer.

Not all sick people qualify for this type of assistance. In one church, for example, a debate broke out over whether a "member" should legitimately be on the list of people to visit, as he had attended services only occasionally, never gave money to the congregation, and never visited other members himself. This implies that, although technically voluntary, participating in this process by donating either money or time to visits serves as a type of insurance policy for one's own future needs: if you don't visit others when they are sick, or at least provide them with some supplies, who will visit or help you when you get sick? This exchange mechanism is founded on very straightforward expectations of reciprocity, common across societies. Family support networks operate according to a similar principle.

Since formal data on visiting the sick are scarce, we again use Malawi Diffusion and Ideational Change Project (MDICP) data, where we asked about this directly. In 2004, which appears to have been close to the height of AIDS-related mortality and illness in Malawi, we asked respondents whether they had visited the sick during the past month. A full 23% of the MDICP sample reported having done so. We specified a set of regression models to allow us to evaluate the religious patterns in practice—net of standard socioeconomic controls (e.g., respondents' age, education and wealth; full models can be found in Appendix I). Once again, our results confirmed our sense that religion plays a central role.

First, we found substantial differences by religious tradition. Most notably, visiting the sick is a distinctively Christian practice in Malawi. For all Christian groups, engagement in this practice hovered around 30%. In contrast, only a very small proportion of Muslims (7%) had visited the sick during the past month, and none of the individuals who did not affiliate with a religious tradition reported participating in this practice.

A second set of results highlighted significant associations by religiosity. For example, a mere 5% of those who seldom attended religious services reported visiting the sick, compared with almost 30% of those who attended services weekly. Finally, visiting the sick was also positively associated with having a large religious network, as measured by the number of people with whom the respondent reported discussing religion.

Taken together, these results confirmed our initial observations that religious congregations in Malawi—Christian ones in particular—are a central institution for helping the sick, one of the principal ways the day-to-day effects of AIDS can be mitigated. In doing so, congregations supplement the care of the extended family network by mobilizing community members to step in and provide assistance. This allows them to address the practical, spiritual, and (we suspect) emotional needs of sick members and friends.

These results also help us understand some broader patterns. One example is the stubborn Christian–Muslim difference in levels of stigma that we described in Chapter 8. For if more than four times as many Christians have visited a sick person in the last month than Muslims (respectively, 30% versus 7%) then it is certainly consistent with the contact hypothesis for Christians to voice less stigmatized views of PLWHA. They have far more contact with PLWHA.

Second, and more broadly yet, to the extent that committees for visiting the sick are part of a more general culture of community engagement in local problems, it suggests that churches, irrespective of denomination, are more animated community spaces than mosques. Even though, as noted in Chapter 1, there are substantial differences across denominations in the level of political engagement or protest, when it comes to local issues related to the welfare of members those differences tend to evaporate. All the Christian denominations in our sample reported some type of established mechanism through which members jointly provide care for the sick, even where these were not particularly active. Even though we might question the motives of some of the participants—perhaps as discussed earlier some visit the sick as an insurance policy rather than out of simple charity—the results are the same: the sick, irrespective of ailment, get visited by, and receive support from, the members of their religious community.

Caring for Orphans

The question of responsibility for orphans in SSA is simultaneously an emotive issue and an urgent practical matter. Between 1990 and 2009—the latest year from which UNAIDS estimates are available—the number of orphans in SSA rose from less than 1 million to 14.8 million (UNAIDS 2007; UNAIDS 2010). Region-wide estimates suggest that about 12% of African children are orphans (UNAIDS, UNICEF, and USAID 2004), and in some of the areas hardest hit by the AIDS epidemic, like Nyanza province in Kenya, the numbers are near 30% (KDHS 2003) (see Appendix J).

The magnitude of these numbers is shocking and begins to make sense only once we dismiss images of a completely parentless child—think *Oliver Twist*, *The Secret Garden*, *A Little Princess*, and countless other childhood classics—and adopt the definitions used in the AIDS literature. There, we find three different types of orphans: paternal orphans (biological father is deceased); maternal orphans (biological mother is deceased); and double-orphans (neither biological parent is alive). In each case, these refer to a person under age 18. Of these three, the most common type is a paternal orphan, primarily a function of the older ages at which men have children. Double-orphans are comparatively rare. While about 6% of Zimbabwean children are double-orphans, in half of the AIDS belt countries we examine here double-orphans constitute less than 1% of the under-18 population.[5]

Of course not all orphans in SSA are AIDS orphans. Children lose parents to other infectious and chronic diseases as well as to accidents and war. No extant data that we know of allow us to make distinctions between AIDS orphans and others across African populations; the "cause of death" that appears on death certificates in developed countries is unavailable for the vast majority of people in SSA. But, as shown in Figure 9.1, the prevalence of orphanhood in SSA corresponds very closely to the prevalence of HIV with a few exceptions. One is in Rwanda, where the 100 days of genocide in 1994 generated an orphanhood problem of massive proportions (nearly 20% of all children), even though HIV prevalence remains relatively low. Another partial exception is Uganda, where relatively high levels of orphanhood are a testament to the rapid reductions in HIV prevalence in recent years. In short, although war, accidents, and other disease all contribute to the high levels of orphanhood that characterize SSA, it is safe to say that AIDS-related adult mortality is the primary cause across the AIDS belt and most of East Africa. As established by previous research, the rising

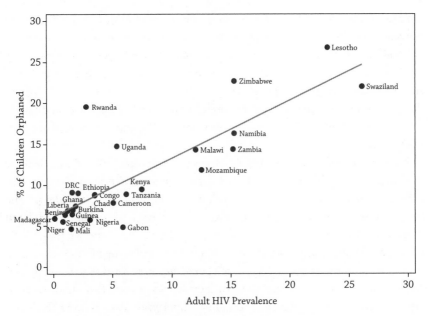

Figure 9.1 Orphanhood and HIV Prevalence in 27 Countries

Note: Orphanhood estimates could not be calculated in Cote D'Ivoire. Data from all other DHS countries used here.

Source: African Demographic and Health Surveys, 2000–2008

number of double-orphans is almost entirely due to AIDS (Heuveline 2004; UNAIDS et al. 2004).

What happens to all these orphans? Where do they end up? Although high-profile visits from Western celebrities to Africa's orphanages might suggest that large numbers of orphans are residing in orphanages—like the one in Malawi from which Madonna pulled her adopted children—in reality things could hardly be more different. Orphanages are a new institution in Africa. Most people are highly suspicious of them and reluctant to send the children of deceased family members to reside there (Rosenthal 2008). Instead, orphans are typically brought up through the traditional child-fosterage system. In the vast majority of cases, this involves configuring and reconfiguring the extended family support system to accommodate orphans—in both the short- and long-term. This system is not unique to orphans. Throughout SSA, there is a long-established and more general system of child circulation or fostering (Bledsoe and Isiugo-Abanihe 1989; Isiugo-Abanihe 1985; Page 1989). Moreover, as we noted earlier, the absence of public safety nets and social security systems turns the extended family into the default institution for addressing all types of family hardships. For example, a newly weaned baby is left with aunts for extended periods of time—it can be years—while the mother, married or unmarried, migrates to the city or a neighboring country for work; struggling parents send their second-grade child to live in the home of a better-off uncle in a neighboring district where her schooling opportunities will be superior and food won't be rationed; after causing trouble at school, parents send their adolescent boy "back to the village," his grandmother's home, believing that the hardships of village life will straighten him out. Historically, orphans have been dealt with in the same way throughout SSA—fostered by members of the extended family (for general reviews of this literature see Goody 2007, and as it relates to AIDS, Madhavan 2004).

The primary view that emerges from the AIDS literature is that the epidemic is producing a surge in orphans and placing an unprecedented burden on families and communities to provide care for children. Swamped and unable to cope, the caregiving structures are liable to breakdown, creating a secondary orphanhood crisis, also of epidemic proportions (Foster, Makuta, Drew, and Kralovec 1997; Foster and Williamson 2000; Hunter 1990; also see dozens of United Nations publications on orphans). There are, of course, grounds for these concerns. Evidence from 10 SSA countries shows that orphans are less likely than the non-orphans with whom they live to be attending school (Case, Paxson, and Ableidinger 2004). Further evidence that orphans living in wealthier households suffer equivalent disadvantages suggests pervasive discrimination against orphans within households—even when resources are not particularly scarce. A new study of the short-term consequences of orphanhood in Tanzania, where about 19% of children have lost a parent, quantifies the health and educational costs of maternal orphanhood clearly: children who lost a mother before age 15 are 2 centimeters shorter and have one full year of schooling less than those whose mothers survived (Beegle, De Weerdt, and Dercon 2010). These health and schooling inequalities can have long-lasting impacts. Evidence from Zimbabwe and South Africa demonstrates that, compared with nonorphans, orphaned adolescents are more likely to have had sex; they initiate sexual activity at earlier ages and are more vulnerable to a range of "adverse sexual outcomes": unplanned pregnancy, HSV-2 (i.e., herpes), and HIV (Birdthistle et al. 2009).

There is a contrasting view, however. It asserts that extended family systems in the region have been surprisingly effective in absorbing orphans, thereby mitigating the full-blown crisis many predicted would result from the sudden and simultaneous burden of so many newly orphaned children (Hosegood, Preston-Whyte, Busza, Moitse, and Timaeus 2007; Monasch and Boerma 2004). Of the millions of AIDS orphans, for example, only a tiny proportion live alone or live in child-headed households—and some of these are only formally child-headed since they remain in their natal homes with family members as neighbors.[6] The overall conclusion, therefore, is that the extended family *works*, albeit imperfectly. Many people take in orphans. Some treat them marginally worse than their own kids. A few treat them much worse. But since almost no one would treat orphans *better* than they treat their own children, we expect to find lower average measures of welfare among orphans. The key question is how much lower.

Religious Messages about Orphans

In observing religious services and interviewing both laypeople and religious leaders, the salience of the orphan problem was immediately relevant to us. Variations of this prayer, which we observed during a large Sunday morning service at a Catholic parish in southern Malawi, were heard on a weekly basis in different churches:

> God, give knowledge to wealthy and all healthy people to help the needy, crippled, hungry and the sick. Those who are suffering from the pandemic disease [AIDS] and other STI diseases. Please give knowledge to those who take care of the orphans here to proceed with the good work.

The prayer highlights both the needs of community members (orphans in particular) and the responsibilities of the sick and wealthy. Wealthy, of course, is a relative term, as most members of this parish would be considered desperately poor by international standards—they are in the dollar-a-day category.

As already noted, throughout SSA orphans typically reside with members of their extended family. Religious congregations frequently provide supplementary support—sometimes in the form of assistance to the orphans themselves but more commonly through general forms of assistance to the entire caregiving household. In churches in Malawi, we observed that offerings are taken two— and often three times—during a single service to support these efforts. On one such occasion, the first plate was devoted to the regular weekly contribution, the second plate to offerings for the sick, elderly, and the orphans, and the third plate to tithes. According to the MRP data, the money collected from these special offerings (the second plate on this occasion) ranged between 200 and 350 KW each week (between 1.50 and 3.00 USD when the data were collected). It was said to be used to provide maize or assist with school fees, uniform expenses, and soap.

Dahl (2009) demonstrates how Christian communities in Botswana have moralized the orphan problem to both address it as a central concern in its own right and offer a pointed critique of what is "bad" about local Tswana culture. Based on an interview with an HIV-positive woman, Dahl's point of departure is this: "It's hard to talk about HIV, but it's a lot easier to talk about the orphan problem" (2009: 25). In promoting their version of Christian love, Dahl observes that Christian leaders and laypeople criticize any and all failings of kin-based

care in reference to the orphan crisis. Relatives who refuse to open their homes
to orphaned family members are the most scandalous villains in this discourse.
"Bad kin" who take in orphans but abuse or neglect them, rather than show care
and love, are a close second.

Our own experiences in Malawi are largely consistent with Dahl's (2009)
observations. We, too, found that warnings against the abuse of orphans were
just as prevalent as messages reminding members of their Christian responsibility to take orphans in. In 2005 we employed a particularly experienced Malawian interviewer to seek out stories of local people who had died and left
children, of others who had fostered children from within or outside the village,
or of others yet who had refused to foster them—this turned out to be an extremely rare event (only one known case, described later in further detail,
across the three research sites). Through these stories, we became acquainted
with the process by which children are fostered. The set of negotiations usually
takes place within the family and involves the orphans' older siblings, aunts,
uncles, and grandparents; sometimes, however, key local leaders like village
headmen and religious leaders are brought in, and their views accompany
final decisions. In theory, orphans are allocated by the extended family to the
household that is most able and willing to take care of them. But in practice,
ability and willingness are negotiable criteria. In other words, there is no clear
algorithm for weighing all the relevant factors to decide who should take
primary responsibility for an orphaned family member. The list of factors is
almost endless and impossible to model: the potential host household's size,
wealth, and physical placement; characteristics of key individuals in the household, including their emotional attributes and gender, and the emphasis they
place on charity and obligation; the set of emotional ties between deceased parents and the surviving child; and the emotional needs of the child. What is clear
to us, however, is that negotiations between members of an extended family
about where to place orphans involve much more than discussions about
housing, that is, where the orphan should sleep at night. The negotiations also
cover a general division of responsibilities between all able-bodied members of
the extended family. All are expected to contribute something, whether mone-
tary or in-kind. Similarly, negotiations also involve debates about how to bal-
ance the ideal that orphans be fostered with their siblings—seen as better for
the orphans' emotional well-being by many local informants—with the burden
that the sudden influx of multiple additional children would undoubtedly
cause.

These points are pertinent to the issue of religion's relationship to orphan
care. One of the key themes we found in our qualitative data about orphanhood
is the extent to which sociocultural and material mechanisms generate willingness to foster orphans. On the sociocultural front, for example, several informants described how certain village and religious leaders publicly laud those

who had fostered, pointing to particular people as worthy of emulation. Another narrative focused on reciprocity. At one of our MDICP field sites, for example, informants recounted cautionary tales about someone who had refused to foster children of deceased relatives; this was the only case known across the three sites. Later, when that person was herself in need, leaders and others were said to have refused her assistance. Like the man earlier in this chapter who hadn't contributed to visiting the sick in the past, by not living up to her side of the bargain, she had disqualified herself from benefiting from the family- and community-based welfare system.[7]

These reports suggested to us that we might find "clusters" of orphans in settings where village or religious leaders actively promoted the fostering of orphans as the right thing to do, whether the justification drew on religious motifs or on a perceived tradition of care within extended families. In either case, the public lauding of those who had actually fostered orphans generated a minimal expectation that refusing to foster an orphan would be more costly in some settings than in others. In such communities, we might even see competition to foster children as a pathway to higher social standing.

As already noted, the practice of orphan care is centered within extended families, but larger religious discourses emphasize the need to show love to orphans by taking responsibility for nonkin. Dahl (2009) found this in Botswana, and we heard very similar messages in Malawi. In one Seventh-Day Adventist church we visited, the leader preached about how the work of God cannot be done by a pastor alone but needs a community:

> The Bible has a lot of say about caring for the poor, the hungry, the widows and the orphans. In James 1 verse 27 we are asked to visit the orphans and widows in their trouble and to keep oneself pure . . . All this is coming from the Bible which contains the message of your God. We have the duty to perform and the duty is for everybody. If we have this duty to be carried out by others then our problems will not end and God will not bless us but send us calamities. This is true religion.

In a nearby African Independent Church (AIC), during a particularly dramatic service we observed a preacher shouting ("as if he would cry") about the sins he observed among his members. Among them: "There is a member of this church who is very rich but doesn't bother to assist the poor, orphans, and those with HIV. Yet he is here, claiming to be a Christian."

While Christian leaders frequently moralized about orphans-related problems, Muslim leaders tended to approach it from a different angle. Messages about orphans were rare in our observations of Friday prayer services in Malawi. But our interviews with local sheikhs revealed that the absence of such messages may not indicate the absence of an orphan problem. Orphan-related themes were just not as deeply embedded in the Muslim leaders' weekly messages. For example, we heard no stories about imams publicly lauding people who had fostered orphans. Likewise, where orphans were talked about, they did not appear to be moralized in the same way: orphans hadn't come to signify AIDS, its impact, and the religious challenge that it poses in the same way that they had in neighboring Christian communities.

What is the cause of this difference? One possible answer is rooted in a gendered perspective. Since orphan care is primarily women's work and women are separated from the main stage of worship more in Islam than in any African Christian denomination with which we are familiar, orphan-related messages are unworthy topics for sermons. Another possible answer takes us back to general discursive styles. The reticence to talk about duties to orphans in general may be related to the imams' general reticence to talk about AIDS-related behavior in sermons—as in the example of Senegalese imams' unwillingness to discuss counseling, discussed in Chapter 8.

These explanations seem reasonable enough and may explain part of the difference. In our view, however, something else is also going on. In fact, the more that we reflected on the Christian–Muslim difference in reported obligations to nonkin, the clearer it became that the differences stem from crucial differences in congregational models of caregiving that affect talk and care not only of orphans but also of visiting the sick.[8] Christian–Muslim differences on these two dimensions of AIDS-related social support are similar. The Christian model of "Godly love" includes visiting the sick and assisting orphans, irrespective of whether they are relatives. Muslim organization and activism on the same front does not emphasize the nonkin aspect. Nor did we observe the same intensity of organizational response on the part of Muslims. This is the reason that many more churches than mosques have developed "orphan care" projects, usually funded through the Malawian Social Action Fund (MASAF). The only partial exceptions to this were in southern Malawi, where the Muslim and Christian leaders are in dialogue with one another and where there are emerging signs that the congregational model implicit in this type of activity is now diffusing to mosques. Either way, right now on the ground the difference exists, and it has implications for the types of AIDS mitigation in which religious communities collectively engage.

Understanding Orphans Empirically

These qualitative data suggest that we should find some religious differences, both across levels of religiosity and between Christians, Muslims, and others, in the actual provision of care for orphans. To do so we follow standard protocol in using data from household rosters: the listing of all people who are resident in the household. Every time there is a household resident under the age of 18 who is not a biological child of the head of household, the head of household is asked whether either parent (mother or father) of this child is deceased. Where either one of them is deceased, the household is marked as an orphan host.

The problem with this type of analysis lies in detecting and interpreting any effects. Fostering an orphan is much less common, and the patterns associated with it are much less clear than, for example, visiting the sick. Finding an orphan in a household typically means only this: a member of the extended family died, leaving children behind. Beyond that, those fostering orphans came to do so under a variety of circumstances. Some eager volunteers leapt at the opportunity; they truly wanted to foster. Others did so begrudgingly, under threat of sanction by their extended family and community members or loathe to be labeled as an immoral eschewer of orphans' needs. Our qualitative data suggest that most fall somewhere between these two extremes: they were deemed most suitable to foster and they chose not to shirk their duty. Unfortunately, no data allow us to differentiate between these three (ideal) types of fostering households.

Despite the heterogeneity among this group, analyses of MDICP data from 2004 demonstrate a number of factors that covary with the presence of orphans. Multivariate models reported in Weinreb, Gerland, and Fleming (2008) show that orphans are less likely to be found in households headed by younger women and in larger households. They are more likely to be found in *poorer* households, where wealth is measured by the number of consumer durables. But they are also more likely to be found in *wealthier* households, where the indicator of wealth is the value of livestock holdings. There are also some religious patterns to the placement of orphans. Consistent with the differential intensity of messages about orphan care being delivered by Christian and Muslim religious leaders, Christians are more likely to host orphans than Muslims, with Church of Central Africa Presbyterian (CCAP), Anglicans, and Baptists being the most likely.

Beyond these differences, a series of spatial analyses of the same data pointed to the emergence of "hot spots"—areas with much higher prevalence of orphan hosting households than one would expect by chance. Since these hot spots are not correlated with village-level HIV prevalence levels or with any other obvious attractions (e.g., a main road or trading center), the most likely explanation for them is the emergence of a motivated and mobilized group of people who are more willing to foster children than their counterparts in other villages. We suspect, though have no solid data with which to prove this, that orphan hot spots are in part the product of local religious leaders, the type that pepper their sermons with encouragement and praise for fostering. For while we agree with Dahl (2009) that it is easier to talk about orphans than HIV, from the perspective of orphans, that isn't a bad thing. To be fostered into a willing household by an eager volunteer almost certainly promises better treatment and prospects than to be fostered into a reluctant and resentful one.

Paralleling the analyses of AIDS-related outcomes presented in previous chapters, Demographic and Health Surveys (DHS) data provide information on the prevalence of orphan fostering. Since fostering is generally "women's work," we do not look at the religious patterning of orphans themselves (data on religion are almost never available for children) but examine the religious patterns in *orphan fostering* among random samples of adult women.[9] Most orphan fostering is done by extended family members, and kin tend to share broad religious traditions (if not affiliation with the same congregation), so we expect fostering patterns to look similar to the religious patterns of HIV prevalence in each country. They do. In countries from which data on both HIV prevalence and orphanhood are available, the patterns of orphan fostering loosely resemble the religious patterns in HIV prevalence (refer to Table 2.1). As with HIV prevalence, we find no evidence that the burden of orphan fostering disproportionately affects any single religious group (see Figure 9.2). In high-prevalence countries

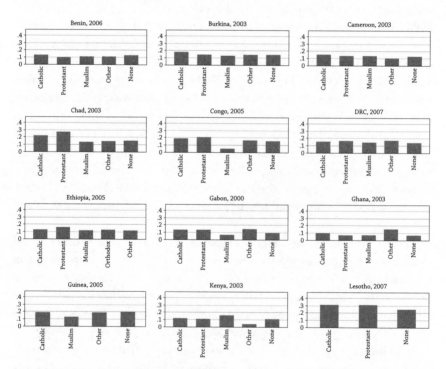

Figure 9.2 Women's Orphan Fostering Responsibilities by Denomination

Note: DHS data Cote D'Ivoire does not allow for the calculation of orphans in households and is, therefore, excluded from these analyses.

Source: African Demographic and Health Surveys, 2000–2008

(e.g., Lesotho, Zimbabwe, Malawi), the burden is distributed fairly equally. In places like Senegal where differences in the fostering burden are visible and significant, they mirror denominational patterns of HIV prevalence discussed in Chapter 2.

Taken together, the results of these analyses resonate strongly with our personal observations from Malawi and Kenya: there is a strong random element in the way that fostering obligations fall on individuals, and these obligations are seldom shirked. This makes it remarkably difficult to tease out religious differences in levels of fostering using sources like DHS data. Even in more detailed data like the MDICP, the patterns are somewhat murky. But the gross patterns we do find are consistent with variability in the intensity of messages about orphanhood and fostering. Just as that intensity varies across religions, so too does the likelihood of child fostering.

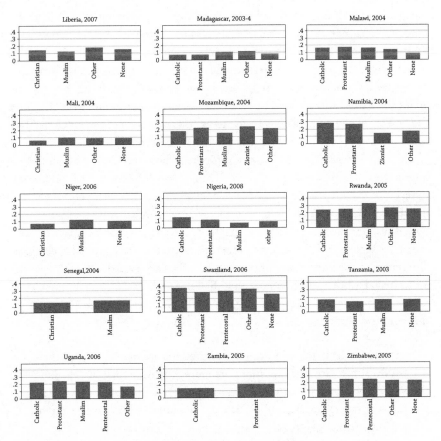

Figure 9.2 Proportion of Adult Women with Orphan Fostering Responsibilities by Denomination

Source: African Demographic and Health Surveys, 2000–2008

Summary

Religion is central to AIDS mitigation in both symbolic and practical ways. In a context of extraordinarily high morbidity and mortality, religious ideas about love, obligation, and charity animate care for the sick and their dependents both before and after death. Christian congregations, in particular, are important organizational spaces for coordinating these caregiving efforts. In the absence of a strong social welfare system, the support that faith communities provide to their members is a critical supplement to family-based support systems. This has always been the case. AIDS has merely highlighted the importance of these systems, especially in high-prevalence countries.

Two main issues arise from these caregiving themes. The first is the extent to which, by highlighting the importance of nonfamilial congregational models of care, AIDS is strengthening religious structures. Our sense is that this is frequently the case in Christian communities and that, though starting from a much lower bar, it is increasingly the case in Muslim communities. Animated by religion—whether actual faith or social pressure rooted in religious networks—communities are augmenting families' ability to cope with AIDS (and other health problems) by using congregational models of caregiving. This in turn has more general implications for religious change. In particular, it raises questions about the extent to which being part of this caregiving movement is changing the face of religion in high-prevalence areas. This inversion of the religion–AIDS causal pathway is the central topic of the next (final) chapter.

The second issue is rooted in the differences between Christians and Muslims. From AIDS-related stigma to caregiving, these differences are pronounced. In terms of magnitude, they dwarf all the religious differences we observe in the interpretation of AIDS and in prevention strategies. What is their origin? Since both Christian and Muslim religious traditions emphasize compassion and charity, it seems unlikely that the differences stem from any general theological differences in the importance of care. Rather, they are rooted in two things: the individual attributes of Christians and Muslims; and the practical differences in how congregational life is organized. One sheikh we interviewed in Malawi made this point explicitly:

> In terms of [general] education the Christians are more educated than the Muslims. Also, the Christians are more organized than the Muslims in terms of their activities, for example, the activities such as, visiting the sick, emerging issues like AIDS, development works on the church, and organizing meetings.

These observations, that Christians are more educated and more organized, are profound. We think that they are deeply embedded in broader Christian-Muslim differences in cultures of organization. Here we follow Kuran (2010). He highlights the relative lack of intermediate institutions in Islamic societies, that is, institutions lying somewhere between the state and the individual. These include NGOs, activist groups, and other constituent parts of civil society. He asserts that the dearth of these intermediate institutions has been one of the central historical impediments to social and economic development in Arab societies. It has also left social welfare in Islam in the hands of the *Waqf*, a type of quasi-governmental religious authority far removed from the congregation (whose many failures Islamist groups have translated into political support; see Berman 2003; Ebaugh 2009).

In the world of AIDS mitigation and beyond, church-related caregiving groups, orphan care groups, and development committees are intermediate institutions, which are critical building blocks of a burgeoning civil society. The differential Christian–Muslim caregiving patterns documented here are consistent with the wider patterns of Christian–Muslim differences in social organization identified by Kuran (2010). As evidenced by our comments about emerging changes in Muslim caregiving practices in Malawi, we think that these patterns are mutable. But right now this structural difference between Christian and Muslim traditions of organization at the most local (i.e., congregational) level has profound effects on caregiving, even given similar levels of HIV prevalence, a shared understanding of AIDS, and a lot of overlap in attitudes to prevention.

|| 10 ||

Effects of AIDS on Religion

Most of our brother Christians showed unbounded love and loyalty, never sparing themselves and thinking only of one another.
Heedless of the danger, they took charge of the sick, attending
to their every need and ministering to them in Christ . . . The
heathen behaved in the very opposite way, at first onset of the
disease, they pushed the sufferers away and fled from their dear-
est, throwing them into the roads before they were dead and
treading on buried corpses as dirt.

—Bishop Dionysius, *Alexandria, 259* CE[1]

Given the centrality of religious life in Africa, it is no surprise that religion,
through its institutions, and the free-flowing discourse it inspires, affects how
people in sub-Saharan Africa (SSA) perceive AIDS, avoid AIDS, and mitigate its
effects within their families and communities. The central question we address
in this chapter reverses that causal direction: to what extent is AIDS affecting
religion or driving religious change?

This is an important question. In Chapter 1 we described how over the course
of the 20th century the percentage of Africans who are Christian increased from
about 10 to almost 50% and the percentage of Africans who are Muslim increased
from about 32 to 42%. We also noted the precipitous rise since the 1970s in the
share of African Christians who are Pentecostal. An enormous body of scholarship on religion in Africa identifies a variety of factors driving these changes.
Missionary efforts throughout the 19th and 20th centuries established hospitals and schools, providing potential converts with both practical and spiritual
motivations to join (Hastings 1996, 2000; Isichei 1995; Ward 1999). The more
recent rise of Pentecostalism is frequently attributed to its focus on healing and
emphasis on women's spiritual gifts. For many, Pentecostal identity provides
them with membership in a global community, whose local network is typically
English-speaking and upwardly mobile (Cox 1994, 2001; Jenkins 2006 Maxwell
2007; Meyer 2004). The question is: is AIDS now among the factors driving religious change in Africa?

Historically, epidemics have triggered substantial changes in religion and religious behavior. Building on general accounts of the social effects of epidemics (Zinsser 1934/2007; McNeil 1977/1998), Stark (1996) and Reff (2005) show how rapid and large-scale conversion to Christianity both in Europe (Rome and Gaul) and the Americas followed closely on the heels of massive plague-driven mortality. They cast epidemics as the primary motor driving the popularization of Christianity.

Yet conversion—and, through conversion, the rise of new religions—is arguably the most extreme religious consequence of plague. The repeated cycles of epidemics within Christendom throughout the medieval and early modern era triggered other types of religious change. Some of these can be found in changing forms of religious expression. As prayer across the major religions slowly developed from a "rudimentary form with short and sparse formulae and chants of a magico-religious nature" (Mauss 1909/2003: 23) into more complicated types of divine solicitations, prayers for protection from illness and hardship became increasingly common.[2] In Catholicism and certain Sufi traditions in Islam, these prayers often called for the intercession of saints, especially saints associated with healing (Schurman Taylor 1998). In Protestantism and more orthodox forms of Islam, prayers were addressed to God directly (Rittgers 2007). Across traditions, prayers for protection were neither fully private nor restricted to churches and mosques. They were often performed publicly in penitential processions, and their frequency increased as epidemics took hold (see Rittgers for an example).

Evidence of other plague-inspired changes can be found in the increasing popularity of peripheral factions within major religious traditions and in the frequency of religious violence. The Black Death, for example—the initial and most destructive wave of the Second Plague Pandemic—dramatically increased the popularity of radical peripheral groups within the Catholic Church such as the Flagellants. This movement first gained popular traction in Italy (Perugia) after a prior plague (Cohn 1970: 128). During the Black Death, it rapidly spread north into German-speaking areas, and it was violently suppressed by papal authorities in the years that followed.

Reflecting a plague-driven crisis of confidence in religious institutions, the Black Death also created the environment in which new anticlerical groups emerged. One notable example is the Lollards in England, who were responsible for the murder of priests, monks, and even the Archbishop of Canterbury (Rex 2002: 50) in the decades following the plague. In this vein, an even more notable case of plague-driven frustration with institutionalized religious responses occurred during the Plague of Moscow in 1771. In an effort to stem the transmission of the virus, the Orthodox archbishop Amvrosii prohibited popular burial practices that involved washing and kissing the dead. Surrounded by mounting deaths that, to paraphrase Stark (1996: 74), "swamped their explanatory and comforting capacities" (20–30% of Moscow's population died that year), the crowds became so incensed that they battered the archbishop to death (Hays 2005: 164).[3]

The big question for us is this: is there evidence that AIDS is effecting changes in the African religious landscape along any of these lines? We do not refer here to some of the more extreme types of violence such as the development of masochistic cults or murder of clerics. (Indeed, during the decade we have been working on this topic, we have seen no evidence of either.) Rather, we focus on the more general types of religious change: changes in religious expression, changes in religiosity, and denominational shifts.

We have already provided ample evidence of signs of change related to religious expression. Chapters 5 and 7 describe new types of religious expression that give an increasingly prominent place to sexual behavior, in some congregations at least. Our discussions of non-ABC strategies in Chapter 7—the promotion of early marriage, the growing acceptability of divorce, and messages about abstaining from alcohol and curbing materialistic desires—may not be completely new but nonetheless reflect a critical level of change within religious discourses. Likewise, Chapters 8 and 9 demonstrate that some congregations, particularly within the Christian tradition, have been emphasizing and supporting social welfare activities as a religious duty.

But how about religious change more generally? For example, does intense exposure to AIDS—a person's own infection or infection of a loved one—make someone become more or less religious? Does it make them more likely to move from one congregation to another, from one denomination to another, or to convert from one religious tradition to another? And on a more macro level, are there signs that certain types of congregations—perhaps those with more developed social surveillance or welfare systems—are becoming increasingly attractive? That they are growing because of AIDS?

There are two reasons for us to expect only minimal religious change in response to AIDS in SSA. First, although the cumulative mortality and suffering associated with AIDS is high, its total social and economic impact is modest relative to that of the premodern epidemics to which AIDS has repeatedly, and misleadingly, been compared. Major epidemics in history include those caused by smallpox, such as the Antonine (165–180 CE) and Cyprian Plagues (251–270 CE), and repeated cycles of Bubonic plague, from the Plague of Justinian (541–542) to the Second Plague Pandemic, which opened with the Black Death (1338–1351 CE) and lasted until the 1770s. Each of these sent up to 50% of the total population to their graves within days of infection (Benedictow 2006; Hays 2005).

Second, as discussed in Chapter 3, the unique features of HIV make the AIDS epidemic very different from others. Even in the absence of antiretroviral therapies (ART), people live for about 10 years after being infected. Unlike the (virtually) instantaneous mortality effects of earlier plagues, the mortality toll of AIDS on communities reflects this approximately 10-year lag; this is one of the reasons that even countries in the heart of the AIDS belt still have growing populations. Third, unlike the historical plagues, AIDS mortality is patterned by age and gender. It is concentrated in certain age groups, though these vary somewhat for men and for women. And finally, since people on the ground rank AIDS much lower on their list of problems than other things like poverty and access to development infrastructure (again, see Chapter 3), its less than central position in people's daily lives suggests that AIDS may not be salient enough to trigger dramatic religious change.

On the other hand, a number of factors lead us to expect important, if modest, religious changes to have resulted from AIDS. The main one is the context of religious change in general: in particular, religious freedoms of the modern era make religious shifts and conversions much easier. As noted in Chapter 2, this is particularly true of Christian areas of SSA, which have an extremely diverse religious market place (Grimm 2010). New churches frequently open and close. New streams of Christianity have been developed locally (African Independent Churches [AICs]) or imported and then Africanized to varying degrees (various evangelical movements). New and old forms of religious expression are syncretizing in new ways. Within African Islam, these trends are somewhat more limited, though one can see it playing out in shifting affiliations between older (typically Africanized) and newer (typically reformist/Salafist, de-Africanizing) traditions.

Another reason for expecting AIDS to have triggered broader religious change is related to the specific mechanisms that link the experience of plague with religious changes. Synthesizing the historical literature on the effects of epidemics on the rise of Christianity in Rome, Stark (1996: 74–75) suggests that three mechanisms were at work. The first, to which we have already referred, was that the epidemics "swamped the explanatory and comforting capacities" of existing religious philosophies, prompting a search for new ones. The second was that "Christian values of love and charity had . . . been translated into norms of social service and community solidarity." This meant that when plagues struck, Christians were encouraged to care for the sick rather than *cede mox, recede longe, redi tarde* (flee fast, flee far, return late), the traditional response (Rittgers 2007: 133). The result is that Christians had "substantially higher rates of survival," which both increased their number directly and also attracted converts (Stark 1996: 74).[4] The third mechanism worked through the effects of high mortality on social connections: it left "large numbers of people without the interpersonal attachments that had previously bound them to the conventional moral order." In other words, the deaths of family and friends allowed survivors to forge new associational ties, including with countercultural groups—Christians in Stark's example.[5]

At least two of these three mechanisms intuitively fit the SSA setting. The main one is related to Stark's (1996) second mechanism: the "norms of social service and community solidarity." As shown in Chapter 9, on aggregate, these are much more developed in Christian congregations than in Muslim ones. This points to at least one reason that Muslims or the religiously unaffiliated might be attracted to some form of Christianity or that members of one low-welfare Christian congregation may switch to a high-care alternative. Also related to this mechanism is differential survival. Here the key difference is much less Christian–Muslim than "safe sect" versus "non-safe sect." Chapter 7 describes the combination of strategies associated with the lowest levels of HIV prevalence. Not only will these communities continue to grow because they bear a lighter share of the mortality burden, but also the relative health of these communities ("fitness" in evolutionary terms) may attract converts, another source of growth.

While conducting fieldwork in Malawi, we heard recurring narratives suggesting that AIDS is having these types of effects on religion. One such narrative is about a married man who, like his friends, is a womanizer. After seeing many of those friends die from AIDS and AIDS-related diseases, he realizes that he must change his ways if he is to avoid the same fate. The man tries to be faithful to his wife but has little success resisting temptation. All the while he struggles with tremendous guilt and worry—he honestly does not want to hurt his wife, whom he loves, or their children. At last, realizing that he cannot resist temptation on his own, the man joins a Seventh-Day Adventist community. He had heard that the Seventh-Day leader is vigilant and that other parishioners do not tolerate movious men. Several years later, the narrative continues, this man is happy and healthy, married and faithful to his wife, and strong enough, with the support of God and the church (his new social network), to resist the temptation of all the beautiful women around him. His spiritual testimony involves praising God that he repented his womanizing ways in time to escape the fate that had befallen many of his friends.[6]

Another common narrative that we heard is about a woman, often a Presbyterian who attends religious services now and again. She grows tired of her husband's wandering ways. She talks with her friends and neighbors about their AIDS-related worries and notices that the women in her village who appear the least worried about being infected by their husbands attend a new Pentecostal congregation that seems to be growing rapidly. All of the Pentecostal husbands have quit drinking. They are spending more time at home in the evenings and less time wandering around the trading centers, where they are likely to find drinking partners and, subsequently, sex partners. The woman begins attending prayer meetings with her Pentecostal friends and after several weeks convinces her husband that they should go together. The church appears to them to be "spirit filled." That is, other members' lives appear to be filled with the health and wealth that, according to church leaders, follow from being faithful to God's blessings. The couple joins. He, like the other husband, changes his ways. And like the other wives, her anxiety about infection plummets. They live happy and healthy lives together.

A number of common themes emerge in these narratives. One is that men and women invoke religious change, including the types of denominational shifting that places them in a safer social pool, as a strategy for avoiding HIV infection. Another one is related to the role that church-centered networks play in the provision of care and support for those already infected and for their families. This could arise for moral reasons: they want to associate with selfless people because they think that selflessness is good. It could equally arise out of more selfish, instrumental reasons—a type of "When I die, I want my family to have that kind of support."[7]

The underlying narrative in all these cases, however, is that religion is an important resource for both men and women, and it is not a fixed resource. People have considerable freedom to choose their religion, or at least their congregation. And within their chosen congregation, people have agency in determining their level of involvement. In some religions they also have some freedom to generate new types of religious expression, either within existing churches (e.g., born-again evangelical fellowships within mainline churches) or in new ones. We think that AIDS is affecting these choices. In particular, it might be fostering growth within congregations that appear to be the most insulated from AIDS and that have the most developed social welfare systems.

We distilled the overarching question about whether AIDS is driving religious change into two sets of empirical questions. First, does exposure to the effects of AIDS at a given time make someone more likely to shift from one denomination or religion to another during a subsequent time period? Second, does exposure to the effects of AIDS at a given time drive people to deepen their religious commitments during a subsequent time period?

The particular model that we're imagining for a religiously diverse SSA setting is represented in Figure 10.1. A type of "decision tree," it reflects a short sequence of decisions that precedes intentional behavior—in this case increasing religiosity or switching religions. We are not assuming that people openly and deliberately follow this type of decision-making sequence. Rather, as a conceptual tool, this approach helps us distinguish one stage of decision making from another and consider the constraints on decisions made at each point in the sequence.

The primary question at the base of this decision tree is, "Do I need a religious change?" It has two possible answers—yes and no. If "yes" there are three options. The first is to change the level of religiosity within one's existing congregation, which includes joining a new or existing fellowship or becoming "born again" (more on that in a bit). The second is to switch congregations but remain within one's larger denomination or, in our categorization, group of churches, including moving from one AIC congregation to another. The third option is a

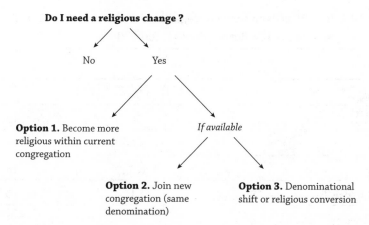

Figure 10.1 Typology of changes in religion or religious behavior that may stem from experience with, or concerns about, AIDS.

denominational change or religious conversion. For the sake of simplicity we treat these three options as mutually exclusive, though in practice an individual may pursue two or three types of religious change simultaneously. We also note that choosing among them is contingent on a number of other factors that are summarized in the "if available" clause. For example, a person may want to switch denominations but may live too far away from any others. Or he may want more opportunities to demonstrate his religiosity (e.g., with more frequent collective prayer or Bible study) but is unable to within his current denomination.

If there is an effect of AIDS on religion, it should be detectable along one of these three dimensions. For example, individuals who have been more exposed to AIDS deaths or who are more worried about their prospects of infection may be more likely to increase their religiosity or make a denominational switch. AIDS might affect these decisions in relation to the types of congregations or denominations that switchers choose to join. Contingent on having decided to make a switch, it should be to a congregation that is (seen to be) more protective against HIV infection than one that is seen to do little.

Congregational and Denominational Shifting

To answer questions about denominational switching, we looked at Malawi Diffusion and Ideational Change Project (MDICP) data on religious affiliation in the five years preceding data collection. We had collected a full listing of all denominations and congregation to which each person had belonged at any time during that period. Of the 1267 women in the sample, 186 (~15%) answered in the affirmative (with significant variation across villages). Some of them had made more than one transition, yielding a total of 225 transitions.

Table 10.1 **Reasons Given for Congregational and Denominational Shifts among MDICP Respondents (1999–2004)**

Reason	%	N
Marriage	42.2	95
Too Much Conflict	8.4	19
Too Strict	8.0	18
Other	8.0	18
Convinced by Family	7.1	16
Convinced by Friends	5.8	13
Too Far	5.3	12
Prefer Lessons	5.3	12
Perceived Miracles	2.7	6
Wanted Spirit-Filled Church	2.7	6
Too Liberal	2.2	5
Wanted Healing	0.9	2
Don't Know	0.9	2
AIDS	0.4	1

Source: MDICP-3, 2004.

Table 10.1 presents basic data on the reasons given for each of these transitions. Of the 225 moving episodes, only 1 was explicitly related to AIDS. Others that we could easily place under the AIDS-related umbrella were also relatively infrequent: two were related to wanting healing, five to claims that the congregation of origin was too liberal, and six to the attraction of perceived miracles in the new congregation. Of course, it is possible to connect some of the other reasons to AIDS (e.g., marriage, too much conflict).[8] But the overall point is that, at least superficially, these data do not support the hypothesis that AIDS is driving large-scale denominational shifts or migrations in conscious ways. If there is an effect, it is either peripheral or more surreptitious.

On the other hand, there are clearly denominational winners and losers in the MDICP research sites. This can be seen in Table 10.2. The first column shows the overall religious breakdown of the sample across major religious group as of 2004. The second shows the religious composition for people who have belonged to the same congregation since their birth. The third shows the religious breakdown of the 408 individuals who had moved from one church to another

Table 10.2 **Religious Affiliation for Lifetime Members and Recent Converts in Malawi**

	Lifetime Members	Converted between 1999 and 2004	Difference
Catholic	19.0	15.0	−4.0
Mission Protestant	21.9	15.7	−6.2
Pentecostal	7.2	20.8	13.6
African Independent Church	15.0	24.0	9.0
Muslim	27.2	6.9	−20.3
New Mission Protestant	9.8	17.7	7.9
N	2768	408	

Source: MDICP-3, 2004.

in the preceding five years. The big winners here are the Pentecostal and AIC congregations. They account for 25% of the sample in 2004 but 45% of all recent converts. Seventh-Day Adventists and Jehovah's Witnesses, though numerically much thinner on the ground, also attract a lot more converts than their initial numbers suggest. Finally, Islam is much less attractive to denominational switchers, though to some extent this may be an artifact of larger religious divisions between Christianity and Islam. It is a more radical step to move from, say, the Catholic Church to Islam than to an AIC.

To what extent is AIDS driving these changes? Beyond tabulating main motives for switching, we identified the characteristics of these denominational shifters in a more systematic way, focusing on both general characteristics such as age, education, and wealth and a number of AIDS-related characteristics. We ran parallel regression analyses on two types of shifting. The first compared the characteristics of the 408 individuals who moved denomination or religion with the 2468 who did not. The second compared the characteristics of the individuals who moved to a Pentecostal or African Indigenous Church (the big winners in Table 10.2) with those who switched to one of the other five traditions.[9]

So what are the characteristics of switchers? A first set of models—comparing the converts with those who stayed in their same religion—shows that other than the fact that they are more likely to be less than 30 years of age there is nothing special about them. They are no more or no less educated or wealthy. In the second set of models—comparing those who moved to a Pentecostal or African Indigenous Church with those who joined a different religion—we see that those who join Pentecostal or AIC congregations are poorer and are also most likely to be in their late 20s.

Somewhat more surprising, no indicator of people's exposure to AIDS or concerns about catching it themselves is significantly associated with denominational switching. For example, during the first wave of the 1998 survey we asked people to estimate the number of people they think have died from AIDS in the area. We also asked them how worried they are about catching AIDS. Neither of these was associated with denominational shifting between 1999 and 2004. In the 2001 wave of the MDICP, we repeated these two questions and asked two new ones: Respondents were asked to estimate the number of people in the area who they thought had died from AIDS in last year and who had become sick with AIDS in the last year. In the 2004 wave, we added more questions. One asked respondents to report the number of siblings with HIV. Another asked about the number of deaths in the household over the last three years. *Not a single one* of these variables—which we think are decent indicators of exposure to AIDS-related mortality or concern about one's own chances of becoming infected—was associated with either of the two types of denominational switching that we identify here: any movement from one denomination to another or, more specifically, moving to a Pentecostal or AIC congregation.[10]

Analyses of the kinds of congregations that converts join are more illuminating. First, as a very rough measure of congregational support for people living with HIV and AIDS (PLWHA), we examined the proportion of members who reported visiting the sick during the past month. As mentioned in Chapter 9, about 24% of MDICP respondents reported having done this in the past month. But this practice is not evenly distributed across congregations: in some congregations ($N = 35$) no members report visiting the sick, whereas in others ($N = 45$) upward of 50% of members say they did this recently. Consistent with our theory that social-service congregations may attract converts, we found that while nonconverts belong to congregations where, on average 23% visit the sick, converts join congregations where the average is 29% (this difference of six percentage points is statistically significant). In other words, there is some evidence that people who change religious congregations are joining congregations in which *more people* are actively engaged with supporting infected members of their community.

The congregational approaches to HIV prevention we describe in Chapter 7 shed additional light on our question about which kinds of congregations attract new members. Table 10.3 compares the distribution of lifetime members to that of converts. If prevention approaches are not driving religious switching, the distribution of these two groups should be nearly identical. We find, however, that converts are proportionally overrepresented in two main categories (the rightmost column of the table): in "moral" only congregations (Mfdb) and in faith healing only congregations (mFdb). They are also marginally overrepresented in congregations where moral approaches are combined with faith healing (MFdb) and in congregations where moral and faith healing are combined with biomedical approaches (MFdB). Conversely, converts are proportionally underrepresented by seven percentage

Table 10.3 **Distribution of Converts and Nonconverts by Congregational Approach to HIV Prevention**

Congregational Prevention Approach	Lifetime Members (%)	Converts (%)	Difference
MFDB	10.8	2.9	−7.8
MFDb	7.4	7.1	−0.2
MFdB	3.9	6.1	2.1
MFdb	13.8	15.6	1.8
MfDB	3.9	4.6	0.6
MfDb	7.9	7.1	−0.8
MfdB	2.2	2.7	0.4
Mfdb	20.0	25.9	5.9
mFDB	0.4	0.5	0.1
mFDb	3.8	1.9	−1.8
mFdb	4.5	8.5	3.9
mfDB	3.2	1.7	−1.5
mfDb	1.8	1.9	0.1
mfdB	2.5	3.1	0.6
mfdb	13.2	9.8	−3.4
Total (%)	100	100	
Total (*N*)	2769	408	

Source: MDICP-3, 2004 and MRP 2005.

points in the "do everything group" (MFDB) and by three percentage points in the "no prevention activities" congregations. We interpret this as evidence that congregational approaches to prevention—particularly the moral and faith healing—act as a magnetic force that attracts religious switchers, even if those switchers do not articulate anything AIDS-related as a primary reason for making this change.

Changing Religiosity

How about religiosity? Does exposure to the effects of AIDS make people more religious within their existing denomination or religious tradition? Does it deepen their religious commitments by arousing a desire to become "born again"?

Our survey data provide suggestive evidence that this is the case. Table 10.4 shows simple cross-tabs on changes in religiosity between waves (2001 to 2004) by HIV status for men and for women. Since there are very few HIV positive cases in this analytical subsample (35 men and 93 women), cell sizes are small, and differences between cells are not statistically significant in any of the combinations seen here. Still, interpreted cautiously and in combination with our qualitative data from in-depth interviews and ethnographic journals, the cross-tabs suggest that people are changing religiously in response to AIDS and that men and women do so differently. While HIV-positive men are less likely than HIV-negative men (14% vs. 22%) to have decreased their reported religious attendance between waves, the opposite is true for women. A full 31% of HIV-positive women reported a decline in religious involvement between 2001 and 2004 compared with 24% of HIV-negative women. For both men and for women, a higher proportion of HIV-positive individuals reported switching religious congregations during the past five years.

More systematic analyses about exposure to AIDS or concerns about becoming infected do not point in this direction. We analyzed two indicators of religiosity: the frequency of church or mosque attendance; and the intensity of other religious activities, including choir, elder's meetings, Bible/Koran study, prayer meetings, visiting the sick, revival meetings, and evangelical work. In each case we looked at the relationship between these two indicators and the same indicators of exposure to AIDS that we used in the analysis of denominational shifting. Measured in the 2001 wave of the MDICP, these included the number of people they thought had died from AIDS in the area in total and in the last year; the number who had become sick from AIDS in the last year; and

Table 10.4 **Changes in Religious Attendance and Congregation for Malawian Men and Women between 2001 and 2004 by HIV Status (%)**

	Men		Women	
	HIV Negative	*HIV Positive*	*HIV Negative*	*HIV Positive*
Decreased Attendance	22	14	24	31
Stable Attendance	57	66	5	48
Increased Attendance	21	20	23	20
Same Congregation	94	92	91	8
Switched Congregation	6	8	9	12
N	511	34	914	93

Sources: Linked MDICP-2, 2001; MDICP-3, 2004.

how worried they were about catching AIDS. We found no significant relationships between any of these indicators of exposure to AIDS and either measure of religiosity.

We also looked at the relationship between exposure to AIDS and becoming "born again," one of the strategies the Malawians—especially "those seeking support for resisting temptations that might bring them death" (Watkins 2004: 687)—employed to avoid infection during the early years of the epidemic. Much has been written about being born again in SSA (e.g., Dijk 1998; Meyer 2004; Prince 2009). We do not describe the process in detail here except to mention that becoming born again is a public commitment of faith that can take place simultaneously with conversion or represent a renewed commitment to religious life within one's tradition of origin (i.e., without conversion or a denominational shift). Because of its public nature, becoming born again provides an extensive spiritual support network including prayer and practical support that Watkins describes as a "defensive 'wall' against outside evil forces" (Watkins: 687). While normally understood as a specifically Christian phenomenon (with origins in Jesus' infamous exchange with Nicodemus in John 3), in Malawi there is an equivalent for Muslims known as "making tauba."[11] As shown in Table 10.5, the prevalence of born-agains cuts across religious traditions in the Malawian context.

We used the MDICP data from 2004 to examine both the prevalence of born-again status (including making tauba among Muslims) and the timing of these events in each of the study's three research sites. Though the three sites are represented about equally in the MDICP, the levels of adult HIV prevalence vary across them: 9% in Balaka, 7% in Mchinji, and 5% in Rumphi. In the four panels of Figure 10.2, each bar represents the *number* of MDICP respondents who

Table 10.5 **Prevalence of Born-Agains by Religious Tradition in Rural Malawi**

Religious Tradition	% Born Again
Catholic	20
Mission Protestant	27
Pentecostal	40
African Independent Church	18
Muslim (*made Tauba*)	25
New Mission Protestant	27
N	3190

Source: MDICP-3, 2004.

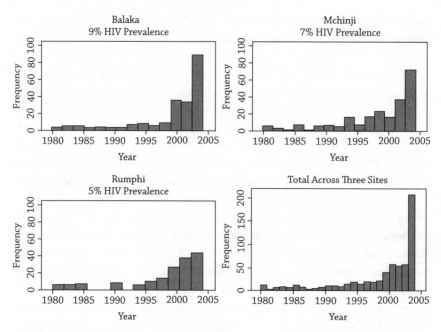

Figure 10.2   Timeline of Born Again Phenomena in Three Malawian Districts
   Source: MDICP, 2004

became born again *during that year*. We see clearly that the born again trend began to take off in the late 1990s, just as AIDS was becoming visible, with sharp increases visible between 2000 and 2004, arguably the peak years of AIDS-related mortality. Cumulatively, we find that the born again trend is proportional to the severity of the AIDS epidemic in the three MDICP sites—it is highest in Balaka and lowest in Rumphi—which further suggests that these two phenomena are linked.

Summary

The AIDS epidemic has brought important changes in how people think about and behave with regard to sex and relationships. We argued here that AIDS is also having an effect on various dimensions of religious life in SSA. While some of these changes are stark (e.g., the increased emphasis on sexual morality within religious teachings), others are more modest.

This inquiry is set against a backdrop of the broader religious changes under way in Malawi and throughout the subcontinent. The most dramatic of these is the marked growth among Pentecostal and AIC congregations and declines within the Catholic and Mission Protestant traditions. It is not difficult to see why these

Pentecostal and AIC congregations are attractive. The unique features that turn these groups into "winners" in the current religious economy are their strict moral code, extensive social support systems, and emphasis on spiritual gifts and healing. All of these are directly relevant to the challenges that accompany AIDS.

We believe that AIDS is among the forces behind these broader changes, even if two factors make its influence on religious change a hard thing to detect at the individual level. First, in examining the changing religious commitments of individuals, we are limited by the relatively short time span of our data. They are long enough to detect rapid, dramatic change but too short to measure subtler effects. Second, we know that religious change is often motivated by a variety of factors and that people vary in their ability to articulate their "true" motivations for any type of behavior or behavior change (Vaisey 2009). Consistent with these insights, we find very few individuals explicitly mentioning "AIDS" or anything AIDS-related as the motivation for their change, even while a substantial proportion of people are changing religion or level of religiosity. However, it is clear that the Pentecostal and AIC churches in general are the most popular destinations, as are congregations emphasizing moral or faith-healing messages about AIDS. Given AIDS's heavy presence in this setting, we doubt that these choices are merely coincidental—that they have nothing to do with AIDS. On the contrary, we see AIDS as a source of additional momentum for this movement.

Examined at supra-individual levels, AIDS's effects on religious life become clearer. At the congregational level, we find both that congregations that are actively engaged in providing social support to PLWHA and those that pursue particular prevention approaches are disproportionately "destination" congregations—that is, they are growing by winning converts (not only by differential mortality and higher fertility). Together this suggests that the AIDS-related activities of specific congregations are part of their appeal to individuals who make religious changes. Moreover, our ecological analyses show that the spread of the born-again phenomenon in Malawi tracks closely with the spread of HIV in rural communities and also matches the severity of the AIDS epidemic in terms of its scale.

Overall, these measurable religious changes are proportional to the scale of the epidemic both in terms of their magnitude and their pace. While the full empirical story of how AIDS is changing SSA's religious landscape will play out over the next several decades, it is clear that this ball is already in play. In SSA, religion affects AIDS. And AIDS has also begun to affect religion.

CONCLUSIONS

Scholars, be cautious with your words for you may incur the penalty
of exile and be banished to a place of evil waters.

—Pirkei Avot *1 v.11*

We began this book with an admittedly ambitious goal: to provide a definitive
empirical account of the relationship between religion and AIDS in sub-Saharan
Africa (SSA). Historical accounts of the role of religion in times of plague, from
the Roman era through the early modern period, provided a fitting backdrop for
this task. All highlight the relevance of religion to Horden's (1999: 49) useful
distinction between the two types of "management" epidemics demand: they
need to be understood, or managed conceptually; and they solicit a response, or
need to be managed practically.

Both conventional wisdom about the role of religion and our own initial
observations from fieldwork in Kenya and Malawi earlier in the AIDS epidemic motivated many of our initial questions. Using a variety of data
sources, we began by identifying religious patterns in HIV prevalence, relevant sexual behavior, and subjective assessments of risk. But we quickly
moved beyond these more traditional epidemiological questions, finding ourselves drawn toward questions about the ways religion imbues the African
AIDS epidemic with meaning, shapes local interpretations of AIDS, and
structures societal responses. Religion's role in how African families and societies have been organizing to meet the needs of an increasing number of
infected individuals and their survivors became a central part of our inquiry.
This, in turn, raised questions about how AIDS is affecting the contours of
religious life in SSA.

To characterize the relationship between religion and AIDS both in broad
strokes and in sufficiently rich detail, we conducted hundreds of interviews with
religious leaders and lay people in Malawi, compared observations from religious services with conversations about AIDS in a variety of other social settings, and drew upon thousands of data points from surveys carried out across
SSA. Throughout, we systematically moved back and forth between analytic

levels, examining relationships among individuals and organizations, with a particular focus on congregations—our key mesolevel vantage point. In this concluding chapter we summarize some of the key patterns we identified in the relationship between AIDS and religion in SSA, elaborating those we deem particularly pertinent for understanding AIDS' pathway in SSA until now and its future prospects on the continent.

Patterns of Prevalence

It is not news that both sexual behavior and HIV prevalence are patterned religiously, but the specific religious contours that we show have not been previously documented. Among them:

- No single religious group appears to be either consistently prone to, or protected from, infection across national contexts.
- A person's religiosity trumps their denominational affiliation as a predictor of sexual behavior and HIV status.
- The overall religious climate of a setting also shapes sexual behavior and HIV status; that is, it alters the relationship between personal religiosity and these outcomes.

These are important findings. They show that religion primarily shapes patterns of HIV infection below the radar of standard analytic approaches. For example, it matters much less whether someone is Protestant, Catholic, or Muslim than how religious they are, how religious is the setting in which they live, and the characteristics of the congregation they attend. Overall this confirms that, at least in terms of its effects, religion is as much an attribute of communities as of individuals. It also suggests that moving beyond broad denominational distinctions is essential for developing convincing empirical and theoretical accounts of how religion matters for other types of social change. Examples include other types of health-related behavior (e.g., child vaccinations, use of family planning), the adoption of new ideas (e.g., gender equality, democratic values) or new technologies (e.g., new seeds, fertilizers, investment opportunities), and behavior in general. In all of these, the general religious climate associated with congregations and communities may matter more than the specific religious identities of individuals.

Moral Talk

We have also shown how religion structures the way that people think and talk about AIDS. Again, on a superficial level there is nothing surprising here. Because AIDS in SSA is about sex, suffering, death, and the struggles of survivors, it provides fertile ground for moralizing narratives. Yet our analysis of the specific moral content of religious messages and contours of the moral debates about AIDS has yielded three unexpected insights.

First, while Christian and Muslim notions of sexual morality in SSA have much in common with their counterparts across the globe, they are also unique in some important ways. Our discussion of abstinence (the first of the ABCs) in Chapter 5 provides a very clear example. We emphasized the "newness" of the very concept in SSA, given the historical backdrop of working childhood, late puberty, early marriage, and early childbearing. We also showed that instrumental messages about abstinence are far more pervasive than religious ones. In other words, abstinence messages are not about a return to "traditional values"; historically speaking, male monogamy and female virginity have seldom been prioritized within most African cultures. Rather, prevention messages more frequently promote abstinence with the promise that it offers a pathway to success in the modern world. Narrowly religious ideas merely provide extra support for this view. Likewise, despite their efforts to promote abstinence among the unmarried members of their congregations or fidelity among the married, most African religious leaders recognize that nonmarital sex is a fact of life and that, therefore, abstinence cannot be the sole basis of HIV prevention efforts. This is why leaders tend to be flexible on the condom question, on marital dissolution, and on other non-ABC approaches to prevention discussed in Chapter 6. Put somewhat differently, leaders' moral preferences are shaped by typically religious ideas about sexual morality. But their actual approaches to prevention also reflect a leaning toward more realistic risk-reduction models that are far more acceptable to their constituencies and to the reality of daily life in their communities.

Second, moral debates about AIDS extend far beyond the realm of sexual behavior. As we show in Chapters 7, 8, and 9, AIDS has given rise to a range of ethical dilemmas, each of which gives rise to religious teachings, if not directives. AIDS-related teachings address when and what type of person to marry, what constitutes reasonable grounds for divorce, how to treat people living with HIV and AIDS (PLWHA), how much of an obligation we have to care for the sick or to take responsibility for orphans—both kin and nonkin. Moralizing discourses about AIDS therefore touch on fundamental building blocks of society: how families and communities are constituted. And religion plays a central role in directing this discourse. In this sense, Binet's (1617/1995) depiction of plagues as a "mistress of virtue" (referenced in the introduction) is still tremendously salient. Far from being tightly circumscribed by sex (with the successful avoidance of infection interpreted as a sign of virtue), the AIDS epidemic cultivates virtue by providing the healthy with ample opportunities to share Godly love with the sick and dying. And in the eyes of many believers, this rather than chastity is *real* religion.

Third, the moralizing narratives about AIDS that center on ideas about God's judgment and punishment provide a clear example of how individuals and communities make sense of death and disease experienced on such a large scale. As discussed in Chapter 3, the stochastic features of HIV transmission mean that despite the now widely recognized patterns in prevalence and mortality, there is a tremendous amount of unexplained variation. People see many cases where a friend, known to have been abstinent until marriage and faithful since, becomes infected. Likewise, others who engage in stereotypically risky behaviors—they are frequently drunk and have multiple sex partners—often show no signs of the disease. In such a context, spiritual explanations make at least as much sense as biomedical ones, especially given that ideas of blind luck and random chance are less widely believed in SSA than in the West. And although Christianity and Islam do not have a monopoly on spiritual explanations—narratives about witchcraft and sorcery are also common—they are the principal players in the interpretive marketplace. For example, to the extent that Christian and Muslim leaders assert that AIDS is a punishment, they clarify that this punishment is directed at communities and not at specific individuals. They also embed this general argument about AIDS in universal teachings about the origins of evil, the meaning of suffering, the consequences of sin, and the opportunity for salvation and redemption.

Official versus Local Responses

Another theme emerging from our analyses is the distance between official positions and local ones, with respect to AIDS-related narratives, positions, and behavior. Official narratives and positions have been highly visible on the international scene. Some of these belong to the "bad guys." Examples include Thabo Mbeki's denial of a syndrome caused by a virus, the Vatican's inflexibility on the issue of condoms, and Uganda's shift away from condoms toward abstinence and fidelity as the cornerstone of its prevention policy. Other official positions and narratives, which represent no less of an official position on AIDS than those of national or religious leaders, belong to the "good guys." Examples here include exaggerated pronouncements about the effects of AIDS by UNAIDS or various nongovernmental organizations (NGOs). In articles and op-eds in both professional publications (e.g., the *Lancet* and *New England Journal of Medicine*) and in the mainstream quality press (e.g., the *New York Times*, the *Washington Post,* and the *Guardian* in the United Kingdom), both types of official position are commonly referenced, though the good guys' narratives are seldom critiqued. The best journalists writing in the best newspapers, such as Sharon La Franiere and Nicholas Kristof in the *New York Times* and Sarah Boseley in the *Guardian*, illustrate the effects of these official positions with carefully selected stories that are poignant and emotive. They pull at our heartstrings. We absorb the narrative. We all know who the good guys and bad guys are.

There is nothing new about dramatizing the story of AIDS in these Manichean terms. Social science has long described how generally accepted ideas about particular social groups, aspects of society, or ideas themselves are generated or "socially constructed." The problem in this case is that the official construction of AIDS in SSA has, with some notable exceptions, largely ignored local interpretations of these issues and local behavioral responses to the underlying problems. We think that this is a terrible mistake. Official positions and narratives certainly comprise part of the story of AIDS. They are also easy to locate and to digest; researchers, activists, journalists, and the like can usually download the reports and read the press releases in English without leaving their desks. But local responses to AIDS are the most relevant to the daily lives of the individuals and communities affected by the virus. By overlooking them completely or by using carefully selected stories to illustrate their effect—for "carefully selected," read "unrepresentative"—the focus on official positions misrepresents AIDS and its effects in general. It also constitutes a significant obstacle to understanding the relationship between religion and AIDS in particular.

Our discussion of condoms provides a particularly clear example of the perils of this disproportionate focus on official narratives. Much has been said about organized religion as a barrier to condom use and therefore an obstacle in the fight against AIDS. Our findings counter this view. It is certainly true that condom use remains remarkably low across SSA, in spite of significant efforts to promote their use through "social marketing" programs. But contrary to popular discourse among Western opinion leaders, religious leaders are not to blame. Doctrinaire opposition to condoms is the exception rather than the rule. In general, religious leaders' positions on condoms are far more nuanced than the popular portrayals suggest. Most do not forbid condom use. They simply treat condoms as an imperfect solution to the reality of the epidemic—imperfect not only because leaders fear that condom promotion may encourage sexual immorality and provide a false sense of security but also because they know (often firsthand) that condoms diminish sexual pleasure and impede fertility (Green 2011; Meyer-Weitz, Reddy, Weijts, van den Borne, and Kok 1998; Tavory and Swidler 2009). In fact, a sizable minority of African religious leaders actually promotes the use of condoms among members of their congregations to the point that they sometimes distribute condoms themselves; this is especially common in the highest-prevalence countries and areas, including in Catholic churches.

Where doctrinaire religious opposition to condoms exists, tensions between that official opposition and actual local responses can easily be found, and they matter. After all, if people in Italy, Spain, or Portugal—where fertility levels are among the lowest in the world in spite of official Catholic opposition to all forms of modern contraception—ignore their religious leaders, why should we assume that people in SSA are any more likely to listen to *their* religious leaders? People in SSA have repeatedly demonstrated that they can resist a range of authoritative discourses, including those backed by coercive power (Comaroff and Comaroff 1997; Scott 1998). Surely, then, they can just as easily ignore bad advice about condoms. In short, the decision to use or not use condoms has much less to do with religion and the directives of national political or religious leaders than with more immediate, situational and relationship-specific concerns. In fact, our sense is that the positions of local religious leaders on condoms—and other aspects of AIDS—are more strongly shaped by local popular opinion than by the official positions of their national or international denominational leaders. Still, the argument that generalized religious opposition to condoms is facilitating the spread of HIV continues to pass as conventional wisdom.

Overall, our decision to differentiate official from local discourses reflects our view of congregational life as the key locus of religious interaction in Africa. Understandings of AIDS develop in congregations—through official teachings and weekly messages, through informal interactions among congregation members, and through interactions between members and leaders. Congregations are also among the primary spaces in which the legitimacy of various approaches to prevention is negotiated and established. We showed strong empirical support for this in our analyses of variation in four types of prevention approaches (Chapter 7). The particular combinations of approaches different congregations employ do not align neatly under denominational umbrellas. Rather, with respect to their approaches to HIV prevention, we find greater heterogeneity within most religious traditions than across them. This underscores the fact that religious leaders and congregational bodies have a great deal of autonomy in how they approach AIDS and that they are influenced by multiple sources in the course of determining their approach. Only one of these is the top-down denominational structure.[1]

The Welfare Gap

Despite the remarkable similarities among Christian blocs and between Christians and Muslims in most aspects of HIV prevalence, understandings of AIDS, and approaches to prevention, there is one important area in which Christian–Muslim differences stand out. The differences between Christians and Muslims in the care of those infected with HIV and those indirectly affected by it are highly significant. We think that these differences have important implications for the health of communities and their religious futures.

We discussed in Chapter 9 how Christian models of care have always, since the early Church, been extrafamilial, focused on a community of believers that transcends kinship ties. In terms of its general discourse, Islam shares this focus on a universal community of believers (the *umma*). But as economic historian Kuran (2010) notes, that general discourse has not translated into larger types of social organization in most Muslim societies. Rather, kinship ties—in particular those associated with unilineal family systems—have remained the predominant type of social bond. The result is a much weaker tradition of nonfamilial congregational care in Islam than in Christianity, a fact that several of our Muslim cleric respondents acknowledged themselves.

This welfare gap between Christians and Muslims in SSA has a wide range of implications. Some of these are directly related to AIDS. Muslims with HIV are less likely to receive assistance from nonfamily members than their Christian counterparts. We argued in Chapter 8 that this relative absence of congregational models of care in African Islam is also one of the causes of the higher levels of AIDS-related stigma we observe among Muslims in SSA—they have much less contact with HIV-positive individuals. Irrespective of this relationship to stigma, the welfare gap suggests that day-to-day life may be far worse for HIV-positive Muslims than for HIV-positive Christians.

The differences in these care practices matter for religious change in general, as argued in Chapter 10. We showed that there is more religious movement into congregations that have developed structures for providing care. In mixed Christian and Muslim communities where the pathways to conversion from one to the other are relatively open, we therefore expect to find that most religious movement involves conversion from Islam to Christianity and, more generally, movement from low welfare congregations to those with comparatively developed welfare systems.

The welfare gap has even broader implications. Putnam (2001) argues that trust (e.g., in neighbors or institutions) is the basis of a community's level of social capital. If either the practice of visiting the sick or the experience of being visited by a group of community members represents an established trust-engendering mechanism, then the sizable Christian–Muslim differences in these practices suggest that African Christianity has a much more salient role in the generation of social capital than does African Islam. It is not difficult to imagine how these differences in social capital would in turn affect patterns of development and change across a number of dimensions, only some of which are related to the struggle against AIDS. For example, the differences suggest that village development committees or local political groups and coalitions are less kin-centered in Christian villages than in their Muslim counterparts. They also hint at the existence of Christian–Muslim differences in the types of local political engagement. We do not know of any academic literature that addresses these types of questions. But inferring macrolevel political outcomes from seemingly insignificant microlevel behavior—in this case, visiting the sick—is consistent with standard sociological approaches to social change (Collins 1981).

There are signs that the historical welfare gap between Christianity and Islam is attenuating. In conversations with Muslim clerics and laypeople throughout Malawi, we found evidence that care groups are being established in Muslim communities. Many of these are explicitly modeled on Christian congregational approaches to care that Muslim leaders and laypeople have observed either in their own or in neighboring communities. Rumors about a Muslim orphanage in Blantyre looking specifically to take in young *Muslim* orphans are circulating within Malawi's rural Muslim communities. However, even if Muslim care groups are being established en masse right now, given that we are now 30 years into the epidemic, we would be very surprised to see meaningful convergence between Christians and Muslims on the caregiving dimension.

Into the Future

Forecasts and predictions about sub-Saharan African societies range from profoundly pessimistic to deeply optimistic. The relationship between AIDS and religion in SSA can be framed accordingly. On one side of the spectrum, we have representations of Africa as a continent filled with disease and death, suffering, and stagnation. These stories center on characters who unreflectively indulge in risk and unthinkingly do the bidding of their illiberal religious leaders. From this perspective, all positive change regarding AIDS, or anything else, is instigated by or at least dependent upon the whims of outsiders—the less religious the better. At the opposite end of the spectrum are representations of Africa as a continent of rapid growth and high potential. The African characters in these stories are skeptical of authority figures in general, whether public health officials, heads of NGOs, or religious leaders; they critically compare the recommendations of all of these leaders to the things that they see happening around them. In relation to AIDS in particular, these African characters and communities figure out how to minimize infection and collaborate in responding to suffering in creative and effective ways. They appreciate the complexity of the epidemic and see risk and prevention as being about much more than the regulation of sexual behavior.

The Africa we have come to know—and the one that emerges from the analyses throughout this book—is much closer to the optimistic representations. Religion in SSA has provided and continues to provide a pathway to thinking about AIDS and to responding to AIDS, both individually and communally. We have shown empirically that many religious approaches to AIDS—in particular those emphasizing what we have called moral lessons—reduce the risk of infection more effectively than anything that non-religious, biomedical approaches have to offer. Likewise, Christian congregations in particular are instrumental in reducing the burden of suffering among the sick and among their dependents. This, too, is accomplished with unambiguous moral messaging originating in religion.

We think these relationships between AIDS and religion will continue in the coming decades, despite the dramatic changes that we expect to see in SSA. It is useful to describe some of those changes, even briefly.

First, the relationships between AIDS and religion are situated within the particular demographic reality of the subcontinent—one of rapid and persistent population growth. In 1975, when the first AIDS deaths were being documented in Central Africa (albeit a few years before AIDS' public appearance on the scientific radar) and Pentecostalism was beginning its precipitous rise, approximately 416 million people lived in SSA. By 2050, SSA's population is projected to exceed 1.5 billion people (UNPD 2007).[2] In other words, the Africa in which AIDS and religion have coexisted thus far and in which they will continue to coexist in the coming decades, is not a place in demographic decline. On the contrary, although SSA has borne a disproportionate share of AIDS-related mortality and will continue to do so, overall population growth rates continue to exceed the world average, even in the highest prevalence countries on the continent and in the world (e.g., Botswana and Swaziland) (Ashford 2006). Despite AIDS, there is much more life than death in SSA. People will continue to use religion to celebrate this in addition to relying upon religion to soothe the suffering and lament the departed.

Second, the relationships between AIDS and religion will also continue as important changes in economic and political life unfold. These sorts of changes are both harder to predict and much more variable across countries. But several features are clear: all countries in SSA are becoming increasingly urban and increasingly middle class (e.g., white-collar professionals, some of whom have a postsecondary education). This increasingly educated subpopulation is drawn to different forms of religious expression and different types of congregations than past generations. The charismatic megachurches in West Africa's urban centers spreading quickly through the region and the global diaspora offer one notable example. These churches appeal to the sensibilities of the new urban middle class (Adogame and Spickard 2010; Akyeampong 2000; Dijk 2004). They also exhibit moral messages of the kind that underpin what we have shown to be the most effective prevention efforts. As both the proliferation and growth of these types of churches continues into the next few decades, we expect to find Africa's burgeoning middle classes to be drawn to the kinds of churches that reduce both the risk of transmission for individuals and the levels of suffering within their communities.

While we acknowledge the possibility that these changes may give rise to a nascent African secularism, we think that its magnitude and impact will be negligible. One reason is that we find it hard to imagine people in Africa, the world's most religious continent, irrevocably or substantially tearing at their own sacred canopy and following Europe's exceptionally secular lead. Much more likely is that any growth in African secularism—there are some indicators of secularization in South Africa, particularly among whites—will be marginal and limited to particular subpopulations. In other words, we think it will follow a more American or Latin American model, where increases in education, wealth, and opportunity have certainly brought about important religious changes but have not been associated with declining religion according to any standard measures.

Second, in the current economic and geopolitical climate, African states' capacity to deliver critical social services (the provision of AIDS-related services) will remain severely limited. There is virtually no chance that a series of strong state-sponsored programs will emerge and undercut the welfare functions of religion across SSA. Given poor revenue generating mechanisms and continued rapid growth in population, African states cannot afford to build or maintain the types of extensive welfare states that first emerged in late 19th century continental Europe. Furthermore, theories about how the state and state structures develop tell us that, even in the absence of severe economic constraints, strong welfare programs are unlikely to emerge in SSA. Compared with the role that the state plays in more developed secular societies with long political and cultural traditions of state-sponsored public services, African states will remain peripheral to AIDS reduction and mitigation efforts because they have no tradition of such activities. In all likelihood, most social welfare functions will remain in local hands: nuclear and extended families and other local institutions, with congregations and religious NGOs providing moral and material backup. We expect this to be the case irrespective of whether Africa's second democratic transition leads to the development of stable democratic governments.

The Last Word

The central empirical point of this book is that religion in Africa has affected AIDS and continues to affect it. Religion influences the way people think about AIDS, their risk of infection, the extent of their suffering, their access to support when infected, and their survivors' welfare. In fact, the magnitude of religious responses to AIDS in terms of prevention efforts and the provision of spiritual, emotional, and practical support for PLWHA is such that without this support, the toll of AIDS on communities in SSA would be infinitely worse.

The central theoretical point of the book is that these influences work much less through individuals than through congregations. The primary social action, in other words, takes place at the mesolevel. It may be affected by the characteristics of individuals or denominations, but it is primarily relational and situational. Religious institutions provide spaces where people can intentionally hang out; where they can talk, watch, and listen; where they can go to learn but also have influence. Religious institutions, in other words, are spaces in which social learning, cultural innovation, and cultural transmission take place. Of course, this insight is not specific to AIDS; congregational spaces facilitate discussion and learning about dozens of other issues as well. But the case of AIDS illustrates these processes in tangible ways. In the SSA context it would be hard to overstate the importance of religious spaces for the dissemination of relevant information and the constitution of new strategies for HIV prevention and AIDS mitigation.

The central public policy message of the book is perhaps the simplest. In SSA, the most effective efforts to reduce the transmission of HIV and to mitigate its effects on families and communities contain a substantial moral component. This should not surprise us. Successful public health interventions in the West have had this same moral dimension, and they *have* changed both behavior and underlying cultural ideas. Today, only bad parents hit their kids—good parents are expected to make them wear bike helmets and buckle up in cars. Today, only bad men hit their wives—good men do the dishes and feel comfortable taking care of the kids. Only bad people drive drunk or smoke in enclosed areas. The list could go on. Our point here is that while the moral dimension of Western public health efforts draws from a liberal secular ethic, in many other parts of the world the moral component draws much more heavily on religion. This is certainly true in SSA.

We recognize that this religious-moral component is off-putting to committed secularists. But we are convinced that ignoring it because it seems antiquated or politically incorrect or because it causes us intellectual or moral discomfort will lead us down the wrong path. It will inevitably push us toward irresponsibly biased social science and public health research that, in turn, will generate interventions built on little more than shifting sands. AIDS deserves better. With millions dead and tens of millions infected, it demands that we give people, including those in Africa, more autonomy to manage AIDS with their own conceptual and practical tools. In Africa, religion is one those tools. In many cases it is a highly effective one. Responsible scholars, policymakers, and journalists alike should recognize and leverage these religious contributions as readily they have denied or ignored them in the past.

LIST OF APPENDICES

Appendix A

DATA SOURCES AND METHODS

This book draws upon a multitude of data sources, which vary tremendously in scope and type. In the following pages, we provide a brief overview of how the data for these studies were collected.

Demographic and Health Surveys

Freely available at: http://www.measuredhs.com

For cross-national analyses of denominational differences in AIDS-related phenomena, we rely heavily on Demographic and Health Surveys (DHS). The DHS are nationally representative household surveys that provide data for a wide range of monitoring and impact evaluation indicators in the areas of population, health, and nutrition. The DHS program is an enormous, worldwide endeavor that has fielded more than 200 surveys in over 75 countries. Standard DHS have large sample sizes (usually between 5,000 and 15,000 households) and are typically conducted every 5 years to allow comparisons over time. The surveys cover a wide range of topics including (but not limited to) family planning, HIV knowledge, attitudes, and behavior, HIV prevalence, and household and respondent characteristics.

Within sub-Saharan Africa (SSA), the DHS has fielded surveys in more than 40 countries. Data on religious affiliation are collected in most of these, though each survey uses a different set of response categories for the question "What religion are you?" We standardized categories of religious affiliation across countries to make these surveys as comparable as possible. Typically, we examine differences in outcomes like HIV prevalence (a percent), years of education (average), and level of knowledge about HIV (a standardized scale). In all cases, we conducted our analyses with and without a set of statistical controls to account for the sociodemographic characteristics that sometimes obscure or exaggerate the actual relationship. In most cases we decided to present only the crude bivariate statistics for ease of interpretation and because more rigorous analyses with statistical controls did not meaningfully alter the relationships we observed. In cases where more nuanced descriptions and interpretations were in order, these are noted in the text and elaborated upon in the appendices that follow.

The strengths of the DHS data for our purposes are obvious: coverage in over two dozen countries; large sample sizes; and the use of standardized questions that are almost always comparable across countries. We are, however, limited by the fact that the DHS asks only one question about religion in its surveys, and an admittedly crude one at that—in some countries (like Zambia), the categories are limited to Christian, Muslim, and Animist. For our cross national-analyses, we made methodological decisions in the analyses and presentation of DHS data that have important consequences for the claims in this book. In deciding what information to present, we are limited to the countries in which the questions were asked. For example, questions measuring knowledge about AIDS and stigma were not asked in all countries. Some countries are excluded on that basis. Second, to make statements about religious differences, we focus our presentation and discussion on the most religiously diverse countries in Africa. In Mali and Niger, for example, 98% of their populations are Muslim, which makes it impossible to make statements about differences across religious traditions.

The Malawi Diffusion and Ideational Change Project

The strongest sources of data for this study come from the Malawi Diffusion and Ideational Change Project (MDICP), which also is the project that initiated our interest in religion and AIDS and that launched our careers. The MDICP is a longitudinal household survey conducted in three distinctive districts of Malawi, one in each of the three regions of the country: Rumphi District, located in the northern region; Mchinji District, located in the central region; and Balaka District, located in the southern region. The sampling strategy for the MDICP was not designed to be representative of the national population of rural Malawi, although the sample characteristics closely match the characteristics of the rural population of the nationally representative Malawi Demographic and Health Survey. The target sample for the first MDICP wave was 500 ever-married women age 15–49 in each of the three districts, plus their husbands. The third survey wave added a sample of approximately 400 adolescents age 15–29 in each district. More detailed information on the sampling strategies employed in the

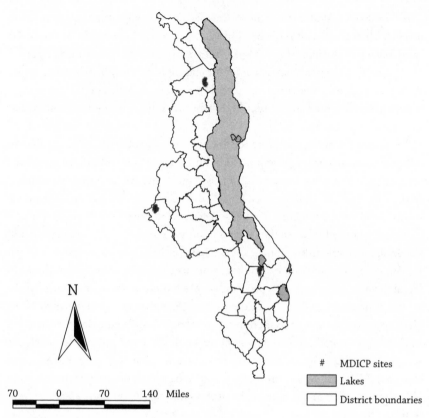

Figure A.1: Map of Three MDICP Research Sites

MDICP is available from the Social Networks website (http://www.malawi.pop.
upenn.edu/).

The first two waves of the MDICP (carried out in 1998 and 2001) focused on
two key empirical questions: the role of social interaction in (1) the acceptance
(or rejection) of modern contraceptive methods and of smaller ideal family size;
and (2) the diffusion of knowledge of AIDS symptoms and transmission mechanisms and the evaluation of acceptable strategies of protection against AIDS.
Beginning with the third wave in 2004, the MDICP expanded in several direc-
tions, including an inventory of beliefs and attitudes about HIV and expanded
religion component—which includes more refined measures of religious affiliation than are available in any other comparable data set, as well as detailed information on religious beliefs and practices. The unique availability of detailed
information on religious beliefs and practices, as well as specific questions about
attitudes toward and interactions with people living with AIDS, makes the
MDICP-3 the ideal data source for exploring the research questions guiding this
study.

The Malawi Diffusion and Ideational Change Project has been funded by the National Institute of Child Health and Human Development (NICHD), grants R01-HD37276, R01-HD044228-01, R01-HD050142, R01-HD/MH-41713-0. The MDICP has also been funded by the Rockefeller Foundation, grant RF-99009#199. The MDICP received ethical approval from institutional review boards at the University of Pennsylvania and the University of Malawi. The project is under the codirection of Drs. Susan Watkins, Jere Behrman, and Hans Peter Kohler. Much of the MDICP data is freely available online (http://www.malawi.pop.upenn.edu/index.html).

Malawi Religion Project

The Malawi Religion Project (MRP) was a multimethod sister project to the MDICP, designed to collect data on religious organizations to examine how these organizations and their "moral communities" influence responses to the epidemic. In 2005, the MRP successfully surveyed the leaders of all the religious congregations respondents interviewed by the third wave of the MDICP reported attending. Each leader was administered a 12-page questionnaire focusing on key aspects of congregational and village life, including AIDS-related issues and problems. The MRP survey data provide a basic numeric description of rural congregations, for example, the *characteristics of the organization* (e.g., number, gender and age composition of the membership, the governance of the congregation, sources of income) and questions about the *impact of AIDS* on the congregation (e.g., estimates of AIDS-related deaths among members, estimates of the burdens of care for orphans and the sick by congregation members). Finally, the MRP asked congregational leaders a battery of questions on AIDS-related attitudes and behavior that were also included in the regular MDICP-3 questionnaire to compare the leaders' views with the characteristics and attitudes of their congregants. In the end, the MRP attempted to collect data from a total of 200 congregations and successfully collected data from 187.[1]

In addition to gathering the perspective of religious leaders, the MRP conducted in-depth interviews with laywomen, MDICP respondents, randomly selecting women to proportionally represent the congregations they attend. The ability to compare leader responses to the perspective of laypersons is another valuable dimension of these data that we use throughout our analyses.

The MRP, funded by the National Institute of Child Health and Human Development, was directed by Susan Watkins, Alexander Weinreb, Mark Regnerus, and Jenny Trinitapoli. More information about the MRP can be obtained online (http://www.malawi.pop.upenn.edu/Level%203/Malawi/level3_malawi_qual-religion.htm).

Linked MRP–MDICP Data Set

The congregational data collected by the MRP in 2005 were then linked to the wealth of individual data collected by the MDICP 2004 (e.g., the respondent's, or the congregation member's, economic status, experience with the death of relatives from AIDS). We used 2004 reports of congregation name, leader's name, congregation village/location, respondent's village, and religious tradition to link the records of individual respondents to the characteristics of their congregation.

Protecting the Next Generation: Understanding HIV Risk among Youth

From 2003 to 2005, researchers at the Guttmacher Institute, in collaboration with in-country partners, fielded an ambitious study that aimed to understand the sexual risk behaviors of youth in SSA. Working in four countries (Burkina Faso, Malawi, Ghana, and Uganda), they collected four distinct types of data, three of which we used here:

1. Focus group discussions (conducted in early 2003; 14–19-year-olds, urban–rural areas, in school and out of school): Transcripts, summary of methodology, and guidelines are available online.
2. In-depth interviews (conducted in late 2003; 12–19-year-olds, urban–rural areas, in school and out of school): Guidelines and summary of methodology are available online.
3. National Survey of Adolescents (conducted in early 2004; 12–19 year olds, household-based sample): Burkina Faso (N = 6489), Ghana (N = 9445), Malawi (N = 7750), and Uganda (N = 6659). Household and adolescent questionnaires are available online. Survey instruments are in English and local languages.

This project was supported by the Bill & Melinda Gates Foundation, the Rockefeller Foundation, and the U.S. National Institute of Child Health and Human Development (grant no. 5 R24 HD043610). Additional information is available online (http://www.guttmacher.org/pubs/PNG-data.html)

World Values Survey

The World Values Survey (WVS) is a worldwide network of social scientists studying changing values and their impact on social and political life. The WVS has carried out representative national surveys in 97 societies containing almost 90% of the world's population. These surveys show pervasive changes in what people want out of life and what they believe. To monitor these changes, the WVS has executed five waves of surveys from 1981 to 2007.

During the 1999–2004 round of data collection, the WVS drew representative samples from 11 countries in SSA. In addition to the affiliation measures available from other surveys, the WVS asked more detailed questions about religious involvement (e.g., church attendance and participation), religiosity (e.g., religious salience), and theological orientation. The WVS methodology consists of the administration of detailed questionnaires in face-to-face interviews. The questionnaires from all five waves (including the incomplete 2005–2006 wave) can be viewed in full on the WVS website (http://www.worldvaluessurvey.org/). Each national team is responsible for its own expenses, and most surveys are financed by local scientific foundations. However, central funding has been obtained in cases where local funding is not possible. The WVS Secretariat is chaired by Ronald Inglehart at the Institute for Social Research at the University of Michigan.

Afrobarometer

Globalbarometer Surveys (GBS) is a comprehensive effort to measure, at a mass level, the current social, political, and economic atmosphere around the world. It provides an independent, nonpartisan, multidisciplinary view of public opinion on a range of policy-relevant issues. Data are available for 55 countries, including 18 African countries that together constitute the Afrobarometer wing of the project. Survey data are gathered via face-to-face interviews by trained interviewers in the language of the respondent's choice. In each country, Afrobarometer relies on national probability samples that represent an accurate cross section of the voting age population. The sample is stratified to ensure that all major demographic segments of the population are covered. Sample size varies from a minimum of 1200 in each country to up to 2400 or more. Afrobarometer data is publicly available online (http://www.afrobarometer.org).

The World Christian Database

The World Christian Database (WCD) provides religious adherence data on 232 world countries and 13,000 ethnolinguistic peoples. The WCD is an initiative of the Center for the Study of Global Christianity at Gordon-Conwell Theological Seminary and is edited by Todd M. Johnson. Religious adherence data in the WCD are drawn from field surveys, statistical questionnaires, interviews, and correspondence with church leaders, census reports, and a range of other sources. Estimates of atheism and agnosticism are also reported in these data. Hsu et al. (2008) found that the World Christian Database's religious adherence estimates were highly correlated with several other major religious adherence data sources, such as the CIA World Factbook and the World Values Survey. They also found some evidence that the World Christian Database reports higher Christian percentage estimates than do other data sources and that it occasionally underestimates Muslim percentages.

Data from Interviews with Senegalese Religious Leaders

In-depth interview data with 87 religious leaders (Muslim, Catholic, and Protestant) from three regions of Senegal were generously shared by David Ansari, who collected these data while on a Fulbright fellowship in Senegal in 2007–2008. These interviews were part of a study investigating the perceptions religious leaders concerning HIV/AIDS as well as sexual health education. The discussions concerned HIV/AIDS-related knowledge broadly, with a focus on questions concerning HIV prevention, stigma, care for HIV positive individuals, and advice for serodiscordant couples. Respondents were recruited through religious organizations concerned with HIV/AIDS (e.g., Jamra and SIDA Service), nongovernmental organizations that worked with religious leaders (e.g., Africa Consultants International and Enda Santé), as well as district and regional offices of the national AIDS program (CNLS) and Ministry of Health. Ansari conducted the interviews in French or in Wolof or Pulaar with the help of a translator.

For more information concerning this research on Senegalese religious leaders' perceptions, please see Ansari's recent publication in *Culture, Health and Sexuality*. Ansari is currently with the Health, Community and Development research program at the Institute of Social Psychology in the London School of Economics.

A NOTE ON AIDS METRICS

We begin by clarifying some key measurement issues. Sociologists, epidemiologists, and other social scientists use several different terms or metrics when studying HIV as an outcome. Common ones include *HIV status*, an *HIV infection*, the *infection rate*, and *HIV prevalence*—the last is the standard measure of the proportion of the population currently infected.

None of these measures is intrinsically better than another. But since each tells us something different, it is important to be clear about the meaning of each one. Much of the imprecision in writing about AIDS stems from misuse of these terms: confusing the infection rate with prevalence is perhaps the most common.

HIV status refers to whether a person is either HIV positive or HIV negative.[1] It is a dichotomous state related to an individual.

An HIV infection is slightly different. Unlike HIV status, which tells us whether a person is positive or negative at a single point in time, an HIV infection should be thought of as a change in HIV status that occurs at a particular point in time. For example, Mary, a 29-year-old respondent in our Malawi study, tested negative for HIV when we interviewed her in 2004. However, when we interviewed her again two years later, she tested positive. Scholars sometimes refer to this change in HIV status as a *seroconversion*—the act of changing from negative to positive. Knowing the time of infection provides scholars with the best chance of figuring out causal patterns. The problem is that, to know when infection occurred, scholars need to follow a sample of individuals over time. This demands special longitudinal data that include repeated collection of biomarker data from the same individuals. Since such data are expensive and time-consuming to collect, they are also rare.

Infection rates or incidence is an aggregate of all new HIV infections. That is, infection rates tell us the number of seroconversions (i.e., new cases of HIV infection) occurring to a group at-risk of infection (i.e., every sexually active person) over a set period of time (demographers and epidemiologists typically measure the latter in terms of *person-years* or *person-months* at risk). Statements about infection rates are among the most error-laden, not only because accurate estimates require the same type of data that from which estimates of HIV infections are derived but also because of confusion between the terms *incidence* and *prevalence*.

HIV prevalence is the most commonly used statistic in the general social science literature on AIDS—a precedent that we follow in this book. Prevalence tells us what percentage of a population (typically adults between the ages of 15 and 49) has HIV at a given point in time. It is frequently used to describe countries (e.g., HIV prevalence in Uganda has been hovering around 6% for the past 10 years) or characterize them in relation to the burden of AIDS (e.g., high-prevalence and low-prevalence countries). Smaller geographical units like villages and districts also have HIV prevalence, as can populations defined by a shared characteristic like age, gender, or religious affiliation (e.g., HIV prevalence for women 15–24 in Kenya is estimated at 10%). For years, in the absence of universal HIV testing, scholars used data from antenatal clinics (pregnant women) or other subpopulations (e.g., army conscripts) to create estimates of HIV prevalence in general populations. Over the last decade it has become clear to all that the models used to extrapolate general prevalence data from these self-selective samples were flawed and almost always overestimated prevalence (Timberg 2006). Consequently, the current gold standard for measuring HIV prevalence requires the collection of biomarker data from a random probability or *population-based* sample.

The principal appeal of HIV prevalence as a metric is that it provides a straightforward snapshot of the burden of HIV in a given place or group. In contrast, data on infection rates or incidence tell us only how many people are becoming infected. The principal flaw of HIV prevalence as a metric—aside from the difficulty of counting all HIV-positive people—is that it can be a somewhat misleading measure in times of change. It is important to understand this since we refer to prevalence data widely throughout this book.

HIV prevalence is measured as a simple percentage, where the numerator is the "number of people of a given age who are HIV positive," and the denominator is the "total number of people in the same given age." Given this, it is clear that HIV prevalence goes up as the numerator increases. The problem is that this increase can occur for two quite different reasons. One is that more individuals become infected—that is, there is an increase in the infection rate, which means that more people are being added to the HIV-positive population than are leaving it though death. The other is that already infected individuals are living longer even though infection rates are stable or even if they are falling themselves. This phenomenon of rising HIV prevalence is exactly what has occurred in Botswana over the last few years. Even while the rate of infection in Botswana appears to have come down, an effective antiretroviral therapy (ART) program has kept more people alive (Stover, Fidzani, Molomo, Moeti, and Musuka 2008). Likewise, as ART is scaled up in other high-prevalence countries in Africa, we will almost certainly see this phenomenon replicating itself. Indeed, one of the underacknowledged ironies of contemporary HIV treatment policy is that it will increase overall HIV prevalence.

There is also a flipside to this weakness: HIV prevalence falls as the numerator shrinks. This, too, can be caused by a couple of things. The first is a reduction in the rate of infection, causing fewer people to join the ranks of the HIV positive. The second is that people who are infected with HIV die relatively quickly. This appears to have been part of the story behind the precipitous pre-ART decline in Uganda's HIV prevalence during the late 1990s.[2] Even with these problems, HIV prevalence is by far the most widely used indicator of AIDS burden in the social science literature.

Appendix C

Percent of Population Believing Most or All Leaders Are Corrupt (versus None/Few)

	President	Elected Leaders	Government Officials	Police	Border Officials	Judges and Magistrates	Local Businessmen	Foreign Businessmen	Teachers	Religious Leaders	Nongovernmental Organizations
Botswana	26	30	33	31	34	21	38	53	17	15	24
Ghana	11	17	29	60	59	43	29	23	16	11	11
Kenya	9	17	32	62	47	32	22	24	14	6	16
Lesotho	17	22	34	33	39	21	23	32	15	11	18
Malawi	44	44	56	56	65	45	44	51	31	23	37
Mali	44	45	52	61	74	63	60	60	26	16	31
Mozambique	21	26	30	51	48	27	31	46	34	21	25
Namibia	17	24	32	38	31	25	23	30	26	18	25

Nigeria	52	56	58	71	63	47	40	38	30	19	29
Senegal	20	27	36	48	56	40	42	37	13	8	20
South Africa	15	25	30	40	38	18	26	38	18	11	21
Tanzania	17	25	31	51	48	35	24	28	9	5	15
Uganda	35	31	52	70	59	43	23	26	14	5	16
Zambia	22	26	32	52	46	32	31	34	22	8	14
Zimbabwe	32	27	43	47	NA	24	56	50	16	10	18
TOTAL	26	31	39	52	50	35	32	35	20	12	21

Source: Afrobarometer, Round 2 (2002–2004).

Appendix D

Percent Religiously Unaffiliated

	% No Religion	N
Benin, 2006	5	23,066
Burkina Faso, 2003	2	16,080
Cameroon, 2004	5	15,897
Chad, 2004	2	7,968
Congo (Brazzaville), 2005	9	10,185
Democratic Republic of Congo, 2007	2	14,743
Cote D'Ivoire, 2005	5	10,645
Ethiopia, 2005	—	20,097
Gabon, 2000	11	8,166
Ghana, 2003	6	10,703
Guinea, 2005	2	11,128
Kenya, 2004	3	11,762
Lesotho, 2004	2	9,880
Liberia, 2007	3	13,004
Madagascar, 2003	9	10,266
Malawi, 2004	1	14,953
Mali, 2006	3	18,689
Mozambique, 2003	—	12,764

	% No Religion	*N*
Namibia	2	13,684
Nigeria, 2003	—	9,958
Niger, 2003	<1	12,728
Rwanda, 2005	1	16,071
Senegal, 2005	—	10,405
Swaziland, 2006	11	9,138
Tanzania, 2004	9	12,959
Uganda, 2006	—	11,028
Zambia, 2005	—	9,786
Zimbabwe, 2005	—	16,082

Note: "—"means zero cases.

Source: African Demographic and Health Surveys.

Individual and Community-Level Predictors of HIV-Positive Status in Malawi

	Women		Men	
	Model 1	*Model 2*	*Model 3*	*Model 4*
Intercept	.00***	.00***	.00***	.00***
Age	1.31***	1.32***	1.40***	1.40***
Age Squared	.99***	.99***	1.00***	1.00***
Value of Livestock (logged)	.99†	.99	.93***	.94***
Secondary Education	1.18	1.18	1.00	.99
Previously Married	2.11***	2.11***	2.56***	2.61***
Total Number of Partners	1.12***	1.08***	1.03***	1.03***
Suspect Partner Unfaithful	1.36***	1.46***	.92	.95
Social Desirability	.89***	.86***	.95	.95
Attendance at Religious Services	.90*	.86***	1.10†	1.14*
Pentecostal	1.31*	1.38**	.93	.86
New Mission Protestant	.36***	.39***	.58***	.58***
African Independent Church	1.34**	1.38***	.55***	.56***
Mission Protestant	1.21†	1.32**	1.02	.99
Muslim	1.24*	.84†	.71***	.65***
Respondent Sick	2.12***	2.20***	NA	NA

	Women		Men	
	Model 1	*Model 2*	*Model 3*	*Model 4*
Village Size	—	1.02***	—	1.00
Average Age in Village	—	.96***	—	1.04***
Proportion Male	—	2.52*	—	.94
Village Religiosity	—	.53***	—	1.36†
Village * Individual Religiosity	—	.44***	—	2.09**
N	1387	1387	1039	1039

Notes: Odds ratios from logistic regression procedure. Denominational coefficients are compared with Catholics.

† p < .10.

* p < .05.

**p < .01.

***p < .001.

Individual and Community-Level Predictors of Recent Extramarital Partner in Malawi

	Women		Men	
	Model 1	*Model 2*	*Model 3*	*Model 4*
Intercept	1.13	.89	.52*	.48**
Age	.89***	.91***	.90***	.90***
Age Squared	1.00†	1.00	1.00***	1.00***
Value of Livestock (logged)	1.13***	.93***	1.01	1.02†
Secondary Education	1.53***	1.59***	1.34***	1.35***
Previously Married	1.56***	1.61***	.58***	.58***
Suspect Partner Unfaithful	1.34***	1.26***	1.25*	1.23*
Social Desirability	1.12***	1.14***	1.03	1.03
Attendance at Religious Services	.77***	.81***	.83***	.85**
Pentecostal	.33***	.31***	1.67***	1.81***
New Mission Protestant	.76*	.67***	1.14	1.18
African Independent Church	.34***	.14***	1.20	1.22***
Mission Protestant	.69***	.67***	1.57***	1.65***
Muslim	1.62***	2.25***	1.86***	1.99***
Respondent Sick	.78***	.77*	NA	NA
Village Size	—	.99***	—	1.00

	Women		Men	
	Model 1	*Model 2*	*Model 3*	*Model 4*
Average Age in Village	—	.96***	—	.94***
Proportion Male	—	.18***	—	.20***
Village Religiosity	—	1.99***	—	.61***
Village * Individual Religiosity	—	.84	—	1.51†
N	1387	1387	1039	1039

Notes: Odds ratios from logistic regression procedure. Denominational coefficients are compared with Catholics.

† p < .10.

* p < .05.

** p < .01.

*** p < .001.

Descriptive Overview of Malawi Religion Project Congregations

	Mean	Std. Dev.	Min	Max
Denomination				
Catholic	0.11	0.32	0	1
Pentecostal	0.17	0.38	0	1
African Independent Church	0.20	0.40	0	1
Muslim	0.12	0.32	0	1
Mission Protestant	0.21	0.41	0	1
New Mission Protestant	0.18	0.39	0	1
Congregational Demographics				
Congregation Size	37.39	52.81	0	370
Congregation Age (in years)	22.12	19.79	1	91
Leader Has at Least Some Secondary Education	0.29	0.45	0	1
Leader Some Religious Training	0.63	0.48	0	1
Network Ties				
Helped by Nongovernmental Organization	0.13	0.34	0	1
Ever Visited by Missionaries	0.37	0.48	0	1
Helped by Mission Work	0.24	0.43	0	1
Ever Visited by Denominational Leaders	0.65	0.48	0	1

	Mean	Std. Dev.	Min	Max
Sexual Culture				
Rampant Unfaithfulness in Congregation	0.16	0.37	0	1
Rampant Teenage Promiscuity	0.16	0.37	0	1
AIDS				
Leader Attended AIDS Workshop	0.47	0.50	0	1
In this congregation, AIDS is:	1.77	0.96	0	3
Not a problem	10.75	—	—	—
Somewhat of a problem	27.42	—	—	—
A big problem	36.02	—	—	—
Single biggest problem	25.81	—	—	—

Note: N = 187.
Source: MRP 2005.

Accompanying Details for QCA Analysis (Figure 7.1)

	Catholic	Mission Protestant	Pentecostal	African Independent Churches	Muslim	New Mission Protestant
MFDB	1	0	1	0	3	0
MFDb	0	6	0	3	1	2
MFdB	2	1	3	1	1	1
MFdb	4	13	6	7	1	1
MfDB	0	3	1	8	1	1
MfDb	2	4	2	2	6	1
MfdB	0	1	1	2	2	0
Mfdb	5	6	2	7	1	19
mFDB	0	1	1	0	0	1
mFDb	2	0	1	0	0	2
mFdb	0	2	10	1	1	0
mfDB	0	0	1	0	2	0
mfDb	1	0	0	0	0	0
mfdB	1	0	0	1	0	1
mfdb	3	3	3	6	3	5
N	21	40	32	38	22	34

Source: MRP 2005.

Predictors of Stigma and Caregiving in Malawi

	Model 1: Support for HIV+ Teacher	Model 2: Visited the Sick
Female	−0.43***	0.53***
	(0.09)	(0.10)
Age	0.00	0.02***
	(0.00)	(0.00)
Livestock (Quartiles)	0.13**	0.01
	(0.04)	(0.04)
AIDS Deaths (Quartiles)	0.10*	0.04
	(0.04)	(0.05)
Attendance (0–3)	0.01	0.79***
	(0.07)	(0.09)
Denomination (vs. Catholic)		
Pentecostal	-0.00	-0.01
	(0.24)	(0.19)
African Independent Church	−0.11	0.06
	(0.21)	(0.15)
Mission Protestant	0.08	0.00
	(0.22)	(0.15)
Muslim	−0.59**	−1.68***
	(0.22)	(0.20)
New Mission Protestant	0.15	0.47**
	(0.23)	(0.17)
Religious Leader Attended AIDS Workshop	−0.10	0.08
	(0.14)	(0.10)

(*continued*)

	Model 1: Support for HIV+ Teacher	Model 2: Visited the Sick
Religious Leader Thinks Movious Got What They Deserved	−0.36*	−0.02
	(0.17)	(0.13)
Religion Network Partners	0.11*	0.03
	−(0.05)	(0.05)
AIDS Network Partners	0.10*	0.11**
	−(0.04)	(0.04)
Support for Teachers	—	−0.00
		(0.12)
Constant	0.91*	−4.52***
	−(0.37)	(0.39)
N	3087	2877

Note: Coefficients and standard errors from logistic regression procedures.

* $p < .05$.

**$p < .01$.

***$p < .001$.

Source: MDICP-3 (2004) and MRP (2005).

Summary of Orphan Prevalence

	Year	*% Nonorphans*	*% Maternal Orphans*	*% Paternal Orphans*	*% Double-Orphans*	*N*
Benin	2006	93.14	1.97	4.35	0.54	46,879
Burkina	2003	93.56	1.64	4.12	0.68	32,707
Cameroon	2003	92.19	2.13	5.10	0.58	25,113
Chad	2004	91.27	2.36	5.21	1.16	15,658
Congo	2005	91.15	2.75	4.96	1.15	14,681
DRC	2007	90.91	2.57	5.41	1.11	25,344
Ethiopia	2005	90.96	2.44	5.59	1.01	34,465
Gabon	2000	95.10	1.72	2.87	0.31	14,957
Ghana	2008	92.50	2.05	4.85	0.60	21,504
Guinea	2005	93.52	1.55	4.00	0.93	19,402
Kenya	2003	90.50	1.67	6.15	1.67	18,556
Liberia	2007	93.04	2.03	4.14	0.79	18,001
Lesotho	2004	73.26	4.95	17.34	4.45	17,861
Madagascar	2008–09	94.11	1.96	3.58	0.35	18,693
Malawi	2004	85.67	3.20	8.07	3.06	31,313
Mali	2006	95.33	1.39	2.83	0.44	38,362
Mozambique	2003	88.15	3.09	7.24	1.15	32,424

(*continued*)

Appendix J

	Year	% Nonorphans	% Maternal Orphans	% Paternal Orphans	% Double-Orphans	N
Namibia	2004	83.67	4.89	9.23	2.21	18,812
Niger	2006	94.48	1.96	3.05	0.51	26,188
Nigeria	2008	94.26	1.70	3.66	0.39	76,560
Rwanda	2005	80.41	3.74	12.36	3.49	23,978
Senegal	2005	93.65	1.55	4.24	0.55	35,212
Swaziland	2006	78.00	5.66	12.48	3.86	10,661
Tanzania	2003	91.08	2.61	5.43	0.88	25,681
Uganda	2006	85.23	3.49	8.32	2.96	26,136
Zambia	2007	85.59	3.49	7.85	3.07	19,365
Zimbabwe	2005	77.30	4.24	12.82	5.64	21,567

Source: Demographic and Health Surveys.

NOTES

Introduction

1. Binet framed this in the opposite way, too, claiming that good health is "the purgatory of our virtues and the mistress of our vices" (Worcester 2007).
2. The existing study was the Malawi Diffusion and Ideational Change Project (MDICP), now called the Malawi Longitudinal Study of Families and Households (MLSFH). Details about this and other data sources can be found in Appendix A.
3. A detailed description of the Malawi Ethnographic Journals Project can be found in Watkins and Swidler (2009).
4. As a teaser we provide an answer to the last of these questions only. Having systematically observed nearly 200 different religious services from a wide variety of religious traditions in 2004, we can definitively say that there was no silence on AIDS in many churches and mosques across Malawi in 2004. Not only did 70% of religious leaders tell us that they preach about AIDS regularly, but also, in the religious services that we and our local collaborators observed, 30% contained explicit references to AIDS and an additional 10% contained general references to *illness* that those in attendance almost certainly interpreted as references to AIDS.
5. We are fans of fieldwork, which to some extent sets us apart from other survey-based researchers who have written about religion and AIDS in Africa. We've always preferred to organize our own data collection, not only for methodological reasons—being able to exert maximum control over the nitty-gritty details of data collection instruments, sampling, and staff, with actual observations acting as a natural check on empirically rootless theorizing—but also for purely fun ones. As romanticized as it sounds, it's enjoyable and energizing to get to know new places intimately, to identify latent patterns and structures in the company of other smart and curious people.
6. It may sound odd to refer to AIDS as "arguably" the most serious global health crisis of our time. But we think this is an accurate characterization. Even in low-income countries, AIDS-related mortality is lower than mortality associated with lower respiratory infections, diarrheal diseases, and coronary heart disease (WHO 2008). It is only in a few countries in the heart of the African AIDS-belt—we return to this in the next chapter—that AIDS can be reasonably considered "the" principal health crisis.

Chapter 1

1. Readers with limited knowledge about religion in Africa may wish to consult Isichei (1995), Hastings (1979, 1996, 1999), and Robinson (2004) for accessible and thorough historical accounts.
2. Resource flows for AIDS-related assistance may dwarf all other aspects of international development spending. Many of these flows are through completely new "financing instruments." The United States President's Emergency Plan for AIDS Relief (PEPFAR), for example, was established in 2004 and committed to spending US$15 billion over its first

five years. Its reauthorization in 2008—to run from 2009 to 2013—increased its budget to a maximum of US$48 billion and broadened its scope to coverage of malaria and tuberculosis in addition to HIV/AIDS. The Global Fund to Fight AIDS, Tuberculosis and Malaria—known simply as the Global Fund—was founded in 2002. ". . . From its founding through December 2009, the Global Fund Board approved proposals totaling US$19.2 billion, and disbursed US$10 billion for HIV, tuberculosis (TB) and malaria control efforts" (Global Fund 2010: 2). Likewise, in 2007 alone, the Bill and Melinda Gates Foundation disbursed US$1.2 billion through its Global Health mechanism and US$2.0 billion across all sectors (Gates Foundation 2007: 46). Since its establishment in 2000, the World Bank's Multicountry AIDS Program (MAP) has disbursed US$1.6 billion. And many other bilateral agencies have dedicated AIDS programs, only some of whose funds are run through multilateral programs.

3. We suspect that this was more serendipitous than intentional.

4. Afrobarometer Surveys, a relatively recent addition to the library of data on SSA, have been fielded in 18 countries in SSA. They are collected from nationally representative samples and ask about a large range of attitudes and behaviors.

5. We make extensive use of DHS data in this book. Briefly, since the late 1980s, DHS surveys have been administered to large, nationally representative samples in most African countries. Multiple rounds—once every four to five years—have been conducted in some countries. The instruments contain a large array of health-related questions but also data on basic sociodemographic characteristics, including religion. More on the DHS can be found in Appendix A.

Chapter 2

1. Cited in Worcester (2007: 47).

2. This may seem surprising. Indeed, to long-term Africa observers who are aware of the importance of religion in Africa, it is surprising, especially given the enormous amount of AIDS-related research that has been conducted in SSA over the last few decades.

3. See Appendix B for a more thorough discussion of the strengths and weaknesses of HIV prevalence as a metric for tracking the AIDS epidemic.

4. Religion and religiosity are not the only suspects here. Variation in national-level HIV prevalence has also been found to be a function of the patterns of marriage and fertility that characterize a country (Bongaarts 2007; Drain, Smith, Hughes, Halperin, and Holmes 2004), its number of prostitutes (Talbott 2007), life expectancy (Oster 2009), economic profile (Nattrass 2009), and medical infrastructure (Drain et al. 2004). In fact, overall, the literature on religion and AIDS is dwarfed by other parts of the AIDS literature.

5. Gray also suggests that ritual washing to improve "penile hygiene" may lessen the risk of transmission. We're skeptical. Muslims' ritual washing does not tend to go anywhere near the penis. Known as *wudu*, it's usually public, clothed, and focused on the head, hands, and feet. Even if it did include the penis, we have not found any empirical evidence to support the assertion that this is a protective mechanism against HIV infection.

6. This is evident at the bivariate level (shown in Pane 3 of Figure 2.1) and holds true net of controls for other factors.

7. As we will discuss at greater length in Chapter 6, compelling evidence that male circumcision reduces HIV transmission is the most plausible alternative hypothesis. Comparing HIV prevalence in countries where male circumcision is high (80% or more), medium (between 20 and 80%), and low (20% or less), we find dramatic differences. In countries where circumcision is widely practiced, HIV prevalence is around 3%. It is nearly four times as high in countries where male circumcision is rare. In multivariate models, controlling for the proportion circumcised explains away the observed association between prevalence of HIV and Muslims, which Gray published in 2004, suggesting this practice as the most plausible mechanism for his initial observations.

8. Some AICs were formed out of schism from Mission Protestant churches—whether out of conflict over the issue of polygamy or disagreements about the preservation of birth and death rituals that had been proscribed by missionaries. While other AICs were African-founded

in response to an unmet demand for Christian leadership, some AIC congregations were separatist. Others were not. Today, some AICs do—and some do not—allow polygamy.

9. In 2004, the MDICP tested for HIV using oral swabs. We used ORASURE saliva test to detect HIV; all positive results were subsequently confirmed using a western blot test on the same specimen. At the time, these tests fit the guidelines of the Malawian Ministry of Health. The MDICP HIV testing protocol was approved by IRBs in Malawi and the United States.

10. Because prevalence for religious "nones" is based on only 23 individuals, we are hesitant to read too much into the high level of HIV prevalence we observe in this group. Only if this finding were replicated across several studies would it be responsible to interpret this as if it were not just a statistical artifact.

11. This is counterintuitive at some level and is certainly contrary to the subtext of some public health messages. A thought experiment may help clarify. Imagine two women. Woman 1 has sex with a different partner every day for a year, but all her partners are HIV negative. Woman 2 has sex once with an HIV-positive partner. Woman 2's probability of contracting HIV is relatively low, but it is necessarily higher than Woman 1's since the latter's probability is zero.

12. HIV transmission is no different from many other diseases or conditions in this respect. Smoking, for example, is a strong risk factor for lung cancer, but we all know of people who defy those odds—they smoke half a century or more and end up dying from something else entirely. The point here is that the general cognitive frame that research in public health chooses to apply to all health-related cause–outcome relationships is one of individuals' control over their risks. We return to this more in our discussion of "self-efficacy" (Chapter 4). In parallel, an analytic focus on individuals as both (1) the sole locus of control and (2) physical objects on whom health outcomes can be measured is easy to implement in standard regression frameworks used to evaluate relationships among variables in contemporary social science. Later in this chapter, and in the following ones, we attempt to escape from the tight strictures of this methodological individualism by focusing on more relational and congregational factors that have, in some sense, a force of their own over and above any characteristics of the individual. In this, we are following an increasing number of researchers who seek to identify a range of supra-individual determinants of health-related behaviors (e.g., Cubbin, Santelli, Brindis, and Bravemen 2005; Entwisle, Casterline, and Hussein 1989; Glanz, Rimer, and Lewis 2002).

13. Many studies on other topics have found support for the moral communities thesis, whether measured as high collective religiosity or religious homogeneity (Breault 1986; Ellison, Burr, and McCall 1997; Pescosolido 1990; Pescosolido and Georgianna 1989; Stark and Bainbridge 1996; Stark, Kent, and Doyle 1982).

14. Our approach here makes an assumption that in SSA, villages remain the most relevant context for thinking about sexual behavior as it relates to HIV infection. Even though sexual networks often cross village boundaries, as do social networks in general, we think this is a reasonable assumption. Observational studies of day-to-day interaction show that for a large majority it tends to be concentrated within villages. Also, village-level differences in HIV prevalence discussed later also imply the existence of distinct village-level patterns.

15. To construct the village-level estimates, we exclude villages that contain less than 10 respondents, since aggregate measures based on very small numbers can cause instability in multilevel models.

16. The relationships are estimated in HLM models and net of a range of socioeconomic controls. Full results of these models are presented in Appendix E.

Chapter 3

1. Appeared in a special form of common prayer as part of a day of "fasting and humiliation" declared by the Church of England as the plague of London began (Bell 1924/1994: 95).

2. It is human nature in general to demand that disaster make sense and be interpretable within a familiar framework or meta-narrative (Berger 1967). In the United States, for

example, the events of and response to September 11, 2001, are recounted by many not as mere historical facts but as part of a larger narrative of resisting evil, pursuing the vindication of freedom and democracy, even at the cost of many lives—all components of a long-standing American narrative (Smith 2003). Some religious Americans add a divine role to the nation's response. In sub-Saharan Africa, in contrast, the same meta-narrative function is not provided by the state—as described in Chapter 2, states do not have that persuasive hold on people's loyalty. Instead, it is provided by competing identities. One of those is religion.

3. Popular perceptions about HIV transmission are often simple. Many equate cheating on a spouse with almost guaranteed infection. When asked to expand on his advice that members should "take care," one AIC pastor states plainly: "You may sleep with someone who has the [virus] that causes AIDS. If that happens, then you have AIDS. If you continue you may spread it to others. Yeah, it happens like that."

4. To be sure, there are other ways of contracting HIV that are not *directly* alter dependent, such as through infected needles, razors, and blood transfusions. But most scholars of HIV transmission consider these routes of infection to be uncommon in SSA. For an exception, see debates involving Devon Brewer, David Gisslequest, and John Potterat on the role of iatrogenic factors in transmission (e.g., Gisselquist, Potterat, Brody, and Vachon 2003).

5. In the next chapter we show that comprehensive knowledge of all prevention methods is far from universal. But here we are talking about some knowledge, which really is in the 90%-plus range in the most recent round of Demographic and Health Surveys (http://measuredhs.com).

6. In the United States, for example, the U.S. Food and Drug Administration (FDA) demands that cigarette packets prominently place "WARNING," followed by one of the following: "Cigarettes are addictive"; "Tobacco smoke can harm your children"; "Cigarettes cause fatal lung disease"; "Cigarettes cause cancer"; "Cigarettes cause strokes and heart disease"; "Smoking during pregnancy can harm your baby"; "Smoking can kill you"; "Tobacco smoke causes fatal lung disease in nonsmokers"; or "Quitting smoking now greatly reduces serious risks to your health."

7. African characters' struggles against uncertainty are often the main motif in African films about Africa (e.g., Ousmane Sembene's *Mandabi, Xala,* and *Moolaadé*). In Western films, African characters also struggle with uncertainty but more heroically (e.g., *Blood Diamond* or *Hotel Rwanda*).

8. Of course, it could be that our expectations are exaggerated. After all, more than 85% of Malawian adults are not infected. However, we think objective measures of prevalence constitute only one small piece of the broader "worry" puzzle. Even though 85% of adults are HIV negative, the intense spotlight on the dangers of infection lead us to expect generalized worry about AIDS to far exceed actual prevalence.

9. We also compared perceived likelihood of infection among laymen (MDICP data) and religious leaders (MRP data). About 4% of men told us it was highly likely that they are currently infected, and 6% said it was likely that they would become HIV positive in the future. On the other hand, 39% of men believe themselves to be at no risk for contracting HIV during their lifetime. Likewise, 1% of religious leaders told us it was highly likely that they are currently infected, 2% said it was likely that they would become HIV positive in the future, and 60% believed that they themselves were at no risk of contracting HIV during their lifetime.

10. See work by Anglewicz and Kohler (2009) for an excellent summary of the relationship between perceptions and actual HIV status. Using the same data we use here, they find a very strong relationship between perceived risk and testing positive for HIV. Importantly, however, most of those who were wrong about their status were not surprised to learn they were positive. On the contrary, most incorrect individuals thought they were infected when, indeed, they were not. This suggests that gaps in understanding, which we deal with at greater length in Chapter 4, fall on the side of overestimating, not underestimating, infection.

11. *Hadith* are reported statements of, or actions associated with, Muhammad. Since they were only formally collated in the 8th and 9th centuries—by which time the collection had grown enormously—the validity of any given *hadith* is dependent on the chain of authenticity linking it back to Muhammad. The one referenced here was authenticated by 'Ibn Majah, whose 9th-century collection is the sixth canonical compilation of *hadith* in Sunni Islam. In other words, it scores high on authenticity.

12. A good indication of this individualism in relation to AIDS can be seen in the way that televangelist and news commentator Pat Robertson was roundly criticized by both secular and religious Americans for making claims about divine judgments and warnings leveled at nations (the United States after 9/11) as well as particular communities (a small Pennsylvania town that ousted school board members who favored teaching intelligent design). Such talk is hard to get away with in the United States—even in religious circles—which illustrates the thoroughness of Americans' sense of religious individualism and the beneficent character of God.

13. When asked whether promiscuous people are getting what they deserve, one AIC bishop responded: "Yes, every time you're indulging yourself in something, there is an end result." In contrast, the Pentecostal elder we quoted earlier in this section disagreed: "We cannot say that they received their reward, because they [may] have done something not related to AIDS"—referring to other pathways of transmission.

14. This is consistent with the arguments of another sheikh, this one on the BBC. Although claiming to be weary of participating in so many funerals, he too doesn't suggest that Allah is bringing judgment (BBC 2005): "I teach that HIV/AIDS is not a punishment from Allah, but something that we can change through our own behavior and culture."

15. In Chapter 6, we describe a set of local prevention strategies that people have developed in an effort to avoid infection. Some of these are based on ideas about the types of people who are likely to be infected. That implies that there is an element of predictability in HIV-positive people's social characteristics. The point that we're making here is that any element of predictability exists only at the aggregate level. At the individual level, there are too many notable exceptions to those rules' observed patterns. By the time HIV-positive individuals are symptomatic, the narrative of their sexual history, migration history, and current status has great explanatory power in their community. But, of course, these narratives are much more limited in terms of their predictive power.

16. Of course, many Americans do ask "why?" and do so with deep emotion. But they tend to do so rhetorically, with little expectation that they can or will receive a real answer. Even the most religious Westerners expect little more than to be reminded that the events are "part of God's plan" for them. In other words, they believe that there is a reason, that the reason is known to God, but they also believe that they can't know it.

17. For many years, talk of sex with monkeys was never far from mind when discussions of the species leap occurs. Although this has provided some great fodder for comedians (see Dave Chappelle for a classic skit: http://www.youtube.com/watch?v=A-lEzYZMo1k), we suspect there's a little more going on here. In particular, since Africans tend to be much more conservative in terms of sexual partnerships and positions than Europeans, it's difficult to treat this theory about a sexual species leap in isolation from either the long-term representation of non-Europeans' voracious sexual appetite (in Voltaire's *Candide*, there's a suggestion that monkeys and native South American women are lovers) or as anything other than the transference of Western bestiality fetishes onto Africans and their animals.

18. UNICEF (2006); Olouch (2006); Hughes (2008).

19. The milder versions of this conspiracy theory describe AIDS as an attempt to reduce population growth that spun wildly out of control; the extreme forms describe AIDS as an extraordinarily evil plot to wipe black Africans off the map.

20. While most religious leaders—elites among Malawians—refrained from such overt, "uncivilized" accusations, in many of our interviews, it lingered just beneath the surface.

21. Peter Duesberg, professor of molecular and cell biology at the University of California–Berkeley and a member of the U.S. National Academy of Sciences, is the most prominent AIDS skeptic. See Duesberg (1996) for an alternative theory about the origin of AIDS. See

Kalichman (2009) for a critical review of Duesberg and other skeptics as well as discussion of their effects on actual AIDS policy, especially in South Africa.

22. The transition into a state of marriage in Africa has often been described as a "process" rather than a single event (i.e., a wedding). This process continues after the actual wedding ceremony, and in many African contexts a couple isn't truly married (in the eyes of their community) until they have a child together (van de Walle 1993). Likewise, in most of Africa, bona fide adulthood is reserved for individuals who have achieved "parent" status. In at least one setting we know of (Cameroon), this follows the birth of a *second* child (Johnson-Hanks 2006).

23. The decoupling of sex and reproduction is a worldwide phenomenon. In the United States, between 20 and 50% of highly religious youth have engaged in premarital and "pre-pre-marital" sex (Regnerus 2007). Among lay Catholics, there is very high approval and use of contraception. Indeed, predominantly Catholic countries are among the lowest fertility countries in the world (Kohler, Billari, and Ortega 2002). In short, there has been a notable shift in sexual and fertility norms in Western countries over the past 100 years. These differences between the ideal-typical African and Western views of sex and fertility are highly relevant for understanding AIDS.

24. As Smith (2004b) notes, partners in monogamous relationships often consider them as exclusive relationships in which HIV cannot be transmitted and as a result avoid condoms. While these relationships may be lower risk than concurrent sexual relationships, they are hardly low risk. The fact remains that to many Africans—Malawians, Nigerians, Ugandans, religious leaders, and laypeople alike—condoms imply infidelity, alternative arguments and ad campaigns notwithstanding.

Chapter 4

1. Ironically, this was claimed by a Malawian who works as an "AIDS educator" but thinks that teaching people about AIDS is a laughable waste of money precisely because everybody already knows about AIDS. Of course, he plans to continue working in this area. By Malawian standards, he's well paid.

2. Widespread misconceptions about HIV transmission are not unique to SSA. In a study of 1283 English-speaking American adults, Herek, Widaman, and Capitanio (2005) report that while 98.3% correctly acknowledged that a person could contract HIV through unprotected intercourse with an infected person, misconceptions about transmission are widespread. For example, 34.3% of respondents incorrectly answered that a person could get AIDS by having unprotected sexual intercourse with an uninfected person, despite the proviso: ". . . we know for sure that neither [partner] is infected with the AIDS virus."

3. Figure 4.2 presents cross-tabulations of comprehensive HIV knowledge and religious affiliation without any statistical controls. While Takyi's (2003) analysis examined only women, we expanded our analyses to include both women and men, except in two countries where data from both sexes were not available. For each country, we ran logistic regression models to predict comprehensive knowledge about AIDS with controls for rural–urban, age, education, and gender. While the urban–rural and education controls "explained away" the Muslim disadvantage in comprehensive AIDS knowledge in nine countries, this significant disadvantage persisted, net of controls, in Benin, Chad, Cote D'Ivoire, Kenya, Mozambique, Nigeria, and Tanzania. We present the simple cross-tabulations here for ease of interpretation.

4. Comparable data on AIDS-related knowledge is not available from women in Senegal's most recent DHS.

5. The Ugandan case is frequently contrasted to South Africa (see, e.g., Epstein 2007; Parkhurst and Lush 2004), where then-president Thabo Mbeki exhibited silence and denialism vis-à-vis AIDS until 2006. In South Africa, national prevalence estimates rose from about 1 to 25% during this same period; in Kwazulu Natal, prevalence among pregnant women visiting antenatal clinics rose from about 4% in 1991 to 27% in 1997 (Stuart, Irlam, and Wilkinson 1999).

Chapter 5

1. Translated in Rittgers (2007: 134).
2. In Francophone Africa, the core ideas—*abstinence, condom, dépistage* [screening/testing], *fidélité*—are not represented alphabetically, but they still guide mainstream prevention efforts.
3. UNICEF statistics available online (http://www.childinfo.org/education_secondary.php) (accessed March 28, 2010).
4. The increasing use of sophisticated marketing techniques can be seen across a range of health interventions, particularly in those directed at adolescents. We return to this point in our discussion of "C," condoms.
5. Examples include "Love Life" in South Africa (Hunter 2010) and minimally adapted versions of the U.S.-based "True Love Waits" in Malawi.
6. The U.S. National Library of Medicine houses an excellent physical and virtual collection of AIDS prevention posters of the sort we describe here (available at: http://www.nlm.nih.gov/hmd/ihm/). AVERT, an international HIV and AIDS charity based in the United Kingdom, has also collected a vast assortment of posters and photographs from AIDS activists and travelers (available at: http://www.avert.org).
7. The abstinence as cool theme also plays out in the use of cultural motifs associated with youth. The refrain in the South African "Love Life" poster campaign, for example, riffs on youth-related texting language. "The got ambition generation: will U b part of it?" asks one of the posters. "The don't want HIV generation: will U b part of it?" asks another.
8. Moral conversations about abstinence frequently involve debates about gender. For example, while waiting for a religious service to start, one of our observers overheard members debating whether the spread of AIDS could be blamed on young women who marry and become sexually active early or on older people—in this case, women—who push them into early marriage:

   > While they were still outside waiting for their friends to come, they were chatting and talking about the youth—especially the girls. These girls once they are matured they get married while they are still at school. "This is now increasing especially here in village," said a certain man. But one man who was among that group argued by saying that it is not young girls' fault: "It's the fault of some foolish women who force the [young girls] to get married. Also these girls do sex while they are schooling, killing their future and digging their own grave." (MRP Sermon Reports)

9. We make no assumptions that attitudes to abstinence—or any other AIDS-related factor—are the same either across or within African countries. We are merely following an old sociological tradition of treating SSA as a more or less distinct culture area, in the same way that people treat Western Europe, South Asia, or the Arab world, as distinct culture areas. In each case, the undeniable differences within these areas do not undermine the fact that they share important cultural and structural commonalities. In this case, we think that these focus group data are useful for illuminating the diversity of opinions about abstinence across Africa and for helping us differentiate between areas of consensus and debate about appropriate and unacceptable ways of navigating the sexual domain during adolescence.
10. As one male participant indelicately put it, "When you are bored, you tend to look for bitches."
11. A variation on this was directed at women: "If you say 'no,' but the guy still insists, you pull his penis. He will discharge, and you will be free." Note that there was no mention of oral sex in any of these transcripts.
12. Stories of girls who rely on a sugar daddy to stay in school or go to college further complicate this particular abstinence narrative. *Sugar daddy* is the popular term for an older man with whom young women have a sexual relationship in return for cash, gifts, money for

school fees, or other material benefits. In the popular AIDS literature, the sugar daddy phenomenon is usually cast as a type of "survival sex." In the more general sociological literature, the "transactional" nature of such relationships is seen to share features with other types of long-term sexual partnerships in SSA settings, courtship in particular (Poulin 2007). There is considerable debate over both the prevalence of this phenomenon and its consequences for the spread of AIDS (Luke 2005; Mensch, Grant, and Blanc 2006; Pisani 2009). Regardless, the key point here is that since the risks of HIV infection are higher for adolescents with older partners, the assumption that abstinence is a pathway through which adolescents can maximize their educational opportunity is flawed. For at least a small subset of adolescents, being sexually active with older, higher-prevalence men may actually increase their odds of staying in school. Note, too, that there are also sugar mommies in SSA—older women who sponsor younger men in exchange for sexual favors—but this appears to be even less common than the sugar daddy phenomenon.

13. Due to these problems with reported sexual behavior—including reported attitudes about abstinence—it is considered more reliable to look at religious variation in adolescent sexual activity by focusing on the differential prevalence of sexually transmitted infections (STIs), including HIV. This would be our preferred approach were such data available. Unfortunately, they are not. At least, there are no available data sources that we are aware of in which sample sizes are large enough to identify statistically significant differences in STI prevalence across religious groups. For example, if 5% of a 2000-person adolescent sample is infected with a given STI, that is 100 people. Even if we lump those 100 people into five major religious groups—Muslims, Catholics, Mission Protestants, Evangelicals and Pentecostals, and members of African Independent Churches—then the differences in infection across these groups will have to be very large for them to attain "statistical significance," that is, for us to be confident that the variation is systematic rather than random. Because of these limitations we rely primarily on survey responses to questions about abstinence and sexual behavior. This does not mean that we simply accept these data as unbiased indicators of the underlying phenomenon that we're interested in. On the contrary, we like to carefully check the reliability of reports to assess the magnitude of under- and overreporting of sexual partners in various data sources. Our consistency checks include using biomarker data (for pregnancy and for STIs, including but not limited to HIV) to identify "virgin" pregnancies and infections (adams, Trinitapoli, and Poulin 2007). Other red flags for the validity of self-reports include high proportions of married persons reporting no sex in the past year (nonmigrant husband or wife) or observing large numbers of individuals who say they not sexually active yet report high levels of worry about being infected with HIV.

14. This same study found that members of conservative religious groups were 20% less likely than their nonreligious counterparts to use a condom when they did become sexually active.

15. Note that "B" intentionally refers to "Be faithful," not "Be monogamous." Bear in mind that polygyny is widely practiced in many areas of SSA, giving men legitimate rights to more than one wife. Also note that there is no consensus about whether polygamy compounds HIV risk by expanding the sexual network or protects against it by maintaining a larger but closed sexual network (Reniers and Watkins 2009).

16. Large flows of male migrants (in demographic terms, sex-selective labor migration) are not exclusively destined for South African mines. High rates of male migration—primarily rural-to-urban but also from one rural area to another—are a more general phenomenon in SSA. This is easiest to see by looking at how the sex ratio, the number of men relative to women, varies across age groups. Our own analyses of Kenyan census data, for example, show that Kenya's Nyanza Province, the highest prevalence region in Kenya, has a dramatically distorted sex ratio at younger adult ages. Instead of having roughly equal numbers of men and women, the sex ratio in Nyanza dips to about 85 men to 100 women in the 20–29 age group. In combination with relatively low age at marriage, this means that a large proportion of young married couples are living apart. Moreover, like South African miners, they are doing so during the ages of peak sexual activity and childbearing.

17. Unfortunately, we didn't ask Davis about the origins of this analogy of an untrustworthy spouse to Judas. So we don't know if it's something he heard from a pastor, some other local leader, or a friend or if this is a connection he made himself.

18. Accurately measuring the prevalence of extramarital sex in any population is a notoriously difficult task (Reniers and Watkins 2009). Strong cultural and religious norms against having nonmarital partners both encourage faithfulness among married persons and make people reluctant to report their infidelities to researchers. All of our analyses include an individual-level measure of "social desirability" bias that accounts, though imperfectly, for this effect.

19. Note that the following results are in addition to—and net of—a couple of general ones: being faithful during the past year is positively associated with religious involvement but does not vary significantly across denominations.

20. For methodological reasons it is important to note that this is not the religious leader who is reporting having more faithful members. The sexual behavior data were collected from a sample of 3000 women and men. Only then did we interview the religious leaders of the churches and mosques with whom those 3000 had claimed to be affiliated, focusing on how they practice religious leadership in general and how they deal with AIDS in particular. By merging those two data sets we could assess how reported sexual behavior varied by religious leader.

21. Detailed results of these models are available in Appendix F. Note that unlike the data on respondents' HIV status—which are observed—those on extramarital sex are reported. This immediately reduces their validity since reports of extramarital affairs, like reports of socially undesirable things in general, tend to be biased downward. We think that these reports are relatively reliable and have no reason to believe that their reliability varies across religious groups. Other results in these models make intuitive sense. In particular: (1) the sociodemographic patterns are consistent with the literature on sexual behavior in this part of the world; (2) denominational differences in reporting an extramarital partner are weak; and (3) Malawian men and women who attend religious services frequently have reduced odds of reporting an extramarital partner (see Appendix F).

22. The aggregated village-level attendance measures can be difficult to interpret, since the theoretical range is from 0 to 4 but the actual range is only from 2.4 to 4 (as illustrated in Table 2.2). On an individual scale, 4 corresponds to weekly attendance and 2 to less than monthly attendance. We distinguished among "high," "medium," and "low" religiosity villages empirically using the interquartile range. In low religiosity villages (bottom quartile), about 65% of villagers report attending religious services weekly. In medium religiosity villages (25th to 75th percentile) about 71% report attending weekly or more often, while in the most religious villages (top quartile) at least 86% of respondents attend this frequently.

23. For a poignant satirical take on this problem in relation to Africa, see Kenyan writer Binyavanga Wainaina's (2005) "How to Write about Africa."

24. A few years ago there were signs that the official position of the Catholic Church on condoms—as a form of contraception it is prohibited—was going to be revised. In 2006, Cardinal Javier Lozano Barragán, head of the Pontifical Council for Health Care, submitted a 200-page document to the Pope for his review. Later that year, Pope Benedict XVI enlisted a group of senior theologians and scientists and commissioned a study of condoms for the prevention of HIV. The committee was tasked with examining the morality of condom use within a marriage where one partner is infected with HIV. While visiting Cameroon in March 2009, however, Pope Benedict XVI squelched optimism that there would be a new Catholic policy on condoms. He argued that the solution to the AIDS problem lies not in condoms but in a "spiritual and human awakening."

25. Compare coverage of the Pope's visit to Cameroon in Kenya (Wesangula 2009), Cameroon (Yufeh 2009), and popular pan-African media sources (Kendemeh 2009; Makori 2009) to coverage in the *Washington Post* (Simpson n.d.), the *Guardian* (Butt 2009), and the BBC (2009).

26. In general, these comments are very similar to some of those triggered by the family planning movement in SSA prior to AIDS. There were fears that making contraception available

to women would liberate them sexually—since they would no longer fear pregnancy resulting from extramarital affairs (Watkins 2000).

27. Debates about the merits of making condoms freely available to teens in the United States have generated arguments along the same lines. Here, too, resistance to the promotion of condom use is framed in both moral and scientific terms. The latter—which garner much less coverage in the media—questions assumptions about the effectiveness of condoms in reducing the spread of HIV. For example, while condoms used properly provide highly effective protection from STIs, their actual effectiveness in a population is lower. This is because actual effectiveness is a product of two things: (1) how frequently condoms are used; and (2) how much more sex is occurring because they are made available. It is not difficult to imagine, for example, a pro-condom campaign increasing the amount of unprotected sex in absolute terms. This would be the case where the increase in the number of unprotected sexual interaction is greater than the increase in condom use. In this case, a pro-condom campaign could actually increase the spread of sexually transmitted infections (STIs). Empirical evidence for all this is relatively thin. But at least one much-cited study suggests that the widespread promotion of condoms reduces HIV transmission effectively in high-risk populations, but not where there is widespread heterosexual transmission, as in the case in SSA (Hearst and Chen 2004).

28. These phrases are common across the region (see Heguye 1995 for Tanzania; Mufune 2005 for Namibia; Selikow 2004 for South Africa) and are reminiscent of phrases used in Britain in the first half of the 20th century (Fisher and Szreter 2003).

29. The exact question is: "Do you think it is acceptable to use a condom with a spouse to protect against HIV/AIDS?"

30. Condom use estimates from the MDICP are based on the answer to, "Did you ever use a condom with this partner?" asked about every sexual partner the respondent had during the past year.

Chapter 6

1. From *The Decameron*, written in the immediate aftermath of the Black Death in Florence.

2. Funnily enough, there is a small stream of nonscholarly critical literature in the West that talks about condoms and latex in the types of terms used to describe some aspects of traditional medicine (e.g., it sees an exaggerated belief in the protective power of latex). There's also a small, self-declared "condom amulet" movement in the United States that consists of women who knit amulet-type pouches in which wearers can store a condom. But neither of these can be thought of as preventive strategies.

3. Both projects we know of are being fielded in Malawi: Tsogolo la Thanzi (http://www.pop.psu.edu/research/projects/tlthf) and Marriage Transitions in Malawi (Beegle, Özler, Poulin, PIs, http://sites.google.com/site/mtmalawiproject/home).

4. It is, of course, problematic to generalize from this small sample of focus-group participants to Africa as a whole. But it is equally important to note that this perspective is consistent with findings from a recent study of young married women in 29 different countries, which describes a lethal combination of limited access to information about HIV and frequent and unprotected sex within marriage that actually increases the risk of infection for married adolescent women (Clark, Bruce, and Dude 2006).

5. We used data from the adolescent sample of the MDICP-3 to calculate the median age at first marriage for the six major religious traditions in Malawi, separately for men and for women. Since these observations are denominational averages this is an "ecological" correlation across a small sample size (six religious traditions × gender, plus women claiming "no" affiliation = 13 observations). But they are instructive nonetheless.

6. Divorce rates in Africa are notoriously difficult to measure for a few reasons. First, marriage and divorce are primarily social arrangements, not legal ones. In addition, estimating the prevalence of divorce using cross sectional data requires sensitivity to a number of factors including the number of divorces, the number of marriages, the speed of remarriage, and the rate of widowhood. As support for this statement, we rely on detailed

analyses conducted by Reniers (2003, 2008) on Malawi and on journalistic accounts from dozens of countries making similar statements.

7. Note that in the contractual terms of Islamic marriage divorce is at least theoretically acceptable where unfaithfulness is interpreted as a breach of the marriage contract that voids the obligations of the other party (Dahl 1997).

8. We used a two-level random effects model that, among other things, controlled for respondents' sociodemographic characteristics (gender, age, household wealth, education), religious identity, and whether they had switched denominations in the last five years.

9. This is only officially. In our Malawi data, Muslim women frequently initiate divorce.

10. See Smith (2001) for an ethnographic evaluation, and African fiction from Sol T. Plaatje's (2006) *Mhudi*—written in 1919—to selected stories in Chimamanda Ngozi Adiche's (2009) *The Thing around Your Neck* for more general descriptions.

11. Frankly, we prefer Hunter's (2010) view of the "materiality of everyday sex and love" to conventional discussions of "transactional sex." But since *transactional sex* is the term that drives the literature—and the ensuing debates—we engage it on its own terms here.

12. Not all small gifts result in a sexual relationship—though the larger ones certainly tend to. More generally, the types of gifts described here are consistent with more general theoretical approaches to gifting, which treat it as an attempt to spotlight a social connection or establish a reciprocal relationship (Blau 1964; Mauss 2000; Zelizer 2005).

13. Quote taken from our analysis of focus group data conducted by AGI. Focus groups were conducted with young men and young women in six countries. More details about these data are provided in Appendix A.

14. The findings from the Lopman et al. (2008) study underscore the difficulty in predicting HIV, as discussed in Chapter 3.

15. This particular poster can be viewed online (www.jhhesa.org/sites/jhhesa.org/files/003622-Drink-Responsibly.pdf).

16. One Muslim leader we interviewed in Malawi in 2001 treats alcohol as one of the key indicators for classifying Muslims as either good (always acting in accordance with Islamic law), being a *fasku* (someone who "does some of the rules but also does things out of Islam"), and a *kafri* (a person who "doesn't do anything about Muslim rules").

17. The same missionary went on to call for 10 years' hard labor as punishment for those who supply Africans with alcohol (not surprisingly given his Anglophone prejudices, these suppliers were primarily "Boers").

18. Note that the number of unaffiliated men in this sample is extremely small: $N = 26$.

Chapter 7

1. An eyewitness to the 1720 Plague of Marseilles describing the "Good Bishop," Henri Francois Xavier de Belsunce de Castelmoron. Cited in Sears (1845: 405).

2. More details on the data for this figure are available in Appendix H.

3. Note, too, that MFDb, adding a pragmatic prodivorce strategy to moral teaching and faith healing, is also most popular in Mission Protestant congregations.

4. We dropped the 16 smallest congregations since HIV prevalence estimates are unstable when based on a very few number of cases. Average prevalence across all congregations in which we have observations on at least 10 respondents is 6.7%, but is highly variable. In several congregations, HIV prevalence is 0%, and in one congregation 50% of the members we tested were HIV positive.

5. We have no way to formally (in statistical terms) tease out these differences here. But later in this chapter and in Chapter 10 we leverage other types of available data to demonstrate that selection processes are not driving this result.

6. This particular religious leader was a busy man. In addition to running a congregation and supporting his own family through farming, he was also part of a family planning group that distributed condoms in both his own home village (where his congregation is) and in his parents-in-law's village.

7. Remember, at the time this interview was conducted (2005) rapid tests were not available in Malawi. Rural residents often had to travel long distances to get tested and then make a separate trip to receive their test results. In other words, this leader had organized a congregational "field trip" for all the members to learn their status.

8. HIV prevalence could be calculated for only 31 of these congregations. In 18 of these, *none* of the members participating in our study tested positive.

9. There is also some evidence that these figures will fall in the near future rather than continue to rise. Due to the global economic crisis, funding for free antiretroviral therapy programs is flat, if not falling. Meanwhile, although the rate of new infections is declining, the absolute number of people with advanced HIV continues to increase (McNeil 2010).

10. It is important to remember that engagement in alternative—that is, nonbiomedical— health therapies is not a uniquely African thing. Just under half of all Americans pursued at least one alternative or complementary therapy in 2004 (the year we collected our first religion-focused round of Malawi data). Indeed, Americans spend approximately $27 billion every year on alternative and complementary medicine (Carey 2006). Just like Africans who are disillusioned with a Western "science" establishment that has failed to eradicate malaria, tuberculosis, and HIV/AIDS, many Americans have also become alienated from some aspects of the modern medical establishment, whether due to the high cost of drugs, harried doctors, perennial concern about whether insurance will cover any given procedure, recollections of misdiagnoses, or the simple conviction that there is more to one's health than what the doctor knows *clinically* (Barnes, Powell-Griner, McFann, and Nahin 2004; Carey 2006). Even the National Institutes of Health recognizes this interest. In 1998 it established the National Center for Complementary and Alternative Medicine.

11. Our argument here is not that African traditional healers are a homogenous bloc. On the contrary, one can find quite different approaches to healing and source-specific illness identification among them (Ingstad 1990). But at the level that we're talking about, we think that it can be treated as a conceptually unified category—that is, practitioners of African traditional medicine share more among themselves than they do with practitioners of Western medicine.

12. We know of no good data from which to calculate the proportion of sub-Saharan Africans with ritual scars, but anecdotally it appears to be high. Even more interesting, there does not seem to be a clear negative relationship between scarring and level of education. In fact, anecdotally we know that, among the younger most educated cohorts, some have taken on scarring as a sign of cultural pride in being African. In other words, this generation is more comfortable publicly acknowledging traditional African practices than their parents are.

13. While traditional healers fall on the "acceptable" side of approaches to health, witchcraft and sorcery represent a darker, more malevolent, and more contested phenomenon. These are widely considered socially undesirable and "uncivilized," which makes them difficult to document, as people avoid talking openly about such issues, especially to Westerners. We do not address witchcraft in any detail here, but direct readers to Adam Ashforth's (2002, 2005) excellent work on the topic, with an emphasis on spiritual insecurity in Soweto, South Africa.

14. Perhaps even more interesting is the fact that "traditional medicine" and "through prayer" are in the same ballpark as "avoid sex with prostitutes" (2%).

15. See Dilger (2007) for a thorough account of claims of spiritual cures for HIV among Ghanaian Pentecostals living in Botswana.

Chapter 8

1. There are two noteworthy examples in the social science literature, neither of which is related to AIDS or Africa. The first deals with the effects of Jewish dietary restrictions. From the perspective of Judaism, those restrictions have both the intended functional effect of reducing Jewish assimilation and the unintended effect of contributing to the perpetuation of anti-Semitic stereotypes and stigma (Douglas 1966). A second example is Harvey Milk's behest that gays and lesbians in the United States should "Come out, come out, wherever you are!" This, too, was based on an intuitive understanding of the contact hypothesis—that

coming out to heterosexual friends and family members reduces prejudice about "gay people" as a group and therefore, in the aggregate, also reduces the stigma associated with being gay.

2. DHS clusters are small, physically bounded spatial units used to facilitate more efficient sampling. It is standard analytic practice in the social sciences to treat them as analogous to a neighborhood.

3. Cluster-level data further illustrate the high levels of heterogeneity within countries. Of the 5862 clusters from which we have biomarker data, 25% of these are "very high prevalence" (prevalence greater than 10%). And 40% of these (*N* = 686) are in low-prevalence countries. This means that 11% of all DHS clusters are high-prevalence areas in low-prevalence countries.

4. The stereotype of the male teacher as a man who preys upon schoolgirls as sexual partners, often exchanging high marks or waived school fees for sexual favors, makes the gender specificity of this question very relevant. Note, too, that some surveys ask questions about stigma that fail to distinguish between HIV and AIDS, because of either an oversight or translation problems. Failing to make these important distinctions leads to a variety of interpretive problems. For example, individuals who would support a functionally healthy HIV-positive teacher in the classroom may get counted as having negative attitudes toward a person with AIDS if they respond: "No, she cannot teach. She is sick, probably dying. A dying person cannot perform her duties in the classroom. She cannot teach." The MDICP's carefully worded and specific questions eliminate problems that have plagued previous studies that have asked about teachers.

5. Other significant predictors of response patterns on these two variables include the following. (1) Individuals from higher socioeconomic status positions (more education and more wealth) are more likely to express support for PLWHAs. (2) Consistent with the contact hypothesis previously discussed, those who have been exposed to more AIDS-related deaths are less likely to hold discriminatory attitudes about teachers and vegetable vendors with HIV. (3) Women are significantly less likely than men to support an infected teacher's right to keep working.

6. See Appendix A for detailed information on the collection of these data.

7. It should also be noted that the home region of most Senegalese Christians is the relatively impoverished province of Casamance, also the site of a Christian rebellion in support of Casamance independence.

8. This statement is paraphrased from a nonrecorded interview.

Chapter 9

1. From Binet's *Consolation* (1617/1995: 35), writing in France during an era of widespread and recurrent plagues (cited in Worcester 2007: 225).

2. Developed countries' commitment to the welfare system is part of a revised social contract that began to emerge in the 19th century. Briefly, in return for a state's rights to taxation and conscription, certain political and civic rights were extended to citizens, including the right to vote and to enjoy basic protections afforded by a publicly funded welfare system. Within this model there are important differences. For example, welfare systems in Nordic countries are the most uniformly public and efficient; those of continental Europe—like equivalents in the United States—are somewhat more mixed (a combination of government and independent, voluntary societies); those of southern Europe are public but highly inefficient. The important point for us is that all of these states have more developed public welfare systems than SSA.

3. Smearing a mud house with fresh mud prevents cracks in the walls from compromising the structure of the building and is an important maintenance task in rural areas.

4. Mortality analyses suggesting that roughly two-thirds of all adult deaths in this region are AIDS-related (Doctor and Weinreb 2003), further imply that a great many of these visits to the sick are the result of AIDS.

5. AIDS-related mortality also introduces a set of questions about care for widows upon the death of a husband. We do not address this in any detail here but point readers to excellent essays by Prince (2007) and Christiansen (2009) on the role of religion in widows' lives.

6. Although nongovernmental organizations might claim credit for seeing to it that few live in child-headed households, we think that this is unlikely. According to a Malawian National AIDS Commission (NAC) report using data from 2004, of the approximately 1 million orphans and vulnerable children (OVC) in Malawi, roughly 47,000 received psychosocial report; 60,000 received nutritional support; and less than 3000 received any financial support (RoM 2005).

7. This case is worth retelling in greater detail, since although it is unrepresentative of the normal pathway for orphans—it was the only case that we heard about where familial fostering did not happen—it spotlights both the interpenetration of different types of social support mechanisms and the costs of placing oneself outside these reciprocal systems. The story is as follows. Two girls were left orphaned by the death of their mother. Their father had already died. Their mother's only surviving sibling was a sister who had moved to her husband's village a couple of hours' bus ride away. Claiming that her husband wouldn't allow it, she refused to take her nieces. Instead, they were adopted by an unrelated village-mate, the deceased mother's best friend. All agreed that this arrangement had worked out well. The girls were well treated. They loved their foster mother and were happy to stay in their natal village. A couple of years later, however, the aunt's own marriage collapsed, and she returned to her natal village looking for shelter. She did not receive it. Having failed the test of reciprocity by refusing to shelter her own nieces, she could no longer count on support herself, whether from her family or from her natal community.

8. Here is a typical field note summarizing an interview with an imam in Balaka district. "Although he didn't seem to think that AIDS was a serious problem in this village, he did say that there are a lot of orphans here and that most of them are living with elder sisters or with aunts and uncles. In the mosque he teaches about caring for orphans and for the people who are suffering frequently as well (again, said that he talks about these things nearly every week.) He said that in this community, people accept these responsibilities and no one denies the responsibility of helping blood relatives or their children."

9. Our analytic approach is admittedly very crude. We exclude children who are not living with any adults, for example, living on streets or in child-headed households, because we have no way to determine a "religion" for these children, who are particularly vulnerable. Though a critical group for intervention, they are small in number, and we don't expect that their exclusion biases the findings we report here.

Chapter 10

1. Quoted in Reff (2005: 74).

2. As paraphrased in Worcester (2007: 229), Binet (1617/1995) insists that "there are so many vows, alms, devotions that would never have been without plague; prayers, masses, and communions." In Chapter 7, we described how even with some access to modern healthcare in SSA, prayer remains an important pathway through which people attempt to prevent illness or seek healing.

3. By focusing on these aspects of plague-driven violence we do not ignore others. For example, delegitimized clergy were much less frequently victims of popular violence than those seen to be responsible for the plague—mainly "Jewish poisoners" (Laqueur 2008: 62) and witches in Europe. Likewise, other effects on European culture have been observed such as the increasing death-related iconography in religious art (Gertsman 2007). For a more general discussion of the cultural effects of plagues and epidemics—part of a much larger literature on the effects of epidemics on human history—see foundational studies by Zinsser (1934/2007) and McNeill (1977/1998). More recent edited collections provide more specific case studies (e.g., Little 2007; Mormando and Worcester 2007).

4. This is not to say that later Christians or Christian leaders always maintained these high standards. Pope Clement VI, for example, rode out the Black Death in his Avignon palace, surrounded by fires that purported to cleanse the *miasma* (corrupted air) that carried the plague. And early Protestant polemics and *responsa* (e.g., Luther's *Whether One May Flee From a Deadly Plague* or Nurnberg magistrates' *A Short Regimen for How One Should Conduct*

Oneself During Plague; see Luther, Lull, and Russell 2005) were motivated by the perceived un-Christian behavior of many fellow residents during cyclical waves of plagues.

5. Histories of plague-driven conversion to Christianity in the same time period and in others provide more general support for Stark's argument (Reff 2005; Stoclet 2007).

6. An alternative narrative begins in the same way but ends more ambivalently. This time, the same womanizing man converts—but not before being infected. For the first year after his conversion, there is no sign of sickness. He is a good member of the community, praying regularly, tithing, and singing with the choir. After he becomes sick, church members visit him on a regular basis, bringing maize and other small gifts as well as offering prayer and encouragement to him and to his family. Although he eventually dies of AIDS, he does so in the company of his loyal and loving family, and after experiencing spiritual healing. His life is then celebrated with a well-attended funeral during which the pastor of his church preaches about faithfulness.

7. There might equally be an opposite effect in some areas. That is, some people may be repelled by what they think are overly developed caregiving structures, put off by the constant demands for contributions of money and time. We saw no signs of this in Malawi.

8. The connection between AIDS and marriage-related religious shifts is a particularly important one, since the events of divorce and widowhood have become more common since the onset of the epidemic and are frequently followed by remarriage. A particularly salient example can be found in the related religious and marital histories of one of our respondents: a Muslim woman who has changed religion three times. She converted to Christianity (Catholicism) when she married her first husband. When her husband died, she remarried and joined her second husband's AIC church. After divorcing her second husband due to AIDS-related concerns, she went back to Islam, though she now attends a different mosque from the one she grew up in.

9. Relationships among variables were estimated in a series of two-level random effects models that allow us to identify variation in the both fixed and random parts of the model across villages in addition to individuals (Raudenbush and Bryk 2001).

10. Although 20% of the overall variance in shifting behavior is at the village level, there are virtually no significant village-level differences in the effects of general social or AIDS-related variables on shifting. There is also very little village-level heterogeneity in the relationship—or lack thereof—between AIDS-related variables and shifting.

11. *Making tauba* refers to heartfelt repentance for past wrongdoing and a commitment to avoid such things in the future. In common usage it parallels becoming born again for Christians. Thus, although a few of our Muslim respondents told us that they make tauba every day, a large majority of Muslims who reported having made tauba could easily recall the year they did so.

Conclusion

1. Others include local community consensus and epidemiological realities.

2. The 2050 figures are from the UN Population Division's "medium projection" (2006 edition of the World Population Prospects). This estimate takes into account the projected effects of ART on mortality as well as decreased vertical (mother-to-child) transmission of HIV. Also, if actual changes in population are in line with the projections, Africa's population will have increased from 10% of the global population in 1975 to approximately 22% of the global population in 2050.

Appendix A

1. There were a total of 31 cases in which a respondent who named a congregation could not be assigned to one of the MRP congregations and is thus missing congregation-level data. See Trinitapoli (2007) for more detailed information about the MRP data collection procedures.

Appendix B

1. HIV status is determined through testing. Tests can be conducted on cells from the cheek, which are collected painlessly with an oral swab, or from blood samples collected with a simple finger prick. Protocols for testing have changed several times in the past four years, but for several years the WHO protocol has recommended serial testing to determine HIV status. First, the individual is given a very sensitive test to detect antibodies. If the test is negative, the individual receives a "negative" diagnosis. If the first test is positive, a second test (more "specific," that is, very unlikely to give a false positive) is given. If this test is also positive, that person is diagnosed as HIV positive. If the first and second tests produce discrepant results—these are rare—a third tie-breaker test is used to determine the individual's HIV status.

2. In theory it is possible to formulate similar criticisms of the HIV prevalence measures in relation to the denominator ("number of people in a given age"). For example, a dramatic decline in birth rates or a war or some other disease that wiped out a big chunk of the population that was not typically susceptible to AIDS (e.g., children or the elderly) would automatically increase HIV prevalence. But there are no notable cases where either of these has occurred of which we are aware, so it seems less important than the numerator-related issues.

REFERENCES

adams, jimi, Jenny Trinitapoli, and Michelle Poulin. 2007. "Letter to the Editor: Regarding Male and Female Circumcision Associated with Prevalent HIV Infection in Virgins and Adolescents in Kenya, Lesotho, and Tanzania." *Annals of Epidemiology* 17:923–25.

Adichie, Chimamanda Ngozi. 2009. *The Thing around Your Neck*. Garden City, NY: Anchor.

Adogame, Afe, and Jim Spickard. 2010. *Religion Crossing Boundaries*. Boston, MA: Brill.

afrol News. 2008. "No Time to "Chill" for Abstinence Campaign." Retrieved March 11, 2010. (http://www.afrol.com/articles/21387).

Agadjanian, Victor. 2001. "Religion, Social Milieu, and the Contraceptive Revolution." *Population Studies* 55:135–48.

Agadjanian, Victor. 2006. "Gender, Religious Involvement, and HIV/AIDS Prevention in Mozambique." *Social Science & Medicine* 61:1529–39.

Agadjanian, Victor, and Cecilia Menjívar. 2008. "Talking about the 'Epidemic of the Millennium': Religion, Informal Communication, and HIV/AIDS in Sub-Saharan Africa." *Social Problems* 55:301–21.

Agadjanian, Victor, and Soma Sen. 2007. "Promises and Challenges of Faith-Based AIDS Care and Support in Mozambique." *American Journal of Public Health* 95:362–67.

Agha, Sohail, Paul Hutchinson, and Thankian Kusanthan. 2006. "The Effects of Religious Affiliation on Sexual Initiation and Condom Use in Zambia." *Journal of Adolescent Health* 38: 550–55.

Ahiante, Andrew. 2003. "HIV/AIDS: Clergymen's Response to Stigmatisation." *Christian Post*, June 26. Retrieved April 16, 2012. (http://www.christianpost.com/news/hiv-aids-clergymen-s-response-to-stigmatisation-70/).

Ahmad, Omar B. 2005. "Managing Medical Migration from Poor Countries." *British Medical Journal* 331:43–45.

AIDS Lunacy. 2007. "AIDS Lunacy." *Los Angeles Times*, September 29. Retrieved September 30, 2007. (http://articles.latimes.com/2007/sep/29/opinion/ed-mozambique29).

AIDSMark. 2007. *A Decade of Innovative Marketing for Health: Lessons Learned*. Washington, DC: Population Services International. Retrieved September 26, 2011. (http://pdf.usaid.gov/pdf_docs/PNADL283.pdf).

Ajami, Fouad. 1992. *The Arab Predicament: Arab Political Thought and Practice Since 1967*. 2nd ed. New York: Cambridge University Press.

Akyeampong, Emmanuel. 1996a. *Drink, Power, and Cultural Change: A Social History of Alcohol in Ghana, c. 1800 to Recent Times*. Portsmouth, NH: Heinemann.

Akyeampong, Emmanuel. 1996b. "What's in a Drink? Class Struggle, Popular Culture and the Politics of Akpeteshie (Local Gin) in Ghana, 1930–67." *Journal of African History* 37:215–36.

Akyeampong, Emmanuel. 2000. "Africans in the Diaspora: The Diaspora and Africa." *African Affairs* 99:183-215.

Allport, Gordon W. 1979. *The Nature of Prejudice: 25th Anniversary Edition*. New York: Basic Books.

Alonzo, Angelo A., and Nancy R. Reynolds. 1995. "Stigma, HIV and AIDS: An Exploration and Elaboration of a Stigma Trajectory." *Social Science & Medicine* 41:303-315.

Anglewicz, Philip, and Hans Peter Kohler. 2009. "Overestimating HIV Infection: The Construction and Accuracy of Subjective Probabilities of HIV Infection in Rural Malawi." *Demographic Research* 20:65–96.

ARHAP for the Bill and Melinda Gates Foundation. 2008. *The Contribution of Religious Entities to Health in Sub-Saharan Africa.* ARHAP for the World Health Organization. Retrieved March 1, 2009. (http://www.arhap.uct.ac.za/downloads/Tues_Olivier_prez.pdf).

ARHAP for Tearfund and UNAIDS. 2008. *The Potentials and Perils of Partnership: Christian Religious Entities and Collaborative Stakeholders Responding to HIV and AIDS in Kenya, Malawi and the DRC.* Retrieved March 1, 2009. (http://www.arhap.uct.ac.za/downloads/TFUN-AIDS_full_June2008.pdf).

ARHAP for the World Health Organization. 2006. *Appreciating Assets: The Contribution of Religion to Universal Access in Africa.* ARHAP for the World Health Organization. Retrieved June 10, 2007. (http://www.arhap.uct.ac.za/downloads/ARHAPWHO _entire.pdf).

Ashford, Lori S. 2006. "How HIV and AIDS Affect Populations." *Population Reference Bureau Report.* Retrieved July 1, 2009. (http://www.prb.org/pdf06/HowHIVAIDSAffectsPopulations.pdf).

Ashforth, Adam. 2002. "An Epidemic of Witchcraft? The Implications of AIDS for the Post-Apartheid State." *African Studies* 61:121–143.

Ashforth, Adam. 2005. *Witchcraft, Violence, and Democracy in South Africa.* Chicago: University of Chicago Press.

Atatah, Clovis. 2004. "Dying with the Stigma of AIDS." *Africa News Service,* December 2. (http://www.postnewsline.com/2004/12/dying_with_the_.html).

Auvert, Bertran, Anne Buvé, Benoît Ferry, Michel Caraël, Linda Morison, Emmanuel Lagarde, et al. 2001. "Ecological and Individual Level Analysis of Risk Factors for HIV Infection in Four Urban Populations of Sub-Saharan Africa with Different Levels of HIV Infection." *AIDS* 15:S15–S30.

Auvert, Bertran, Dirk Taaljard, Emmanuel Lagarde, Joëlle Sobngwi-Tambekou, Rémi Sitta, and Adrian Puren. 2005. "Randomized, Controlled Intervention Trial of Male Circumcision for Reduction of HIV Infection Risk: The ANRS 1265 Trial." *PLOS Medicine* 2:1112–22.

Ayikukwei, Rose, Duncan Ngare, John Silde, David Ayuku, Joyce Baliddawa, and James Greene. 2007. "Social and Cultural Significance of the Sexual Cleansing Ritual and Its Impact on HIV Prevention Strategies in Western Kenya." *Sexuality & Culture* 11:32–50.

Badri, Malik. 1997/2000. *The AIDS Crisis: An Islamic Socio-Cultural Perspective.* Kuala Lumpur: International Institute of Islamic Thought.

Badri, Malik. 2007. Keynote Address, 3rd International Muslim Leaders' Consultation on HIV/AIDS in Addis Ababa, Ethiopia, July 23–27. Pp. 14–16 in *The Islamic Approach to HIV/AIDS: Enhancing the Community Response.* IMAU: Kampala.

Baker, Joseph O., and Buster G. Smith. 2009. "The Nones: Social Characteristics of the Religiously Unaffiliated." *Social Forces* 87:1251–1263.

Balise, Joseph. 2008. "Botswana Government to Introduce 30% Levy on Alcohol (Update1)-Bloomberg." *Bloomberg.* Retrieved April 21, 2011. (http://www.bloomberg.com/apps/news?pid=newsarchive&sid=aFfjLHH2JptM&refer=africa).

Barnes, Patricia, Eve Powell-Griner, Kim McFann, and Richard Nahin. 2004. CDC Advance Data Report #343. Complementary and Alternative Medicine Use among Adults: United States, 2002. May 27. Retrieved September 26, 2011. (http://news.bbc.co.uk/2/shared/spl/hi/picture_gallery/05/africa_malawi_village/html/5.stm).

Barz, Gregory. 2005. *Singing for Life: HIV/AIDS and Music in Uganda.* London: Routledge.

Bates, Robert H. 2008. *When Things Fell Apart: State Failure in Late-Century Africa.* New York: Cambridge University Press.

BBC. 2005. "BBC NEWS | In Pictures | Malawi Village." Retrieved September 19, 2011 (http://news.bbc.co.uk/2/shared/spl/hi/picture_gallery/05/africa_malawi_village/html/5.stm).

BBC. 2006. "Cardinal Backs Limited Condom Use." *BBC,* April 21. Retrieved April 13, 2010. (http://news.bbc.co.uk/2/hi/europe/4929962.stm).

BBC. 2007. "Shock at Archbishop Condom Claim." *BBC,* September 26. Retrieved April 22, 2010. (http://news.bbc.co.uk/2/hi/7014335.stm).

BBC. 2009. "Pope Tells Africa 'Condoms Wrong.'" *BBC*, March 17. Retrieved April 26, 2009. (http://news.bbc.co.uk/2/hi/7947460.stm).

Bearman, Peter S., and Hannah Brückner. 2001. "Promising the Future: Virginity Pledges and the Transition to First Intercourse." *American Journal of Sociology* 106:859–912.

Beegle, Kathleen, Joachim De Weerdt, and Stefan Dercon. 2010. "Orphanhood and Human Capital Destruction: Is There Persistence into Adulthood?" *Demography* 47:163–80.

Behrman, Greg. 2004. *The Invisible People: How the U.S. Has Slept through the Global AIDS Pandemic, the Greatest Humanitarian Catastrophe of Our Time*. New York: Free Press.

Bell, Walter George. 1924/1995. *The Great Plague in London*. London: Folio Society.

Benedictow, Ole J. 2004. *The Black Death 1346–1353: The Complete History*. Rochester, NY: Boydell and Brewer.

Benefo, Kofi D. 2007. "Determinants of Zambian Men's Extra-Marital Sex: A Multi-level Analysis." *Archives of Sexual Behavior* 37:517–29.

Berger, Peter L. 1967. *The Sacred Canopy: Elements of a Sociological Theory of Religion*. Garden City, NY: Doubleday.

Berman, Sheri. 2003. "Islamism, Revolution, and Civil Society." *Perspectives on Politics* 1:257–72.

Bham, Moulana E. 2008. "AIDS: A Moral Perspective—Is AIDS a Punishment of Allah?" Retrieved February 28, 2010. (http://www.ima.org.za/publications/AIDS.pdf).

Binet, Etienne. 1617/1995. *Consolation et réjouissance des maladies et personnes affligées*. Edited by Claude Louis-Combet. Grenoble: Jérôme Million.

Bird, Richard M., and Sally Wallace. 2003. *Taxing Alcohol in Africa: Reflections from International Experience*. Toronto: International Tax Program, Institute for International Business, Joseph L. Rotman School of Management, University of Toronto. Retrieved June 30, 2010. (http://ideas.repec.org/p/ttp/itpwps/0304.html).

Birdthistle, Isolde, Sian Floyd, Auxilia Nyagadza, Netsai Mudziwapasi, Simon Gregson, and Judith R. Glynn. 2009. "Is Education the Link between Orphanhood and HIV/HSV-2 Risk among Female Adolescents in Urban Zimbabwe?" *Social Science and Medicine* 68:1810–18.

Bishop, Meghan, and Karen Foreit. 2010. *Serodiscordant Couples in Sub-Saharan Africa: What Do Survey Data Tell Us?* Washington, DC: Futures Group, Health Policy Initative, Task Order 1.

Blau, Peter Michael. 1964. *Exchange and Power in Social Life*. New York: John Wiley.

Bledsoe, Caroline, and Uche Isiugo-Abanihe. 1989. "Strategies of Child-Fosterage Among Mende Grannies in Sierra Leone." Pp. 442–74 in *Reproduction and Social Organization in Sub-Saharan Africa*, edited by Ron J. Lesthaeghe. Berkeley: University of California Press.

Boerma, J. Ties, Simon Gregson, Constance Nyamukapa, and Mark Urassa. 2003. "Understanding the Uneven Spread of HIV within Africa: Comparative Study of Biologic, Behavioral, and Contextual factors in rural populations in Tanzania and Zimbabwe." *Sexually Transmitted Diseases* 30:779.

Bongaarts, John. 2006. "The Causes of Stalling Fertility Transitions." *Studies in Family Planning* 37:1–16.

Bongaarts, John. 2007. "Late Marriage and the HIV Epidemic in Sub-Saharan Africa." *Population Studies* 61:73–83.

Botswana Harvard AIDS Institute. 2012. "About: Timeline." Retrieved March 6, 2012. (http://www.hsph.harvard.edu/bhp/about/timeline.html).

Bouare, Oumar. 2007. "Internal Migration and the Spread of HIV/AIDS in South Africa." *Social Sciences* 2:405–11.

Breault, Kevin D. 1986. "Suicide in America: A Test of Durkheim's Theory of Religious and Family Integration (1933–1980)." *American Journal of Sociology* 92:628–56.

Bryceson, Deborah Fahy. 2002. *Alcohol in Africa: Mixing Business, Pleasure, and Politics*. Portsmouth, NH: Heinemann.

Burdette, Amy M., Christopher G. Ellison, Darren E. Sherkat, and Kurt A. Gore. 2007. "Are There Religious Variations in Marital Infidelity?" *Journal of Family Issues* 28:1553-81.

Burgard, Sarah A., and Susan M. Lee-Rife. 2009. "Community Characteristics, Sexual Initatiation, and Condom Use among Young Black South Africans." *Journal of Health and Social Behavior* 50:293–309.

Burgat, Francois, and William Dowell. 1997. *The Islamic Movement in North Africa*. Austin: University of Texas Press.

Burt, Ronald. 1995. *Structural Holes: The Social Structure of Competition*. Cambridge, MA: Harvard University Press.

Burt, Ronald S. 2005. *Brokerage and Closure: An Introduction to Social Capital*. New York: Oxford University Press.

Butt, Riazat. 2009. "Pope Claims Condoms Could Make African Aids Crisis Worse | World News | guardian.co.uk." *Guardian*, March 17. Retrieved April 26, 2009. (http://www.guardian.co.uk/world/2009/mar/17/pope-africa-condoms-aids).

Caldwell, John C., Pat Caldwell, and Pat Quiggin. 1989. "The Social-Context of AIDS in Sub-Saharan Africa." *Population and Development Review* 15:185–234.

Caldwell, John C., I. Olatunji Orubuloye, and Pat Caldwell. 1999. "Obstacles to Behavioural Change to Lessen the Risk of HIV Infection in the African AIDS Epidemic: Nigerian Research." Pp. 113–24 in *Resistances to Behavioural Change to Reduce HIV/AIDS Infection in Predominantly Heterosexual Epidemics in Third World Countries*, edited by John C. Caldwell, et al. Canberra: Health Transition Centre, National Centre for Epidemiology and Population Health, Australian National University.

Carey, Benedict. 2006. "When Trust in Doctors Erodes, Other Treatments Fill the Void." *New York Times*, February 3, p. A1.

Case, Anne, Christina Paxson, and Joseph Ableidinger. 2004. "Orphans in Africa: Parental Death, Poverty, and School Enrollment." *Demography* 41:483–508.

Chandra, Anjani, William D. Mosher, and Casey C. Copen. 2011. "Sexual Behavior, Sexual Attraction, and Sexual Identity in the United States: Data from the 2006–2008 National Survey of Family Growth." *National Health Statistics Report* 36:1–36, March 11. Hyattsville, MD: National Center for Health Statistics. (http://www.cdc.gov/nchs/data/nhsr/nhsr036.pdf).

Chatterji, Minki, Nancy Murray, David London, and Philip Anglewicz. 2005. "The Factors Influencing Transactional Sex among Young Men and Women in 12 Sub-Saharan African Countries." *Biodemography and Social Biology* 52:56-72.

Chirwa, Wiseman C. 1997. "Migrant Labour, Sexual Networking and Multi-partnered Sex in Malawi." *Health Transition Review* 7S:5–15.

Christakis, Nicholas A., and James H. Fowler. 2011. *Connected: The Surprising Power of Our Social Networks and How They Shape Our Lives—How Your Friends' Friends' Friends Affect Everything You Feel, Think, and Do*. New York: Back Bay Books.

Christiansen, Catrine. 2009. "The New Wives of Christ: Paradoxes and Potentials in the Remaking of Widow Lives in Uganda." Pp. 85–118 in *AIDS and Religious Practice in Africa*, edited by Felicitas Becker and Wenzel Geissler. Boston, MA: Brill.

Clark, Shelley. 2004. "Early Marriage and HIV Risks in Sub-Saharan Africa." *Studies in Family Planning* 35:149–160.

Clark, Shelley, Judith Bruce, and Annie Dude. 2006. "Protecting Girls from HIV/AIDS: The Case against Child and Adolescent Marriage." *International Family Planning Perspectives* 32:79–88.

Cohen, Jon. 2004. "HIV Transmission: Allegations Raise Fears of Backlash against AIDS Prevention Strategy." *Science* 306:2168–69.

Cohn, Norman. 1970. *The Pursuit of the Millennium: Revolutionary Millenarians and Mystical Anarchists of the Middle Ages*. New York: Oxford University Press.

Collins, Randall. 1981. "On the Microfoundations of Macrosociology." *American Journal of Sociology* 86:984–1014.

Colombant, Nico. 2005. "Gambia Bishop Breaks Religious Opposition to Condom Use." *Voice of America*. Retrieved September 26, 2011. (http://www.aegis.org/news/voa/2005/VA050414.html).

Comaroff, Jean. 1980. "Healing and the Cultural Order: The Case of the Barolong Boo Ratshidi of Southern Africa." *American Ethnologist* 7:637–57.

Comaroff, Jean, and John Comaroff. 1997. "Postcolonial Politics and Discourses of Democracy in Southern Africa: An Anthropological Reflection on African Political Modernities." *Journal of Anthropological Research* 53:123–46.

Cox, Harvey. 2001. *Fire from Heaven: The Rise of Pentecostal Spirituality and the Reshaping of Religion in the 21st Century*. Cambridge, MA: Da Capo Press.

Cox, Harvey J. 1994. "Healers and Ecologists: Pentecostalism in Africa." *Christian Century* 111:1042–46.

Cubbin, Catherine, John Santelli, Claire D. Brindis, and Paula Braveman. 2005. "Neighborhood Context and Sexual Behaviors among Adolescents: Findings From the National Longitudinal Study of Adolescent Health." *Perspectives on Sexual and Reproductive Health* 37:125–34.

Dahl, Bianca. 2009. "The 'Failures of Culture': Christianity, Kinship, and Moral Discourses about Orphans during Botswana's AIDS Crisis." *Africa Today* 56:23–43.

Dahl, Tove S. 1997. *The Muslim Family: A Study of Women's Rights in Islam*. Oslo, Norway: Scandinavian Universities Press.

Dijk, Rijk van. 1998. "Pentecostalism, Cultural Memory and the State: Contested Representations of Time in Pentecostal Malawi." Pp. 155–81 in *Memory and the Postcolony: African Anthropology and the Critique of Power*, edited by Richard Werbner. London: Zed Books.

Dijk, Rijk van. 2002. "Modernity's Limits: Pentecostalism and the Moral Rejection of Alcohol in Malawi." Pp. 249–65 in *Alcohol in Africa: Mixing Business, Pleasure, and Politics*, edited by Deborah Fahy Bryceson. Portsmouth, NH: Heinemann.

Dilger, Hansjörg. 2007. "Healing the Wounds of Modernity: Salvation, Community and Care in a Neo-Pentecostal Church in Dar Es Salaam, Tanzania." *Journal of Religion in Africa* 37:59–83.

Dionne, Kim Yi, Patrick Gerland, and Susan Watkins. Forthcoming. "AIDS Exceptionalism: Another Constituency Heard from." *AIDS and Behavior*.

Doctor, Henry V., and Alexander A. Weinreb. 2003. "Estimation of AIDS Adult Mortality by Verbal Autopsy in Rural Malawi." *AIDS* 17:2509–13.

Douglas, Mary. 1966. *Purity and Danger: An Analysis of the Concepts of Pollution and Taboo*. London: Taylor Press.

Douglas, Mary. 1992. *Risk and Blame: Essays in Cultural Theory*. London: Routledge.

Drain, Paul K., Jennifer S. Smith, James P. Hughes, Daniel T. Halperin, and King K. Holmes. 2004. "Correlates of National HIV Seroprevalence: An Ecologic Analysis of 122 Developing Countries." *Journal of Acquired Immune Deficiency Syndromes* 35:407–20.

Druckerman, Pamela. 2007. *Lust in Translation: The Rules of Infidelity from Tokyo to Tennessee*. New York: Penguin Press.

Duesberg, Peter H. 1996. *Inventing the AIDS Virus*. Washington, DC: Regnery Publishing Co.

Ebaugh, Helen Rose. 2009. *The Gulen Movement: A Sociological Analysis of a Civic Movement Rooted in Moderate Islam*. New York: Springer Press.

Ebrahim, Mahomed, and Suraiya Nawab. 2008. "HIV/AIDS Prevention: An Islamic Perspective Experience from South Africa." Pp. 91–100 in *Federation of Islamic Medical Associations (FIMA) Year Book 2007*, edited by Hossam E. Fadel, Aly A. Misha'l, Abdul Fadl Mohsin Ebrahim, and Hakan Ertin. Amman: Jordan Society for Islamic Medical Sciences. Retrieved June 1, 2010. (http://fimaweb.net/cms/index.php?option=com_content&view=article&id=89:fima-year-book-2007&catid=49:fima-yearbook&Itemid=205).

Economist Intelligence Unit. (EIU). 2009. *Index of Democracy 2008*. Retrieved July 8, 2009. (http://graphics.eiu.com/PDF/Democracy%20Index%202008.pdf).

Ellison, Christopher G., Jeffery A. Burr, and Patricia L. McCall. 1997. "Religious Homogeneity and Metropolitan Suicide Rates." *Social Forces* 76:273–99.

Entwisle, Barbara, John B. Casterline, and Hussein A.A. Sayed. 1989. "Villages as Contexts for Contraceptive Behavior in Rural Egypt." *American Sociological Review* 54:1019–34.

Epstein, Helen. 2002. "The Hidden Cause of AIDS." Retrieved June 25, 2010. *New York Review of Books*, May 9. (http://www.nybooks.com/articles/archives/2002/may/09/the-hidden-cause-of-aids/?pagination=false).

Epstein, Helen. 2005. "God and the Fight against AIDS." *New York Review of Books,* April 28. Retrieved September 26, 2011. (pdf://epstein_2005–0246095628/epstein_2005.pdf).

Epstein, Helen. 2007. *The Invisible Cure: Africa, the West, and the Fight against AIDS*. New York: Farrar, Straus and Giroux.

Esacove, Anne W. 2010. "Love Matches." *Gender & Society* 24:83–109.

Eyawo, Oghenowede, Damien de Walque, Nathan Ford, Gloria Gakii, Richard T. Lester, and Edward J. Mills. 2010. "HIV Status in Discordant Couples in Sub-Saharan Africa: A Systematic Review and Meta-Analysis." *Lancet Infectious Diseases* 10:770–77.

Ezra, Kate (curator). 2007 (Jan. 11–Feb. 17). "Pandemic in Print: African HIV/AIDS Posters." A.D. Gallery, Columbia College, Chicago.

Feierman, Steven. 1985. "Struggles for Control: The Social Roots of Health and Healing in Modern Africa." *African Studies Review* 28:73–147.

Ferguson, James. 1990. *The Anti-Politics Machine: "Development," Depoliticization, and Bureaucratic Power in Lesotho.* Cambridge, UK: Cambridge University Press.

Fisher, Kate, and Simon Szreter. 2003. "'They Prefer Withdrawal': The Choice of Birth Control in Britain, 1918–1950." *Journal of Interdisciplinary History* 34:263–91.

Foster, Geoff, Choice Makuta, Roger Drew, and Etta Kralovec. 1997. "Factors Leading to the Establishment of Child-Headed Households: The Case of Zimbabwe." *Health Transition Review* 7S2:155–68.

Foster, Geoff. and John Williamson. 2000. "A Review of Current Literature on the Impact of HIV/AIDS on Children in Sub-Saharan Africa." *AIDS* 14S3:S275–84.

Foster, George M. 1976. "Disease Etiologies in Non-Western Medical Systems." *American Anthropologist* 78:773–82.

Frazer, Donald. 1914. *Winning a Primitive People: Sixteen Years' Work among the Warlike Tribe of the Ngoni and the Senga and Tumbuka Peoples of Central Africa.* New York: E.P. Dutton and Company.

Gama, Hobbs. 2003. "Malawi: Churches Now Espouse Condom Use in War on AIDS." *African News Update,* September 4. Retrieved September 26, 2011. (http://www.afrika.no/Detailed/4354.html).

Garner, Robert C. 2000. "Safe Sects? Dynamic Religion and AIDS in South Africa." *Journal of Modern African Studies* 38: 41–69.

Gates Foundation. 2007. *Bill & Melinda Gates Foundation Annual Report 2007.* Retrieved February 21, 2012. (http://www.gatesfoundation.org/nr/public/media/annualreports/annualreport07/index.html).

Gatheru, Claire. 2002. "Clerics to Fight HIV/AIDS Stigma." *Africa News Service,* June 10. Retrieved March 13, 2009. (http://allafrica.com/stories/200206100024.html).

Gerland, Patrick. 2005. *Effects of Social Interactions on Individual AIDS-Prevention Attitudes and Behaviors in Rural Malawi.* Ph.D. dissertation, Office for Population Research, Princeton University, Princeton, NJ.

Gertsman, Elina. 2007. "Visualizing Death: Medieval Plagues and the Macabre." Pp. 64–89 in *Piety and Plague: From Byzantium to the Baroque,* edited by Franco Mormando and Thomas Worcester. Kirksville, MS: Truman State University Press.

Ghys, Peter D., Erica Kufa, and M.V. George. 2006. "Measuring Trends in Prevalence and Incidence of HIV Infection in Countries with Generalized Epidemics." *Sexually Transmitted Infections* 82:i52–i56.

Gifford, Paul. 1995. *The Christian Churches and the Democratization of Africa.* Portsmouth, NH: Brill Academic Publishers.

Gifford, Paul. 1998. *African Christianity: Its Public Role.* Bloomington: Indiana University Press.

Gisselquist, David, John J. Potterat, Stuart Brody, and Francois Vachon. 2003. "Let It Be Sexual: How Health Care Transmission of AIDS in Africa Was Ignored." *International Journal of STD and AIDS* 14:148–61.

Githieya, Francis Kimani. 1997. *The Freedom of the Spirit: African Indigenous Churches in Kenya.* New York: Oxford University Press.

Glanz, Karen, Barbara K. Rimer, and Frances Marcus Lewis. 2002. *Health Behavior and Health Education: Theory, Research, and Practice.* 3d ed. San Francisco: Jossey-Bass.

Global Fund. 2010. *Global Fund 2010 Innovation and Impact.* Retrieved March 24, 2010. (http://www.theglobalfund.org/en/publications/progressreports/2010).

Goffman, Erving. 1963. *Stigma: Notes on the Management of Spoiled Identity.* Englewood Cliffs, NJ: Prentice-Hall.

Goldberg, Michelle. 2007. "How Bush's AIDS Program Is Failing Africans." *American Prospect,* July 10. Retrieved April 27, 2010. (http://www. prospect.org /cs/articles?article=how_bushs_aids_program_is_failing_africans).

Goody, Esther N. 2007. *Parenthood and Social Reproduction: Fostering and Occupational Roles in West Africa.* Cambridge, UK: Cambridge University Press.

Gould, W.T.S., and M.S. Brown. 1996. "A Fertility Transition in Sub-Saharan Africa?" *International Journal of Population Geography* 2:1–22.

Government of Malawi. (GoM). 2005. "Health Systems Strengthening and Orphan Care and Support." [Malawi Round 5 Proposal Form]: Geneva: The Global Fund. Retrieved October 10, 2011. (www.theglobalfund.org/grantDocuments/MLW-R05-HA_Proposal_0_en).

Gray, Peter B. 2004. "HIV and Islam: Is HIV Prevalence Lower among Muslims?" *Social Science & Medicine* 58:1751–56.

Gray, Ronald H., Maria J. Wawer, Rob Brookmeyer, Nelson K. Sewankambo, David Serwadda, Fred Wabwire-Mangen, Tom Lutalo, et al. 2001. "Probability of HIV-1 Transmission per Coital Act in Monogamous, Heterosexual, HIV-1 Discordant Couples in Rakai, Uganda." *Lancet* 357:1149–53.

Green, Edward C. 2003. *Rethinking AIDS Prevention: Learning from Successes in Developing Countries*. Westport, CT: Praeger Publishers.

Green, Edward C. 2011. *Broken Promises: How the AIDS Establishment Has Betrayed the Developing World*. San Francisco: PoliPoint Press.

Green, Edward, Daniel Halperin, Vinand Nantulya, and Janice Hogle. 2006. "Uganda's HIV Prevention Success: The Role of Sexual Behavior Change and the National Response." *AIDS and Behavior* 10:335–46.

Greene, Jody M., Susan T. Ennett, and Christopher L. Ringwalt. 1999. "Prevalence and Correlates of Survival Sex among Runaway and Homeless Youth." *American Journal of Public Health* 89:1406–09.

Gregson, Simon, Tom Zhuwau, Roy M. Anderson, and Stephen K. Chandiwana. 1999. "Apostles and Zionists: The Influence of Religion on Demographic Change in Rural Zimbabwe." *Population Studies* 53:179–93.

Grimm, Brian. 2010. "Briefing on US International Freedom Policy." March 19. Retrieved June 1, 2011. (http://pewforum.org/Government/Briefing-on-US-International-Religious-Freedom-Policy.aspx).

Gross, Terry. 2005. "Most Reverend Archbishop Njongonkulu Ndugane: NPR." *Fresh Air*. Retrieved September 13, 2011. (http://www.npr.org/templates/story/story.php?storyId=4509892).

Gyimah, Stephen Obeng. 2007. "What Has Faith Got to Do With It? Religion and Child Survival in Ghana." *Journal of Biosocial Science* 39:923–37.

Gyimah, Stephen Obeng, Baffour K. Takyi, and Isaac Addai. 2006. "Challenges to the Reproductive-Health Needs of African Women: On Religion and Maternal Health Utilization in Ghana." *Social Science & Medicine* 62:2930–44.

Hajnal, John. 1965. "European Marriage Pattern in Historical Perspective." Pp. 101–43 in *Population in History: Essays in Historical Demography,* edited by David V. Glass and D.E.C. Eversley. London: Edward Arnold.

Handa, Sudhanshu, Steve Koch, and Shu Wen Ng. 2009. "Child Mortality in Eastern and Southern Africa." *Population Review* 49:8–35.

Hapgood, David. 1965. *Africa: from Independence to Tomorrow*. New York: Antheneum.

Hardee, Karen, Jay Gribble, Stephanie Weber, Tim Manchester, and Martha Wood. 2008. *Reclaiming the ABCs: The Creation and Evolution of the ABC Approach*. Population Action International. Retrieved March 1, 2010. (http://www.populationaction.org /Publications/Report/Reclaiming_the_ABCs/ABCs_8.5x11.pdf).

Hastings, Adrian. 1979. *A History of African Christianity 1950–1975*. New York: Cambridge University Press.

Hastings, Adrian. 1996. *The Church in Africa, 1450–1950*. New York: Oxford University Press.

Hastings, Adrian. 1999. *A World History of Christianity*. Grand Rapids, MI: W.B. Eerdmans.

Hastings, Adrian. 2000. "African Christian Studies, 1967–1999: Reflections of an Editor." *Journal of Religion in Africa* 30:30–44.

Hatzfeld, Jean. 2007. *Life Laid Bare: The Survivors in Rwanda Speak*. New York: Other Press.

Hays, Jo N. 2005. *Epidemics and Pandemics: Their Impacts on Human History*. Santa Barbara, CA: ABC-CLIO.

Hearst, Norman, and Sanny Chen. 2004. "Condom Promotion for AIDS Prevention in the Developing World: Is It Working?" *Studies in Family Planning* 35:39–47.

Helleringer, Stéphane, and Hans Peter Kohler. 2005. "Social Networks, Perceptions of Risk, and Changing Attitudes towards HIV/AIDS: New Evidence from a Longitudinal Study Using Fixed-Effects Analysis." *Population Studies: A Journal of Demography* 59:265–82.

Heguye, Eli S. 1995. "Young People's Perception of Sexuality and Condom Use in Kahe." Pp. 107–122 in *Young People at Risk: Fighting AIDS in Northern Tanzania*, edited by Knut-Inge Klepp, Paul Biswalo, and Aud Talle. Oslo: Scandinavian University Press.

Herek, Gregory M., Keith F. Widaman, and John P. Capitanio. 2005. "When Sex Equals AIDS: Symbolic Stigma and Heterosexual Adults' Inaccurate Beliefs about Sexual Transmission of AIDS." *Social Problems* 52:15–37.

Heuveline, Patrick. 2004. "Impact of the HIV Epidemic on Population and Household Structure: The Dynamics and Evidence to Date." *AIDS* 18:S45–S53.

Hill, Zelee E., John Cleland, and Mohamed M. Ali. 2004. "Religious Affiliation and Extramarital Sex among Men in Brazil." *International Family Planning Perspectives* 30:20–26.

Hooper, Edward. 1999. *The River*. Boston: Little Brown and Company.

Horden, Peregrine. 1999. "Disease, Dragons, and Saints: The Management of Epidemics in the Dark Ages." Pp. 45–76 in *Epidemics and Ideas: Essays on the Historical Perception of Pestilence*, 2d ed., edited by Terence Ranger and Paul Slack. Cambridge, UK: Cambridge University Press.

Hosegood, Victoria, Eleanor Preston-Whyte, Joanna Busza, Sindile Moitse, and Ian M. Timaeus. 2007. "Revealing the Full Extent of Households' Experiences of HIV and AIDS in Rural South Africa." *Social Science & Medicine* 65:1249–59.

Hughes, Dana. 2008. "Sun, Safaris and Sex Tourism in Kenya." *ABC News*, October 7, http://abcnews.go.com/Travel/story?id=5935427&;page=1#.T0HKVPkpCGc

Hsu, Becky, Amy Reynolds, Conrad Hackett, and James Gibbon. 2008. "Estimating the Religious Composition of All Nations: An Empirical Assessment of the World Christian Database." *Journal for the Scientific Study of Religion* 47:678–693.

Hunt, Ezra M. 1880. "Our Present and Our Needed Knowledge of Epidemics." *Public Health Papers and Reports* 6:93–106.

Hunter, Mark. 2002. "The Materiality of Everyday Sex: Thinking beyond 'Prostitution.'" *African Studies* 61:99–120.

Hunter, Mark. 2010. *Love in the Time of AIDS: Inequality, Gender, and Rights in South Africa*. Bloomington: Indiana University Press.

Hunter, Susan S. 1990. "Orphans as a Window on the AIDS Epidemic in Sub-Saharan Africa: Initial Results and Implications of a Study in Uganda." *Social Science & Medicine* 31:681–90.

Huntington, Samuel P. 1993. *The Third Wave: Democratization in the Late Twentieth Century*. Edmond: University of Oklahoma Press.

Iliffe, John. 2005. *The African AIDS Epidemic: A History*. Athens: Ohio University Press.

Ingstad, Benedicte. 1990. "The Cultural Construction of AIDS and Its Consequences for Prevention in Botswana." *Medical Anthropology Quarterly* 4:28–40.

Isichei, Elizabeth Allo. 1995. *A History of Christianity in Africa: From Antiquity to the Present*. Grand Rapids, MI: W.B. Eerdmans.

Isiugo-Abanihe, Uche C. 1985. "Child Fosterage in West Africa." *Population and Development Review* 11:53–73.

Janz, Nancy K., and Marshall H. Becker. 1984. "The Health Belief Model: A Decade Later." *Health Education and Behavior* 11:1–47.

Jenkins, Philip. 2002. *The Next Christendom: The Rise of Global Christianity*. New York: Oxford University Press.

Jenkins, Philip. 2006. *The New Faces of Christianity*. New York: Oxford University Press.

Johnson-Hanks, Jennifer. 2006. *Uncertain Honor: Modern Motherhood in an African Crisis*. Chicago: University Of Chicago Press.

Jolly, Susan, and Hazel Reeves. 2005. *Gender and Migration: Overview Report*. Institute of Development Studies: BRIDGE. Retrieved May 16, 2011. (http://www.bridge.ids.ac.uk/reports/CEP-Mig-OR.pdf).

Kaldellis, Anthony. 2004. *Procopius of Caesarea: Tyranny, History, and Philosophy at the End of Antiquity*. Philadelphia: University of Pennsylvania Press.

Kalichman, Seth C. 2009. *Denying AIDS: Conspiracy Theories, Pseudoscience, and Human Tragedy.* New York: Copernicus Books/Springer.

Kalipeni, Ezekiel, and Eliya M. Zulu. 1993. "Gender Differences in Knowledge and Attitudes toward Modern and Traditional Methods of Child Spacing in Malawi." *Population Research and Policy Review* 12:103–21.

Kamwi, Richard, Thomas Kenyon, and Gary Newton. 2006. "PEPFAR and HIV Prevention in Africa." *Lancet* 367:1978–79.

Kelly, Kevin, and Warren Parker. 2000. *Communities of Practice: Contextual Mediators of Youth Response to HIV/AIDS.* Johannesburg: Sentinel Site Monitoring and Evaluation Project, Stage Two Report. Retrieved March 10, 2010. (http://www.cadre.org.za/node/105).

Kendemeh, Emmanuel. 2009. "Cameroon: Pope Delivers Message of Sacrifice and Faithfulness." *allAfrica.com*, March 19. Retrieved April 26, 2009. (http://allafrica.com/stories/200903190608. html).

Kenya Demographic and Health Survey. (KDHS). 2003. *Kenya Demographic and Health Survey 2003: Preliminary Report.* Calverton, MD: National Council for Population and Development, Central Bureau of Statistics, and Macro International Inc.

Kisting, Denver. 2010. "Namibia: 'Discrimination rather than No Bursaries at All.'" *allAfrica.com*, June 28. Retrieved July 15, 2010. (http://allafrica.com/stories/201006290178.html).

Klaits, Frederick. 2010. *Death in a Church of Life: Moral Passion during Botswana's Time of AIDS.* Berkeley: University of California Press.

Kohler, Hans-Peter, Francesco C. Billari, and José Antonio Ortega. 2002. "The Emergence of Lowest-Low Fertility in Europe during the 1990s." *Population and Development Review* 28:641–80.

Kohler, Hans-Peter, Jere R. Behrman, and Susan C. Watkins. 2001. "The Density of Social Networks and Fertility Decisions: Evidence From South Nyanza District, Kenya." *Demography* 38:43–58.

Komakech, Richard. 2003. "Clergy to Lead Anti-AIDS-Stigma Drive." *Africa News Service*, November 29. Retrieved September 20, 2009. (http://allafrica.com/stories/200311290002.html).

Krapf, Rev. Dr. Johann L. 1860. *Travels, Researches and Missionary Labours During an Eighteen Year Residence in Eastern Africa.* London: Trubner and Co.

Ku, Leighton C., Freya L. Sonenstein, and Joseph H. Pleck. 1992. "The Association of AIDS Education and Sex Education with Sexual Behavior and Condom Use among Teenage Men." *Family Planning Perspectives* 24:100–106.

Kuran, Timur. 2010. *The Long Divergence: How Islamic Law Held Back the Middle East.* Princeton, NJ: Princeton University Press.

Laqueur, Walter. 2008. *The Changing Face of Anti-Semitism: From Ancient Times to the Present Day.* New York: Oxford University Press.

Lafraniere, Sharon. 2005a. "AIDS and Custom Leave African Families Nothing." *New York Times*, February 18. Retrieved July 15, 2010. (http://www.nytimes.com/2005/02/18/international/africa/18property.html).

Lafraniere, Sharon. 2005b. "AIDS Now Compels Africa to Challenge Widows' 'Cleansing.'" *New York Times*, May 11. Retrieved July 15, 2010. (http://www.nytimes.com/2005/05/11/international/africa/11malawi.html).

Lancet Editorial. 2006. "HIV Prevention Policy Needs an Urgent Cure." *Lancet* 367:1213.

Lancet Editorial. 2006. "Condoms and the Vatican." *Lancet* 367:1550.

Laumann, Edward O. 2004. *The Sexual Organization of the City.* Chicago: University of Chicago Press.

Leclerc-Madlala, Suzanne. 1997. "Infect One, Infect All: Zulu Youth Response to the AIDS Epidemic in South Africa." *Medical Anthropology* 17:363–80.

Leclerc-Madlala, Suzanne. 2003. "Transactional Sex and the Pursuit of Modernity." *Social Dynamics: A Journal of African Studies* 29:213.

Liddell, Christine, Louise Barrett, and Moya Bwdawell. 2005. "Indigenous Representations of Illness and AIDS in Sub-Saharan Africa." *Social Science & Medicine* 60:691–700.

Lieberman, Evan S. 2009. *Boundaries of Contagion: How Ethnic Politics Have Shaped Government Responses to AIDS.* Princeton, NJ: Princeton University Press.

Liebowitz, Jeremy. 2002. "The Impact of Faith-Based Organizations on HIV/AIDS Prevention and Mitigation in Africa." *Health Economics and HIV/AIDS Research Division (HEARD)*. Retrieved December 2, 2006. (http://www.ukzn.ac.za/heard/research/ResearchReports/2002/FBOs%20paper_Dec02.pdf).

Link, Bruce G., and Jo C. Phelan. 2001. "Conceptualizing Stigma." *Annual Review of Sociology* 27:363–85.

Little, Lester K. (Ed.). 2007. *Plague and the End of Antiquity: The Pandemic of 541–750*. Cambridge, UK: Cambridge University Press.

Longest, Kyle C., and Stephen Vaisey. 2008. "Fuzzy: A Program for Performing Qualitative Comparative Analyses (QCA) in Stata." *Stata Journal* 8:79–104.

Lopman, Ben, Constance Nyamukapa, Phyllis Mushati, Zivai Mupambireyi, Peter Mason, Geoff P. Garnett, and Simon Gregoson. 2008. "HIV Incidence in 3 Years of Follow-Up of a Zimbabwe Cohort—1998–2000 to 2001–03: Contributions of Proximate and Underlying Determinants to Transmission." *International Journal of Epidemiology* 37:88–105.

Luther, Martin, Timothy F. Lull, and William R. Russell. 2005. *Martin Luther's Basic Theological Writings*. Minneapolis, MN: Fortress Press.

Luke, Nancy. 2005. "Confronting the 'Sugar Daddy' Stereotype: Age and Economic Asymmetries and Risky Sexual Behavior in Urban Kenya." *International Family Planning Perspectives* 31:6–14.

Luke, Nancy. 2006. "Exchange and Condom Use in Informal Sexual Relationships in Urban Kenya." *Economic Development and Cultural Change* 54:319–48.

Lux, Steven, and Kristine Greenaway. 2006. *Scaling Up Effective Partnerships: A Guide to Working with Faith-Based Organizations in the Response to HIV and AIDS*. Geneva: Ecumenical Advocacy Alliance. Retrieved September 26, 2011. (http://www.e-alliance.ch/hiv_faith_guide.jsp).

Lwanda, John. 2003. "Constructions of *Ufiti* (Witchcraft) in 21st Century Malawi: Youth, State and HIV/AIDS." Paper presented at the 46th African Studies Association meeting, Boston, MA, October 30–November 2.

Madhavan, Sangeetha. 2004. "Fosterage Patterns in the Age of AIDS: Continuity and Change." *Social Science & Medicine* 58:1443–54.

Makori, Henry. 2009. "Are World Media Fighting Pope Benedict XVI?" allAfrica.com, March 24. Retrieved April 26, 2009. (http://allafrica.com/stories/200903240854.html).

Maman, Suzanne, Rebecca Cathcart, Gillian Burkhardt, Serge Omba, and Freida Behets. 2009. "The Role of Religion in HIV-Positive Women's Disclosure Experiences and Coping strategies in Kinshasa, Democratic Republic of Congo." *Social Science and Medicine* 69:965–70.

Manglos, Nicolette D., and Jenny Trinitapoli. 2011. "The Third Therapeutic System: Faith Healing Strategies in the Context of a Generalized AIDS Epidemic." *Journal of Health and Social Behavior* 52:107–122.

Mansaray, N., A.M. Kosia, and E. Mikiu. 1992 (July 19–24). "Religious Leaders as AIDS Educators in Sierra Leone." *International Conference on AIDS* 8:D437 (abstract no. PoD 5301) Retrieved February 27, 2012. (http://aegis69.aegis.org/DisplayContent/DisplayContent.aspx?sectionID=234746).

Maren, Michael. 1997. *The Road to Hell: The Ravaging Effects of Foreign and International Charity*. New York: Free Press.

Maslove, David, Anisa Mnyusiwalla, Edward Mills, Jessie McGowan, Amir Attaran, and Kumanan Wilson. 2009. "Barriers to the Effective Treatment and Prevention of Malaria in Africa: A Systematic Review of Qualitative Studies." *BMC International Health and Human Rights* 9:26-36.

Mauss, Marcel. 2000. *The Gift: The Form and Reason for Exchange in Archaic Societies*. Reissue. New York: W.W. Norton & Company.

Maxwell, David. 2007. *African Gifts of the Spirit: Pentecostalism & the Rise of a Zimbabwean Transnational Religious Movement*. Athens: Ohio University Press.

May, Philip A., J. Phillip Gossage, Lesley E. Brooke, Cudore L. Snell, Anna-Susan Marais, Loretta S. Hendricks, Julie A. Croxford, and Denis L. Viljoen. 2005. "Maternal Risk Factors for Fetal Alcohol Syndrome in the Western Cape Province of South Africa: A Population-Based Study." *American Journal of Public Health* 95:1190–99.

McNeil, Donald G. 2010. "At Front Lines, AIDS War Is Falling Apart." *New York Times*, May 9. Retrieved May 16, 2010. (http://www.nytimes.com/2010/05/10/world/africa/10aids.html).

McNeill, Fraser G., and Deborah James. 2008. "Singing Songs of AIDS in Venda, South Africa: Performance, Pollution and Ethnomusicology in a 'Neo-Liberal' Setting." *South African Music Studies* 28:1–30.

McNeill, William H. 1977/1998. *Plagues and Peoples*. New York: Anchor Books.

Meda, Nicolas, Ibra Ndoye, Souleymane M'Boup, Alpha Wade, Salif Ndiaye, Cheikh Niang, et al. 1999. "Low and Stable HIV Infection Rates in Senegal: Natural Course of the Epidemic or Evidence for Success of Prevention?" *AIDS* 13:1397.

Mensch, Barbara S., Monica J. Grant, and Ann K. Blanc. 2006. "The Changing Context of Sexual Initiation in Sub-Saharan Africa." *Population and Development Review* 32:699–727.

Mensch, Barbara S., Paul C. Hewett, and Annabel S. Erulkar. 2003. "The Reporting of Sensitive Behavior by Adolescents: A Methodological Experiment in Kenya." *Demography* 40:247–68.

Meyer, Brigit. 2004. "Christianity in Africa: From African Independent to Pentecostal-Charismatic Churches." *Annual Review of Anthropology* 33:447–74.

Meyer-Weitz, A., P. Reddy, W. Weijts, B. van den Borne, and G. Kok. 1998. "The Socio-Cultural Contexts of Sexually Transmitted Diseases in South Africa: Implications for Health Education Programmes." *AIDS Care* 10:S39–55.

Middleton, John, and Edward H. Winter. [1963] 2004. *RL E: Anthropology and Ethnography: Witchcraft and Sorcery in East Africa*. Reprint. London: Routledge.

Monasch, Roeland, and J. Ties Boerma. 2004. "Orphanhood and Childcare Patterns in Sub-Saharan Africa: An Analysis of National Surveys from 40 Countries." *AIDS* 18:S55–65.

Moonze, Larry. 2003. "AIDS Stigma Is Due to the Church." *Africa News Service*, July 19. Retrieved September 10, 2008. (http://allafrica.com/stories/200307210206.html).

Morgan, S.Philip, Sharon Stash, Herbert L. Smith, and Karen Oppenheim Mason. 2002. "Muslim and Non-Muslim Differences in Female Autonomy and Fertility: Evidence from Four Asian Countries." *Population and Development Review* 28:515–537.

Mormando, Franco, and Thomas Worcester (Eds.). 2007. *Piety and Plague: From Byzantium to the Baroque*. Kirksville, MS: Truman State University Press.

Morris, Brian. 1986. "Herbalism and Divination in Southern Malawi." *Social Science & Medicine* 23:367–77.

Morris, Martina, Ann E. Kurth, Deven T. Hamilton, James Moody, and Steve Wakefield. 2009. "Concurrent Partnerships and HIV Prevalence Disparities by Race: Linking Science and Public Health Practice." *American Journal of Public Health* 99:1023–31.

Mosher, William D., Linda B. Williams, and David P. Johnson. 1992. "Religion and Fertility in the United States: New Patterns." *Demography* 29:199–214.

Moszynski, Peter. 2008. "Kenyan Muslim Clerics Decide to Campaign against Use of Condoms." *BMJ (Clinical Research Ed.)* 336:1154.

Mufune, Pempelani. 2005. "Myths about Condoms and HIV/AIDS in Rural Northern Namibia." *International Social Science Journal* 57:675–686.

Mullan, Fitzhugh. 2005. "The Metrics of the Physician Brain Drain." *New England Journal of Medicine* 353:1810–18.

Murphy, Elaine M., Margaret E. Greene, Alexandra Mihailovic, and Peter Olupot-Olupot. 2006. "Was the 'ABC' Approach (Abstinence, Being Faithful, Using Condoms) Responsible for Uganda's Decline in HIV?" *PLoS Medicine* 3:e379.

Musallam, Basim F. 1983. *Sex and Society in Islam: Birth Control before the Nineteenth Century*. Cambridge, UK: Cambridge University Press.

National AIDS Commission. 2003. *Estimating National HIV Prevalence in Malawi from Sentinel Surveillance Data: Technical Report*. Lilongwe, Malawi: POLICY Project, Retrieved October 1, 2004. (http://www.policyproject.com/pubs/countryreports /MALNatEst2003.doc).

National AIDS Control Council. (NACC). 2007. *National HIV Prevalence in Kenya*. Nairobi: National AIDS Control Council and National AIDS and STD Control Programme. Retrieved July 8, 2009. (http://www.fpfk.or. ke/aids/images/Resources/Resources/national_hiv_prevalence_in_kenya._released_jun_2007.pdf).

Nattrass, Nicoli. 2009. "Poverty, Sex and HIV." *AIDS and Behavior* 13:833–40.

Ndungane, Njongonkulu. 2004. "The Challenge of HIV/AIDS to Christian Theology." Retrieved September 26, 2011. (http://www.uwc.ac.za/arts/Rel-Theo/AIDS-Ndungane.doc).

Nicholas, Lionel, and Kevin Durrheim. 1995. "Religiosity, AIDS, and Sexuality Knowledge, Attitudes, Beliefs, and Practices of Black South-African First-Year University Students." *Psychological Reports* 77:1328–30.

Nunberg, Geoffrey. 2007. *Talking Right: How Conservatives Turned Liberalism into a Tax-Raising, Latte-Drinking, Sushi-Eating, Volvo-Driving,* New York Times-Reading, Body-Piercing, Hollywood-Loving, Left-Wing Freak Show. New York: PublicAffairs.

Obermeyer, Carla M. 1992. "Islam, Women, and Politics-the Demography of Arab Countries." *Population and Development Review* 18:33–60.

Offen, Karen. 1999. *European Feminisms, 1700–1950: A Political History*. Stanford, CA: Stanford University Press.

Olouch, Fred. 2006. "Kenya: Sex Tourism Thrives Unabated." *News from Africa*, April 6. Retrieved June 10, 2009. (http://www.newsfromafrica.org/newsfromafrica/articles/art_10656.html).

Oppenheimer, Valerie Kincade. 1988. "A Theory of Marriage Timing." *American Journal of Sociology* 94:563–91.

Orubuloye, I. Olatunji, John C. Caldwell, and Pat Caldwell. 1993. "The Role of Religious Leaders in Changing Sexual Behaviour in Southwest Nigeria in an Era of AIDS." *Health Transition Review* 3:93–104.

Ositelu, Rufus Okikiolaolu Olubiyi. 2002. *African Instituted Churches*. London: LIT Verlag Münster.

Oster, Emily. 2007. "HIV and Sexual Behavior Change: Why Not Africa?" NBER Working Paper #13049. (http://www.nber.org).

Page, Hillary J. 1989. "Childrearing Versus Childbearing: Coresidence of Mother and Child in Sub-Saharan Africa." Pp. 401–41 in *Reproduction and Social Organization in Sub-Saharan Africa*, edited by Ron J. Lesthaeghe. Berkeley: University of California Press.

Pager, Devah, and Lincoln Quillian. 2005. "Walking the Talk? What Employers Say Versus What They Do." *American Sociological Review* 70:355–80.

Parkhurst, Justin O. 2002. "The Ugandan Success Story? Evidence and Claims of HIV-1 Prevention." *Lancet* 360:78–80.

Parkhurst, Justin O., and Louisiana Lush. 2004. "The Political Environment of HIV: Lessons from a Comparison of Uganda and South Africa." *Social Science & Medicine* 59:1913–24.

Pavitt, Nigel. 1989. *Kenya: The First Explorers*. New York: St. Martin's Press.

Pellow, Deborah. 1999. "Sex, Disease, and Culture Change in Ghana." Pp. 17–42 in *Histories of Sexually Transmitted Diseases in Sub-Saharan Africa*, edited by Philip W. Setel, Milton Lewis, and Maryinez Lyons. Westport, CT: Greenwood Press.

Pescosolido, Bernice A. 1990. "The Social Context of Religious Integration and Suicide: Pursuing the Network Explanation." *Sociological Quarterly* 31:337–57.

Pescosolido, Bernice A., and Sharon Georgianna. 1989. "Durkheim, Suicide, and Religion: Toward a Network Theory of Suicide." *American Sociological Review* 54:33–48.

Pew Research Center. 2010. "Tolerance and Tension: Islam and Christianity in Sub-Saharan Africa." Washington DC: Pew Research Center. Retrieved April 20, 2010. (http://pewresearch.org/pubs/1564/islam-christianity-in-sub-saharan-africa-survey).

Pfeiffer, James. 2002. "African Independent Churches in Mozambique: Healing the Afflictions of Inequality." *Medical Anthropology Quarterly* 16:176–99.

Pfeiffer, James. 2004. "Civil Society, NGOs, and the Holy Spirit in Mozambique." *Human Organization* 63:359–72.

Philpott, Daniel. 2004. "Christianity and Democracy: The Catholic Wave." *Journal of Democracy* 15:32–46.

Pierson, Delavan L. (Ed.). 1922. *Missionary Review of the World*, vol. 45. Funk & Wagnalls.

Pisani, Elizabeth. 1999. *Acting Early to Prevent AIDS: The Case of Senegal*. Geneva: Joint United National Program for HIV/AIDS.

Pisani, Elizabeth. 2009. *The Wisdom of Whores: Bureaucrats, Brothels and the Business of AIDS*. New York: W.W. Norton & Company.

Plaatje, Sol T. 2006. *Mhudi*. New York: Penguin Global.

Population Services International and AIDSMark. 2009. *A Decade of Innovative Marketing for Health: Lessons Learned*. Washington, DC: Population Services. Retrieved August 1, 2009. (http://pdf.usaid.gov/pdf_docs/PNADL283.pdf).

Poulin, Michelle. 2009. "School-Girl Networks and School-Girl Identity: Maintaining Social Status in a Poor Country." Paper presented at the American Sociological Association of America Annual Meeting, San Francisco, CA, August 10.

Poulin, Michelle. 2010. "Reporting on First Sexual Experience: The Importance of Interviewer–Respondent Interaction." *Demographic Research* 22:237–88.

Poulin, Michelle J. 2007. "Sex, Money, and Premarital Relationships in Southern Malawi." *Social Science & Medicine* 65:2383–93.

Preston-Whyte, Eleanor. 1999. "Reproductive Health and the Condom Dilemma: Identifying Situational Barriers to HIV Protection in South Africa." Pp. 139–55 in *Resistances to Behavioural Change to Reduce HIV/AIDS Infection in Predominantly Heterosexual Epidemics in Third World Countries,* edited by John C. Caldwell, Pat Caldwell, John Anarfi, Kofi Awusabo-Asare, James Ntozi, I. Olatunji Orubuloye, et al. Canberra, Australia: Health Transition Centre.

Prince, Ruth. 2007. "Salvation and Tradition: Configurations of Faith in a Time of Death." *Journal of Religion in Africa* 37:84–115.

Prince, Ruth. 2009. "Christian Salvation and Luo Tradition: Arguments of Faith in a Time of Death in Western Kenya." Pp. 49–84 in *AIDS and Religious Practice in Africa*, edited by Felicitas Becker and P. Wenzel Geissler. Leide, The Netherlands: Brill.

Putnam, Robert D. 2001. *Bowling Alone: The Collapse and Revival of American Community.* New York: Simon & Schuster.

Ragin, Charles. 2000. *Fuzzy-Set Social Science.* Chicago: University of Chicago Press.

Rankin, Sally H., Teri Lindgren, William W. Rankin, and Joyce Ng'oma. 2005. "Donkey Work: Women, Religion, and HIV/AIDS in Malawi." *Health Care for Women International* 26:4–16.

Raudenbush, Stephen W., and Anthony S. Bryk. 2001. *Hierarchical Linear Models: Applications and Data Analysis Methods.* 2d ed. Thousand Oaks, CA: Sage.

Redding, Colleen A., Joseph S. Rossi, Susan R. Rossi, Waye F. Velicer, and James O. Prochaska. 2000. "Health Behavior Models." *International Electronic Journal of Health Education* 3:180–93.

Reff, Daniel T. 2005. *Plagues, Priests, Demons: Sacred Narratives and the Rise of Christianity in the Old World and the New.* Cambridge, UK: Cambridge University Press.

Regnerus, Mark. 2007. *Forbidden Fruit.* New York: Oxford University Press.

Reniers, Georges. 2003. "Divorce and Remarriage in Rural Malawi." *Demographic Research* 1:175–206.

Reniers, Georges. 2008. "Marital Strategies for Regulating Exposure to HIV." *Demography* 45:417–38.

Reniers, Georges, and Jeffrey Eaton. 2009. "Refusal Bias in HIV Prevalence Estimates from Nationally Representative Seroprevalence Surveys." *AIDS* 23:621–29.

Reniers, Georges, and Susan Watkins. 2009. "Polygyny and the Spread of HIV in Sub-Saharan Africa: A Case of Benign Concurrency." *AIDS* 23:299–307.

Republic of Malawi. (RoM). 2005. *Malawi HIV and AIDS: Monitoring and Evaluation Report.* Lilongwe: Department of Nutrition, HIV and AIDS, Office of the President and Cabinet.

Rex, Richard. 2002. *The Lollards.* New York: Palgrave Macmillan.

Rittgers, Ronald K. 2007. "Protestants and Plague." Pp. 132–155 in *Piety and Plague: From Byzantium to the Baroque*, edited by Franco Mormando and Thomas Worcester. Kirksville, MO: Truman State University Press.

Robbins, Joel. 2004. "The Globalization of Pentecostal and Charismatic Christianity." *Annual Review of Anthropology* 33:117–43.

Robinson, David. 2004. *Muslim Societies in African History.* Cambridge, UK: Cambridge University Press.

Rosenstock, Irwin M. 1966. "Why People Use Health Services." *Milbank Memorial Fund Quarterly* 44:94–127.

Rosenstock, Irwin M., Victor J. Strecher, and Marshall H. Becker. 1988. "Social Learning and the Health Belief Model." *Health Education Quarterly* 15:178–83.

Rosenthal, Anat. 2008. "Raising Our Children: Community Strategies for Coping with Orphans and Vulnerable Children in Rural Malawi." Ph.D. dissertation, Department of Anthropology, Hebrew University, Jerusalem.

Rugalema, Gabriel. 2004. "Understanding the African HIV Pandemic: An Appraisal of the Contexts and Lay Explanation of the HIV/AIDS Pandemic with Examples from Tanzania and

Kenya." Pp. 191–203 in *HIV & AIDS in Africa: Beyond Epidemiology*, edited by Ezekiel Kalipeni, Susan Craddock, Joseph R. Oppong, and Jayati Ghosh. Oxford: Blackwell.

Ruiter, Stijn, and Nan Dirk De Graaf. 2006. "National Context, Religiosity, and Volunteering: Results from 53 Countries." *American Sociological Review* 71:191–210.

Sabar-Friedman, Galia. 1997. "Church and State in Kenya, 1986–1992: The Churches' Involvement in the 'Game of Change.'" *African Affairs* 96: 25–52.

Scott, James C. 1998. "Compulsory Villagization in Tanzania: Aesthetics and Minitiarization." Pp. 223–61 in *Seeing like a State: How Certain Schemes to Improve the Human Condition Have Failed*, edited by James C. Scott. New Haven, CT: Yale University Press.

Schurman Taylor, Christopher. 1998. *In the Vicinity of the Righteous: Ziyara and the Veneration of Muslim Saints in Late Medieval Egypt*. New York: Brill Academic Publishers.

Sears, Robert (Ed.). 1845. *The Guide to Knowledge, or Repertory of Facts, Forming a Complete Library of Entertaining Information in the Several Departments of Science, Literature, and Art*. New York: E. Walker and Co.

Selikow, Terry-Ann. 2004. "'We Have Our Own Special Language.' Language, Sexuality and HIV/AIDS: A Case Study of Youth in an Urban Township in South Africa." *African Health Sciences* 4:102–108.

Shelton, James D. 2006. "Confessions of a Condom Lover." *Lancet* 368:1947–49.

Simpson, Victor L. 2009. "Pope Says Condoms Worsen HIV Problem." *Washington Post*, March 18. Retrieved April 26, 2010. (http://www.washingtonpost.com/wp-dyn/content/article/2009/03/17/AR2009031703369.html).

Smith, Christian. 2003. *Moral, Believing Animals: Human Personhood and Culture*. New York: Oxford University Press.

Smith, Daniel Jordan. 2001. "'These Girls Today Na War-O': Premarital Sexuality and Modern Identity in Southeastern Nigeria." *Africa Today* 48:98–120.

Smith, Daniel Jordan. 2004a. "Premarital Sex, Procreation, and HIV Risk in Nigeria." *Studies in Family Planning* 35:223–35.

Smith, Daniel Jordan. 2004b. "Youth, Sin, and Sex in Nigeria: Christianity and HIV/AIDS-related Beliefs and Behaviour among Rural-Urban Migrants." *Culture, Health & Sexuality* 6:425–37.

Smith, Kirsten P., and Susan Cotts Watkins. 2005. "Perceptions of Risk and Strategies for Prevention: Responses to HIV/AIDS in Rural Malawi." *Social Science & Medicine* 60:649–60.

Stammers, Trevor. 2005. "As Easy as ABC? Primary Prevention of Sexually Transmitted Infections." *Postgraduate Medical Journal* 81:273–75.

Stark, Rodney. 1996. "Religion as Context: Hellfire and Delinquency One More Time." *Sociology of Religion* 57:163–73.

Stark, Rodney. 1996. *The Rise of Christianity: A Sociologist Reconsiders History*. Princeton, NJ: Princeton University Press.

Stark, Rodney. 1997. *The Rise of Christianity: How the Obscure, Marginal Jesus Movement Became the Dominant Religious Force in the Western World in a Few Centuries*. San Francisco: Harper Collins.

Stark, Rodney, and William Sims Bainbridge. 1996. *A Theory of Religion*. New Brunswick, NJ: Rutgers University Press.

Stark, Rodney, Lori Kent, and Daniel P. Doyle. 1982. "Religion and Delinquency: The Ecology of a 'Lost' Relationship." *Journal of Research in Crime and Delinquency* 19:4–24.

Stoclet, Alain J. 2007. "Consilia Humana, Ops Divina, Superstitio: Seeking Succor and Solace in Times of Plague, with Particular Reference to Gaul in the Early Middle Ages." Pp. 135–49 in *Plague and the End of Antiquity: The Pandemic of 541–750*, edited by Lester K. Little. Cambridge, UK: Cambridge University Press.

Stoneburner, Rand L., and Daniel Low-Beer. 2004. "Population-Level HIV Declines and Behavioral Risk Avoidance in Uganda." *Science* 304:714–18.

Stover, John, Boga Fidzani, Batho Chris Molomo, Themba Moeti, and Godfrey Musuka. 2008. "Estimated HIV Trends and Program Effects in Botswana." *PLoS ONE* 3:e3729.

Stuart, James M., James H. Irlam, and David Wilkinson. 1999. "Routine Reporting or Sentinel Surveys for HIV/AIDS Surveillance in Resource-Poor Settings: Experience in South Africa, 1991–97." *International Journal of STD and AIDS* 10:328–30.

Summers, Todd. 2002. *The Global Fund to Fight AIDS, TB, and Malaria Challenges and Opportunities: A Report of the Committee on Resource Mobilization and Coordination*. Washington, DC: Center for Strategic and International Studies. Retrieved August 1, 2009. (http://www.kaisernetwork.org/health_cast/uploaded_files/Globalfundbook.pdf).

Surur, Feiruz, and Mirgissa Kaba. 2000. "The Role of Religious Leaders in HIV/AIDS Prevention, Control, and Patient Care and Support: A Pilot Project in Jimma Zone." *Northeast African Studies* 7:59–79.

Swarns, Rachel L. 2002. "South African Village, Fearing AIDS, Trusts God More than Drugs." *New York Times*, August 10, 2002. Retrieved September 26, 2011. (http://www.nytimes.com/2002/08/10/international/africa/10AFRI.html).

Swidler, Ann, and Susan Cotts Watkins. 2007. "Ties of Dependence: AIDS and Transactional Sex in Rural Malawi." Retrieved June 30, 2010. (http://escholarship.org/uc/item/7t14c4h0).

Swidler, Ann, and Susan Watkins. 2009. "Teach a Man: The Ironies of Sustainability in Rural Malawi." *World Development* 37:1183–96.

Takyi, Baffour K. 2003. "Religion and Women's Health in Ghana: Insights into HIV/AIDS Preventive and Protective Behavior." *Social Science and Medicine* 56:1221–34.

Talbott, John R. 2007. "Size Matters: The Number of Prostitutes and the Global HIV/AIDS Pandemic." *PLoS ONE* 2:e543.

Tavory, Iddo, and Ann Swidler. 2009. "Condom Semiotics: Meaning and Condom Use in Rural Malawi." *American Sociological Review* 74:171–89.

Thiong'o, Ngugi wa. 1986. *Decolonising the Mind: The Politics of Language in African Literature*. Portsmouth, NH: Heinemann.

Thomas, Linda E. 1994. "African Indigenous Churches as a Source of Socio-Political Transformation in South Africa." *Africa Today* 41:39–56.

Thomas, William I. and Dorothy Swaine Thomas. 1928. *The Child in America: Behavior Problems and Programs*. New York: Knopf.

Thornton, Arland. 2005. *Reading History Sideways: The Fallacy and Enduring Impact of the Developmental Paradigm on Family Life*. Chicago: University of Chicago Press.

Timberg, Craig. 2006. "How AIDS in Africa Was Overstated: Reliance on Data from Urban Prenatal Clinics Skewed Early Projections." *Washington Post*, April 6.

Todd, J., I. Cremin, N. McGrath, J.-B. Bwanika, A. Wringe, M. Marston, I. Kasamba, et al. 2009. "Reported Number of Sexual Partners: Comparison of Data from Four African Longitudinal Studies." *Sexually Transmitted Infections* 85:i72–i80.

Treichler, Paula A. 2004. *How to Have Theory in an Epidemic: Cultural Chronicles of AIDS*. Durham, NC: Duke University Press.

Trinitapoli, Jenny. 2006. "Religious Responses to AIDS in Sub-Saharan Africa: An Examination of Religious Congregations in Rural Malawi." *Review of Religious Research* 47:253–70.

Trinitapoli, Jenny. 2007. *The Role of Religious Congregations in the AIDS Crisis of Sub-Saharan Africa*. Ph.D. dissertation. Department of Sociology, The University of Texas at Austin.

Trinitapoli, Jenny. 2009. "Religious Teachings and Influences on the ABCs of HIV Prevention in Malawi." *Social Science & Medicine* 69:199–209.

Trinitapoli, Jenny, and Mark D. Regnerus. 2006. "Religion and HIV Risk Behaviors among Married Men: Initial Results from a Study in Rural Sub-Saharan Africa." *Journal for the Scientific Study of Religion* 45:505–28.

Uecker, Jeremy E. 2008. "Religion, Pledging, and the Premarital Sexual Behavior of Married Young Adults." *Journal of Marriage and the Family* 70:728–44.

UNAIDS. 2007. *2007 AIDS Epidemic Update*. Geneva: UNAIDS. Retrieved September 26, 2011. (http://data.unaids.org/pub/EPISlides/2007/2007_epiupdate_en.pdf).

UNAIDS. 2008. *Country Situation: South Africa, July 2008*. Retrieved March 3, 2010. (http://data.unaids.org/pub/FactSheet/2008/sa08_soa_en.pdf).

UNAIDS. 2009. *2009 AIDS Epidemic Update*. Geneva: UNAIDS. Retrieved September 26, 2011. (http://www.unaids.org/en/media/unaids/contentassets/dataimport/pub/report/2009/jc1700_epi_update_2009_en.pdf).

UNAIDS. 2010. *UNAIDS Report on the Global AIDS Epidemic, 2010*. Geneva: UNAIDS. Retrieved September 26, 2011. (http://www.unaids.org/documents/20101123_globalreport_em.pdf).

UNAIDS, UNICEF, and USAID. 2004. *Children on the Brink 2004: A Joint Report of New Orphan Estimates and a Framework for Action*. New York: UNAIDS. Retrieved June 21, 2010. (http://www.unicef.org/publications/index_22212.html).

UNICEF. 2006. *The Extent and Effect of Sex Tourism and Sexual Exploitation of Children on the Kenyan Coast*. New York: UNICEF. Retrieved September 26, 2011. (http://www.linkbc.ca/torc/downs1/extent%20of%20sex%20tourism%20in%20kenyan%20coast.pdf).

UNICEF. 2007. *What Religious Leaders Can Do about HIV/AIDS: Action for Children and Young People*. New York: UNICEF. Retrieved August 1, 2009. (http://www.unicef.org /publications/files/Religious_leaders_Aids.pdf).

UNICEF. 2009. *The State of the World's Children: Celebrating 20 Years of the Convention on the Rights of the Child*. Geneva: UNICEF. Retrieved January 20, 2010. (http://www.unicef. org/rightsite/sowc/fullreport.php).

United Nations Population Division. (UNPD). 2008. "World Marriage Data 2008." Retrieved April 19, 2010. (http://www.un.org/esa/population/publications/WMD2008/Main.html).

United Nations Population Division. (UNPD). 2007. *World Population Prospects: The 2006 Revision*. New York: United Nations, Department of Economic and Social Affairs.

United Nations Population Division. (UNPD). 2009. *World Population Prospects: The 2008 Revision*. New York: United Nations, Department of Economic and Social Affairs (advanced Excel tables). Retrieved September 26, 2011. (http://esa.un.org/unpd /wpp2008/index.htm).

United Nations Population Division (UNDP) Somalia. 2007. "Female Religious Leaders Lead the Fight against AIDS." Retrieved February 10, 2010. (http://www.so.undp.org/index.php/Somalia-Stories/Female-religious-leaders-lead-the-fight-against-AIDS.html).

United Nations Population Division (UNDP) Sudan. 2009. "Sinkat Religious Leaders Join the Fight against HIV/AIDS at Locality Level." Retrieved March 26, 2010. (http://www.sd.undp.org/story%20sinkat.htm).

USAID. 2010. "USAID HIV/AIDS Country Profile for Ghana-September 2010." Washington, DC. Retrieved March 1, 2011. (http://www.usaid.gov/our_work/global_health/aids/Countries/africa/ghana.html).

USAID and PSI. 2006. *Kenya (2005): HIV/AIDS TRaC Study Evaluating Abstinence among Urban Youth (10–14 years)*. Washington, DC: Population Services International, Research Division (Social Marketing Research Series).

Vaisey, Stephen. 2009. "Motivation and Justification: A Dual-Process Model of Culture in Action." *American Journal of Sociology* 114:1675–715.

Valente, Thomas W., Susan C. Watkins, Miriam N. Jato, Ariane Van Der Straten, and Louis-Philippe M. Tsitsol. 1997. "Social Network Associations with Contraceptive Use Among Cameroonian Women in Voluntary Associations." *Social Science & Medicine* 45:677–87.

Van de Walle, Etienne. 1993. "Recent Trends in Marriage Ages." Pp. 117–152 in *Demographic Change in Sub-Saharan Africa*., edited by Karen A. Foote, Ken Hill, Linda G. Martin, National Research Council (U.S.) Panel on the Population Dynamics of Sub-Saharan Africa. Washington, DC: National Academies Press.

Van de Walle, Nicolas. 2001. *African Economies and the Politics of Permanent Crisis, 1979–1999*. Cambridge, UK: Cambridge University Press.

Van Hoyweghen, Saskia. 1996. "The Disintegration of the Catholic Church of Rwanda: A Study of the Fragmentation of Political and Religious Authority." *African Affairs* 95:379–401.

Viljoen, Denis L., J. Phillip Gossage, Lesley Brooke, Colleen M. Adnams, Kenneth L. Jones, Luther K. Robinson, et al. 2005. "Fetal Alcohol Syndrome Epidemiology in a South African Community: A Second Study of a Very High Prevalence Area." *Journal of Studies on Alcohol* 66:593–604.

Waal, Alex De, and Helen Young. 2005. "Steps towards the Stabilization of Governance and Livelihoods in Darfur, Sudan." Report for USAID. Retrieved September 26, 2011. (http://pdf.usaid.gov/pdf_docs/Pnadc781.pdf).

Waal, Alexander De. 1997. *Famine Crimes: Politics & the Disaster Relief Industry in Africa*. Bloomington: Indiana University Press.

Wainaina, Binyavanga. 2005. "How to Write about Africa." *Granta 92: The View from Africa*. Retrieved September 26, 2011. (http://www.granta.com/Magazine/92/How-to-Write-about-Africa/Page-1).

Ward, Kevin. 1999. "Africa." Pp. 193–233 in *A World History of Christianity*, edited by Adrian Hastings. Grand Rapids, MI: William B. Eerdmans.

Watkins, Susan Cotts. 2000. "Local and Foreign Models of Reproduction in Nyanza Province, Kenya." *Population and Development Review* 26:725–59.

Watkins, Susan Cotts. 2004. "Navigating the AIDS Epidemic in Rural Malawi." *Population and Development Review* 30:673–705.

Watkins, Susan Cotts, and Ann Swidler. 2009. "Hearsay Ethnography: Conversational Journals as a Method for Studying Culture in Action." *Poetics* 37:162–84.

Wawer, Maria J., Ronald H. Gray, Nelson K. Sewankambo, David Serwadda, Xianbin Li, Oliver Laeyendecker, et al. 2005. "Rates of HIV-1 Transmission per Coital Act, by Stage of HIV-1 Infection, in Rakai, Uganda." *Journal of Infectious Diseases* 191:1403–09.

Weinreb, Alexander A. 2002. "Lateral and Vertical Intergenerational Exchange in Rural Malawi." *Journal of Cross-Cultural Gerontology* 17:101–38.

Weinreb, Alexander A. 2006. "Substitution and Substitutability: The Effects of Kin Availability on Intergenerational Transfers in Malawi." Pp. 13–38 in *Allocating Public and Private Resources across Generations: Riding the Age Waves*, edited by Anne H. Gauthier, Cyrus Chu, and Shripad Tuljapurkar. Springer-Verlag Publishers.

Weinreb, Alexander. 2010. "Social Interaction in Rural Malawi: An Observational Study." Unpublished manuscript, Population Research Center, UT.

Weinreb, Alexander, Patrick Gerland, and Peter Fleming. 2008. "Hotspots and Coldspots: Household and Village-Level Variation in Orphanhood Prevalence in Rural Malawi." *Demographic Research* 19:1217–48.

Wesangula, Daniel. 2009. "Daily Nation: Pope's Message to Africa." *Daily Nation*, March 21. Retrieved April 26, 2009. (http://www.nation.co.ke/News/africa/-/1066/549308/-/13qiwhqz/-/index.html).

Whitehead, Ann. 1999. "'Lazy Men,' Time-Use, and Rural Development in Zambia." *Gender and Development* 7:49–61.

Williams, Brian G., James O. Lloyd-Smith, Eleanor Gouws, Catherine Hankins, Wayne M. Getz, John Hargrove, et al. 2006. "The Potential Impact of Male Circumcision on HIV in Sub-Saharan Africa." *PLOS Medicine* 3:e262. Retrieved September 26, 2011 (internal-pdf://HIV_williams_2006–4260859904/HIV_williams_2006.pdf).

Williams, Glen, Amanda Milligan, and Tom Odemwingie. 1997. *Common Cause: Young People, Sexuality, HIV and AIDS in Three African Countries*. Oxford, UK: Actionaid.

Willis, Justin. 2002. *Potent Brews: A Social History of Alcohol in East Africa, 1850–1999*. James Currey.

Wilson, Rodney. 1997. *Economics, Ethics, and Religion: Jewish, Christian, and Islamic Perspectives*. New York: New York University Press.

Wojcicki, Janet Maia. 2002. "Commercial Sex Work or Ukuphanda? Sex-for-Money Exchange in Soweto and Hammanskraal Area, South Africa." *Culture, Medicine and Psychiatry* 26:339–70.

Wolffers, Ivan, Irene Fernandez, Sharuna Verghis, and Martijn Vink. 2002. "Sexual Behaviour and Vulnerability of Migrant Workers for HIV Infection." *Culture, Health & Sexuality* 4:459–73.

Worcester, Thomas. 2007. "Plague as Spiritual Medicine and Medicine as Spiritual Metaphor: Three Treatises by Etienne Binet, S.J. (1569–1639)." Pp. 224–237 in *Piety and Plague: From Byzantium to the Baroque*, edited by Franco Mormando and Thomas Worcester. Kirksville, MO: Truman State University Press.

World Bank. 1997. *Confronting AIDS: Public Priorities in a Global Epidemic*. Oxford, UK: Oxford University Press.

World Health Organization. (WHO). 2008. *The Top Ten Causes of Death. Fact Sheet No. 310*. Retrieved September 26, 2011. (http://www.who.int/mediacentre/factsheets/fs310_2008.pdf).

Wuthnow, Robert. 1989. *Meaning and Moral Order*. Berkeley: University of California Press.

Yamba, C. Bawa. 1997. "Cosmologies in Turmoil: Witchfinding and AIDS in Chiawa, Zambia." *Africa: Journal of the International African Institute* 67: 200–221.

Yeatman, Sara, and Jenny Trinitapoli. 2008. "Beyond Denomination: The Relationship between Religion and Family Planning in Rural Malawi." *Demographic Research* 19:1851–82.

Yufeh, Brenda. 2009. "Cameroon: The Pope Blesses the Sick." *allAfrica.com*, March 20. Retrieved April 26, 2009. (http://allafrica.com/stories/200903200654.html).

Zablotska, Iryna B., Ronald H. Gray, David Serwadda, Fred Nalugoda, Godfrey Kigozi, Nelson Sewankambo, et al. 2006. "Alcohol Use before Sex and HIV Acquisition: A Longitudinal Study in Rakai, Uganda." *AIDS* 20:1191–996.

Zelizer, Viviana. 2005. *The Purchase of Intimacy*. Princeton, NJ: Princeton University Press.

Zinsser, Hans. 1934/2007. *Rats, Lice, and History*. New Brunswick, NY: Transaction Publishers.

Zungu-Dirwayi, Nompumelelo. 2004. *An Audit of HIV/AIDS Policies in Botswana, Lesotho, Mozambique, South Africa, Swaziland and Zimbabwe*. Cape Town: HSRC Press.

INDEX